Unraveling

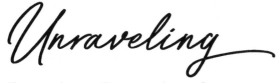

Unraveling

Remaking Personhood
in a Neurodiverse Age

. . .   .

MATTHEW J. WOLF-MEYER

University of Minnesota Press
Minneapolis
London

The University of Minnesota Press gratefully acknowledges the financial assistance provided for the publication of this book by Binghamton University.

Published by the University of Minnesota Press
111 Third Avenue South, Suite 290
Minneapolis, MN 55401-2520
http://www.upress.umn.edu

ISBN 978-1-5179-0913-0 (hc)
ISBN 978-1-5179-0914-7 (pb)
A Cataloging-in-Publication record for this title is available from the Library of Congress.

Printed on acid-free paper

The University of Minnesota is an equal-opportunity educator and employer.

UMP KEP

For Katherine, in laughter and tears

CONTENTS

Blind Man and World

> Consider a blind man with a stick. Where does the blind man's self begin? At the tip of the stick? At the handle of the stick? Or at some point halfway up the stick? These questions are nonsense, because the stick is a pathway along which differences are transmitted under transformation, so that to draw a delimiting line *across* this pathway is to cut off a part of the systemic circuit which determines the blind man's locomotion.
>
> —Gregory Bateson, *Steps to an Ecology of Mind*

Gregory Bateson, twentieth-century anthropologist, cyberneticist, philosopher, and institutional gadfly, provides this thought experiment as an incitement to think through how the body and its senses are conceptualized in a cybernetic framework. Bateson was an uncommon thinker in his time, moving between psychology, anthropology, and philosophy before interdisciplinarity became the buzzword that it is today. Across a diverse body of work, Bateson was compelled by how societies, communities, and families are reproduced through the production of particular kinds of persons and subjectivity. Moreover, as captured in this thought experiment, he was expressly invested in destabilizing the human body as an isolated and isolatable object. He suggested that dominant conceptions of the human body are unnecessarily delimiting in how they imagine the body to exist in the world. He was not, by any stretch of the imagination, invested in disability as a concept. Yet disability pulls him toward this example. For Bateson, the figure of the blind man and his walking stick helps expose how our bodies are more than the organic parts that compose them. Our bodies also include the necessary prosthetics we use to navigate our everyday worlds. He suggests, using this conjoined blind man with stick, that we are all determined by the tools that we use to know the world, to apprehend differences and patterns, to navigate our social environments. Why does Bateson pick an imaginary blind man with a stick to make this point? Could he have just as easily done it with a person stirring a pot of soup with a spoon? Or a person dressed for cold weather, with some flesh exposed to the elements while other flesh is kept warm? It seems for Bateson, sensorial impairment casts into stark relief what might otherwise be unremarkable: the visually impaired figure has a necessary dependency on the walking stick to attain "normalcy" in a way that is not shared with a stirring spoon or climate-appropriate clothing. The everyday use of tools by "normal" bodies can be seen as a mere convenience, but the use of an obvious prosthetic points to the necessary relationship between bodies and tools. Disability and impairment serve as a threshold for a wide variety of thinkers to conceptualize what is normal and abnormal. They emphasize what bodies need social affordances, prosthetics, and medical treatment. They also serve as ways for thinkers to work through what the category of "human" is, and what it might be.

Scholars in the field of disability studies have been invested in how disability has been made and how it serves as means to know the world and the ableist biases of societies, communities, and families. Rather than depend on the imagined figure of disability, disability studies scholars use lived experiences to work through the ways that impairments, social affordances, and environments work together to produce particular forms of subjectivity. This cripistemology, to use a term coined by Merri Lisa Johnson and Robert McRuer, works to unravel ableist, normative conceptions of bodies and personal experience.[1] Disability studies has long been associated with the humanities—literary studies, history, cultural studies, philosophy, and queer theory foremost among them—and the social sciences. One of the motivating aspects of this scholarship is the political project that works against ableism and ableist biases. Bateson's use of the blind man with a stick might seem quite different to a reader with a disability; it might seem to traffic in an implicit ableism that relies on fantasies of disability more than its lived experience. Although Bateson might be read as insensitive to these politics, his interest in destabilizing the body, individuality, personhood, subjectivity, and society might also be read as seeking a reconfiguration of the social to make more kinds of life livable. This is in part why I keep returning to this parable. I see in it a critical reimagining of the human and our worlds.

Anthropologists have long been invested in this kind of discussion of the human and its variations, but only recently has there developed a sustained conversation about how disability might play a role in this project. Faye Ginsburg and Rayna Rapp have suggested that the figure of "disability has a distinctive quality: It is a category anyone might enter through aging or in a heartbeat, challenging lifelong presumptions of stable identities and normativity." Moreover, they argue that disability "is a universal aspect of human life."[2] Yet despite disability's inevitability and universality, anthropology has come rather late to the topic. This delay may very well be due to the discipline's implicit interest in describing a normative subject, a universal human person that is obvious in every society, albeit with the possibility for profound differences in how personhood and subjectivity are elaborated. It may also be due to the inherent instability in the category of disability itself, with an impairment in one society for one person in one situation not being accepted as a disability for another person in another situation, largely due to social affordances, medical attention, and institutional recognition. It may also have to do with the lack or abundance of stigma associated with an impairment, and the ways that individuals and families either hide disabilities from public view or utilize them as the basis for recognition, community, and political change. It may also have to do with the tension between the particular, which ethnography focuses on, and the general, especially in the context of disability as a category. Or it may be due to the nature of necessity in the figure of disability and how, unless necessity becomes apparent through the use of prosthetics, social affordances, or institutional accommodation, the empirical apparatuses of the social sciences tend to ignore phenomena. The blind man with a stick compels attention precisely because the prosthetic of the stick points to the necessary relationship that the man has with it in order to navigate a world that has been built for people unlike him.

Beyond Bateson's reliance on disability for his thought experiment, it is this assumed necessity between the blind man and his stick that pulls me back to thinking through the category of the "normal." The man comes into being through his necessary relationship with the stick. This is not to say that he does not exist prior to the stick, but that in his relationship to the stick, he becomes a new kind of subject. He becomes a blind man and a stick, and through that relationship becomes something approaching "normal." But why stop at the end of the stick? Why not include the ground on which he walks, the obstacles he navigates around, the sounds and smells he encounters, the people and interactions he has? It is not simply technological prosthetics that extend our bodies into the world but all of the external objects, institutions, persons, and nonhumans that facilitate our being in the world. Our worlds are the necessary preconditions for us as persons and subjects. Disability helps point attention toward those sites where human being in the world falters because of a lack of attention to the necessary relation bodies have to their environments and the implicit and explicit forms of facilitation that occur to make moving in the world and relations between persons possible. It is not simply that disability brings into relief the category of the human and the normative assumptions that are built into the figure of the able-bodied person; disability provides an immanent critique of the social worlds humans have built that make some kinds of lives livable and make others difficult or impossible.

Bateson's blind man and stick might capture our actual worldly experiences. The blind man might also be accepted as connected to the various processes that make social relations possible. Beyond ambulation through space, what about communication? What about interactions between bodies?

Unraveling is my attempt to work through Bateson's thought experiment, substituting "neurological disorder" for "disability" as a means to reconceptualize the affective connections that make life possible through the diverse and changing landscape of worldly facilitations and animations that are rendered invisible by science and brought into relief through disabled people's experiences of the world. The category of neurological disorders is large and grows continually as science and medicine associate more and more human experiences with neurological differences or impairments. The cases I focus on—aphasia, coma, autism, deafness—sit uneasily under the rubric of neurological disorder. Over their histories, they have moved in and out of the auspices of the brain. But it is precisely this unease, this shifting nature of the neurological, that motivates my investment in them and in the lives of individuals who confront the category of the neurological and its attendant reductionism. If any of these disorders strikes you as more than merely neurological, you're not wrong. That is precisely why I group them together. I reconceptualize subjectivity as not merely relational but affective, nested in and produced through an admixture of physiological, interactive, and material experiences of the world that move beyond recognition and enculturation. Affective subjectivity has the potential to disrupt the growing tendency of neurological reductivism, and of biological reductivism more generally. Affective approaches to subjectivity point to how the making and unmaking of persons has depended on the differentiation of full subjects from those who are stigmatized, marginalized, and imperiled by institutionalized forms of subjectivity that are based on exclusionary assumptions about human capacities. It is no mistake that Bateson uses the figure of the blind man with a stick. Disability unravels our conceptions of our bodies, our social relations, our worlds. Knitting our bodies, our social relations, and our worlds back together depends on considering how disabilities are produced and enforced institutionally; this reknitting depends on how our bodies and relations might be used as the basis for founding emergent ways of being in the world and of being human.

INTRODUCTION

Let's Build a New Nervous System

> There is room, I believe for all sorts of language. Not only for those thousands of versions of English, but also for the literate formations of people who have been persuaded they are not speaking English at all—and are therefore silenced.
>
> —Paul West, *The Shadow Factory*

I write about my second child, Ignatius—whom we all call Iggy—with some trepidation. When I finished the first draft of this book in the summer of 2017, he had just turned two. He was, like so many two-year-olds, curious, social, and fun. But unlike his older brother, Felix, he was slow to come to language. We first noticed that something was different with Iggy when, at around age one, he was introduced to solid foods. His breastfeeding had been difficult, and after consultations with physicians about the possibility that he might have a tongue tie—all of whom dismissed our concerns—we eventually gave up seeking a surgical remedy for his troubled feeding. When he choked repeatedly on soft foods and purees that his older brother had had no difficulties with at the same age, we eventually sought early intervention from the state, whereupon we were visited by a team of experts—speech pathologists, occupational and physical therapists, special education specialists. They recommended that he receive speech therapy to help with his feeding problems.

Throughout this time, doctors labeled him as having failure to thrive. He was literally off the growth charts, both in weight and height.

This was especially troubling because his brother, four years earlier, was off the charts in the other direction: he was heavy and big. Yes, kids are different, but this different? We were concerned. This was magnified because the medical–industrial complex in the United States often sees failure to thrive as a result of neglect on the part of parents and caregivers. We worried that not taking him to the physician who had treated him roughly during an earlier examination would lead the hospital to refer us to child protective services. We worried that taking him back to a physician with whom he had had a bad experience would cause him to develop an aversion to any kind of interaction with a health care worker.

It wasn't until age three that he was diagnosed with childhood apraxia of speech, a neurological condition characterized by disorders of motor planning. Apraxia of speech usually gets diagnosed much later in children, but because we had a first child with typical development, we had a baseline to compare Iggy's development against. The diagnosis made sense. He had difficulties eating and talking, but he didn't have other cognitive issues. He had taught himself the alphabet at age two, putting together an alphabet train puzzle with the help of parents and caregivers. He obviously couldn't attend day care, as he was at high risk of choking, so we hired nannies and changed our schedules to spend as much time caring for him as we could, given our professional commitments and social obligations. At age three and a half, he was recommended for occupational therapy for ongoing low-muscle-tone issues, even though he had finally gotten onto the normative growth charts. We were aware that he would likely always have motor planning difficulties that could interfere with his gross motor planning; he might have a speech impediment; he might have who knows what else as a comorbidity of his apraxia. It should have been a relief to realize that Iggy's difficulties were organic, even if they were still unknown, but it wasn't.

I wrote this book about communication impairments, neurological disorders, and the history of neuroscience before Iggy was diagnosed with anything other than a nebulous eating difficulty. This is not a book about my son, about our family, or about our interactions with the medical–industrial establishment in the United States. Yet on some level it can't help but be about us and our experience.

Years earlier, in 2010, around the time I first started working on this book, my father had been diagnosed with Alzheimer disease. We had lived apart for more than a decade, and most of my interactions with him were through the telephone. But for a month before we moved from Michigan to California in 2008, my partner and I lived with my parents between our apartment's lease running out and before we took possession of our new home. He could communicate clearly, but it was as if he had become unmoored in time. He knew where he was and he knew who we were, but I'm not sure that he knew when we were. His dementia had softened him. After years of his obvious awareness of his growing and deepening symptoms spawning a self-protective aggression, he seemed to finally be at some kind of peace with himself.

We would have conversations where I wasn't entirely sure that he followed me. Yet he retained a lot of his prior knowledge. He knew, for instance, that I had recently completed my doctorate, that my partner and I were moving across the country, that he was no longer going to work or allowed to drive a car. But there were things that he didn't know. His lifetime career of being a family doctor seemed to provide him with the conversational skills to cover for his ignorance and forgetfulness. Unsure what my doctorate was in or what it was about, he would allow me to introduce both subjects to one of his visiting friends; he would sit back to enjoy the explanation—again, as if for the first time.

This is not a book about my father or my relationship with him. Although I began to conceive of the project during his earliest troubles, at the time, it was a project wholly interested in the then-exploding diagnosis of autism. I was interested, in a sympathetic way, in how the transparent ability to communicate the self was taken as fundamental in psychiatry and neurology as well as in the social sciences and humanities. Such a position necessarily troubled nonnormative ways of communicating, troubled other kinds of selves.

My trepidation about writing about my son, my father, and my family is twofold. First, this book is both impersonal and personal. It is no more about me and my family than it is about anyone's experiences, because we are all caught in the same world that sees particular kinds of verbal communication as the norm, so other forms of communication are abnormal. Anyone who has raised a child or cared for a parent or sibling who struggles with communication will know how tenuous communication is and how exclusionary normative models of communication can be. Second, inasmuch as my experiences are generalizable, this book draws on specific historical accounts of individuals, families, scientists, academics, and activists that help build a theory of subjectivity and personhood that challenges reductive ways of conceptualizing the individual, communication, and human and worldly relationships. To think of my son's and my father's experiences as reducible to their brains is to miss the complex social world they exist within and that is determined through and by the symbolic valence of the brain in limiting the interpretation of their experiences.

Language, Communication, and the Neurological

Unraveling is my effort to move beyond the brain as an explanatory object. The brain and the idea of the neurological have become so pervasive as the basis of consciousness, the self, personhood, identity, individuality, and life itself that they have come to obscure the fundamental relationships between bodies and the worlds that they inhabit. I focus throughout this book on the neurological as a category in an effort to displace it—or at least to unravel it. I focus on the structural creation of neurological disorder in relation to unmarked assumptions about neurological order as the basis of full personhood.

Neuroscience has been knitted together from a diverse set of disciplines and thinkers, who have tied together symbolic-cultural psychoanalysis and information and environmentally focused cybernetics with laboratory-based behavioral and physiological sciences, all of which share a basis in the material experience of living. Yet each sees only part of the consequences of its models of personhood and subjectivity.[1] The neurological—the idea of the brain as the basis of the self—needs to be unraveled, or needs to be taken apart, unbraided, to reveal other possible configurations of the human and the world. To accomplish this goal means reconsidering how the neurological has been knitted together over time, particularly in the United States, and specifically in the period after World War II, when neuroscience and psychiatry ascended to their places of social importance. Here I examine the lives of individuals who are put into the category of neurological disorder by the medical–industrial complex—although their trajectories are quite different, as are their diagnoses—and situate them alongside trends in neuroscience and psychiatry to see how the neurological and disorder might be conceptualized otherwise and separately.[2] If we start with the assumption that cognition is a material process, that the nervous system is connected to the world it inhabits rather than walled off inside the body, then the idea of the brain as a quiet, lone machine, making the self inside the skull, begins to falter.

This book builds an affective theory of subjectivity that is fundamentally cybernetic.[3] Affect theory points to how the capacities of bodies are made and inhibited by their environments. Cybernetics draws attention to the necessary relationship between patterns and the forms that they produce. A cybernetic theory of affective subjectivity focuses on how the capacities of individuals are produced through their situational contexts, which favor some ways of being in the world over others. This cybernetic approach to affective subjectivity draws together theory and experience from neuroscientists, psychiatrists, psychologists, physicians, disability rights activists, and individuals and families who confront dominant ideas about communication and normalcy.[4] On one side are experts in the laboratory and clinical sciences who have helped to contribute to exclusionary modes of thought about brains, communication, and subjectivity. Rather than discard that science, I suggest that returning to it critically can help expose the elements that are generative for remaking personhood and subjectivity in this moment, roughly a half century after the advent of modern neuroscience and psychiatry.[5] On the other side are individuals and families who write memoirs of their experiences with the medical–industrial complex, particularly as they encounter difficulties associated with communication impairments. Their experiences, like those of scientists, are both theoretical and practical; like laboratory practices, they are experimental and help point toward a more capacious model for conceptualizing subjectivity.

This book is unified by my interest in what are recognized as neurological disorders—that is, diseases attributed to the brain that are expressed in one's personhood, self, or mind.[6] In focusing on neurological disorders, I am especially invested in the assumptions that motivate thinking about disorders as being a problem of the individual, as being nested in particular physiological or social experiences that are reducible to the experience of an individual and ultimately located in that individual's brain. By thinking through neurological disorders, institutionalized expectations of individual expressions of normalcy, orderly behavior, and development come into conflict with the lived experiences of individuals, their families, and the institutions that compose their care networks, including hospitals, schools, workplaces, and kin.

Since at least the 1990s, neurological disorders have erupted as widely held concerns in the United States, from the rise of autism diagnoses to the increased incidence of dementia and Alzheimer disease in our aging population.[7] But the history of neurological disorders is much longer than that; the history of neurological disorders draws on ideas about schizophrenia, hysteria, depression, and anxiety.[8] The general lack of cures for neurological disorders trouble and motivate medical action, which have led to the use of psychosurgery (like lobotomy), the use of electroshock therapies, and the general acceptance of psychopharmaceuticals.[9] The lack of clear causes for neurological disorders troubles and motivates scientific research, which has led to changing conceptions of their material, social, and hereditary origins. Neurological disorders share a central symptom: the apparent lack of being able to communicate in an untroubled and transparent way. That one criterion of autism is the lack of a capacity to understand the meaning of social interactions troubles therapeutic and educational goals. How can meaning be valued by an individual when meaning is unrecognizable in the first place?[10] That people with aphasia cannot communicate their experiences of the world or intentions through speech troubles ideas about self-expression and the interior experience of selfhood. Aphasia provokes the question of whether there is a self without the ability to communicate.[11] That deafness troubles one's ability to communicate and be communicated with in spoken language runs counter to expectations that individuals equally access shared language and symbolic repertoires.[12] Disorders unravel the orderly expectations of society, troubling ideas about subjectivity and personhood. Neurological disorders exist as disorders because the order of society creates them as such, and this order is implicitly imposed on "normal" brains.[13]

In the cases that I present, communication often develops situationally, growing out of the capacities of the communicators and their contexts. One of the questions that such cases raise is whether these instances of communication are also instances of language. This is a complex problem that has been solved historically by subjecting the communication in question to a set of criteria, such as whether it abides by syntactic and grammatical regularity or mutual comprehensibility among a community. Although anthropologists have contributed to an increasingly fine sense of the role of context in language,[14] many scholars have nevertheless presumed the possibility of such defining criteria for differentiating human language from nonhuman communication.[15] An alternative approach is offered by linguistic anthropologists who look at how such ideas about language (what they call language ideologies) shape what kinds of linguistic activity counts as language and what does not.[16] These scholars have repeatedly demonstrated how the judgment that some linguistic variety is or is not a real language has served political purposes, both by rationalizing social orders and by shaping linguistic practice. One of the implications of this critical work has been the investigation of the boundaries of language as an anthropological category: Does a language necessarily have rule-governed syntactic forms? What about mutual comprehensibility across a community of speakers? Anthropologists of disability and deafness have been at the forefront of these questions, especially in their exploration of home sign and emergent interactional communities.[17] This work suggests that some of the fundamental criteria for defining what counts as a language in contemporary scholarship, such as syntactic regularities and communities of practice, are also involved in naturalizing and institutionalizing distinctions between humans who are considered holders of personhood and humans—often categorized as disabled—who are not.

Inspired by this work, I am skeptical of attempts to determine which interactions among disabled people, or between disabled people and their caregivers, do or do not involve language. Instead, I take an approach inspired by Gregory Bateson, who views communication as the conveyance of affect between individuals, between individuals and their societies, between environments and the bodies that inhabit them.[18] Bateson puts aside the symbolic as the primary repository of human meaning to explore the variety of communications and interactions that actually occur, utilizing gestures and sound. Bateson's approach allows us to see how dominant expectations about language determine what is accepted as a signal and what is discarded as noise, both in face-to-face interactions and across institutions. Communication is about information and interaction; it might also traffic in the symbolic, but it need not. Focusing on idiosyncratic forms of communication helps to dislodge the anthropocentric, ableist biases that privilege particular linguistic and gestural forms as the only valid form of communicative interaction.

Moving away from historically situated, rule-governed, and shared conceptions of language also helps decenter the role of intent in communicative actions.[19] Dominant models of subjectivity based on language (and on language use as rooted in individual intent) depend on liberal models of agency that accept communicative acts as founded in the interior experience of an individual who seeks to communicate that experience of the world or the self with an interlocutor. In these models, language works to codify individual experience. Communication is based on the sharing of that experience in language. Conceptualizing language as foremost an interactional engagement between actors, and secondarily as a meaning-making activity that is a shared process rather than a static, signifying event, emphasizes the epiphenomenal aspect of interpretation, placing weight not on the speaker but on the interpreter.[20] What an interpretation is, how it is reached, and what its effects are, are all integral to ascribing intent to the speaker, and they are all actions undertaken by the interpreter. In this way, interpretation reads intention backward into the speaker. Placing emphasis on the interpreter and interpretation in these ways voids the speaker of intent and more clearly shows how intention and behavior become loci for medical and familial concern, and how concerns about intention indicate broader concerns about personhood, subjectivity, and the place of language and communication in American society throughout the twentieth and early twenty-first centuries.

What Is a Person? What Is Subjectivity?

At the heart of this book are four interrelated words: individual, person, self, and subject. If individuals are the base unit of U.S. society— something that can be known through censuses and through birth, marriage, and death certificates, all of which recognize the existence of, if not the qualities of, an individual—then persons are those individuals imbued with particular rights and responsibilities as agreed on by society and secured by the state.[21] In this way, individuals are abstract. It is not until they are made into persons that they acquire social recognition. This can occur through naming or other socially accepted forms. In the United States, this process of making persons increasingly occurs through fetal sonograms, in utero sexing, and baby showers, despite the fetus being unborn and physically dependent on the mother's body.[22] In this way, an individual can be a person without being a self or subject.

In the United States, personhood is a binary proposition: an individual is either a person or not. Full personhood comes with institutional recognition; we have little means to adjudicate partial personhood. Parents and guardians are asked to make decisions on behalf of individuals seen as not full persons, particularly children and adults with impairments.[23] But the guiding assumption is that an individual is a person unless he or she lacks specific capacities, particularly around self-determination and communicative powers. Children grow into full persons, and the aged sometimes move away from full personhood as dementia and loss of bodily control and sensory impairments develop.[24] In both cases, personhood is extended to children and the aged, either based on the promise that they will emerge into full persons or based on the promise that they have been a person in the past. The history of American liberalism is littered with attempts to articulate full personhood on behalf of marginalized populations, including women, nonwhites, and the disabled. But what if we began with the premise that no one is a full person and that personhood is always ascribed as a means to socially mark those with whom connections are perceived as being possible?[25] Paradoxically, saying that no one is a full person means that more individuals count as persons. Moreover, starting with such a position allows us to see how personhood is a project—one that is necessarily incomplete and dependent on interdependencies. This is not to suggest that we inaugurate new forms of categorical and partial personhood. Rather, it is to recognize that full personhood is never an intrinsic quality of an individual. Personhood is always a judgment on the part of those who ascribe it as a status to some and not to others.

The subject, produced through processes of subjection and as an effect of the internalization of recognition, is taken as being dependent on personhood.[26] The feeling of selfhood is the result of successful subjection; as Lorna Rhodes phrases it, subjectivity is the "internalization of external relations."[27] Such a view depends on the ability to internalize the external, implying that only those with such a reflexive capacity are full subjects. As Rhodes shows in her work with inmates in supermax prisons, the institutional recognition that prisoners are less than full persons leads to their treatment in inhumane ways. This leads in time to prisoners developing forms of subjectivity that reinforce their status as inhuman and capable of violent and antisocial acts. This depriving an individual of personhood allows for the treatment of that individual as less than human, as more bestial or animal, a logic of care that has operated in prisons, schools, asylums, hospitals, and residential care facilities, intersecting with ideas of race and ethnicity, with sexuality and gender, with class, age, and disability. Across the families and individuals I discuss, the categorization of individuals as particular kinds of people—autistic, nonverbal, deaf—leads to particular forms of treatment by those in power. To meet institutionalized standards of behavior and to be recognized as persons, individuals can be coerced into normative forms of subjectivity that accord with cultural expectations, which include acceptance of medical treatments, normative forms of self-presentation and communication, acceding to governmental expectations of care, and discriminating against particular forms of community and kinship.

However, there can be subjectivity without personhood; there can be feeling and connectivity without institutional or social recognition. Taking the more-than-human experience of the world seriously—how it is built, how it is experienced, how it connects people and makes forms of communication possible—points to modes of subjection that exist outside of recognition and personhood.[28] Attempts to diagnostically recognize individual experiences of disorder may lead to the treatment of symptoms; however, they can also lead to the simplification of a diverse set of experiences that cannot be fully captured by a diagnostic category. In this way, recognition can be a misrecognition.[29] This externally derived basis for personhood, subjectivity, and the self point to how they are all epiphenomenal. They are the effects of social interactions, reactions, and expectations of "normal" behavior on the part of institutions and institutional actors.[30] Subjectivity is an affective process, a function of intimate investments in reciprocal bonds between persons, human or nonhuman, whether through spoken communication or through some other form of modular animation and facilitation. Focusing on families and networks of facilitating care provides ways to conceptualize alternatives to the normative and exclusionary practices of person making in the United States, particularly those focused on communication as an expression of an interior self.[31]

Facilitation, Animation, Modularity, and the Cybernetic Subject

At the heart of this book is a set of ideas—facilitation, animation, and modularity—that challenge the ways that individuals tend to be thought of in the liberal tradition. Liberalism is predicated on the individual as an able-bodied, self-transparent, communicating subject.[32] At its heart, liberalism has depended on this set of capacities. Individuals who are taken as not having these capacities are intrinsically barred from full participation in society. Over time, this has included nonwhites, women, children, and the disabled. Focusing on facilitation, animation, and modularity shows how the individualism at the heart of the liberal project is ideological and obscures the activities that make lives livable for individuals, families, and communities.[33]

Facilitation is a processural interaction between bodies. Facilitation aims toward an end that only can be reached—or that can be reached more immediately—through interactions between actors. In articulating facilitation in this way, I draw on the experience of individuals who rely on facilitated communication (FC) to communicate. I discuss this at length in chapter 3, where I focus on the Goddard family and their use of FC for their adult daughter, Peyton. After decades of Peyton's not being able to speak, the Goddards experiment with using FC, which involves a caregiver holding Peyton's arm so that she can type on a Lightwriter, a speaking keyboard. FC is seen as controversial by some people, particularly those who are committed to the language ideology that communication is a transparent expression of the unmediated self. The source of criticism of FC is the conception of the facilitator supplying the content of the communication and using the impaired individual as a medium for the facilitator's interests.[34] In this way, FC is seen by some as a direct manipulation of the disabled individual to serve the ends of the facilitator. But for many who use FC, mediated communication is the only possible means to communicate, and, as I discuss in chapter 3, FC shows how all communication is mediated. My discussion of facilitation extends the work of Jens Rydstrom and Don Kulick, who use the term "facilitation" to describe the interpersonal practices in enabling sexual interactions between clients in assisted living communities for the disabled in Denmark and Sweden.[35] Like Rydstrom and Kulick, I see facilitation as enabling the expression of desire and a communication of the self. However, I want to conceptualize facilitation more expansively as existing within all interactions between bodies. Facilitation can occur both positively and negatively based on the experiences of the bodies and persons involved.

This view of facilitation depends on a conception of the possibility of connectivity as existing prior to the facilitation between bodies. Connection underlies interactions and binds bodies to their environments. My conception of connectivity is fundamentally affective and draws on Spinoza's monism.[36] If we begin with the principle that all organic and inorganic matter is connected in complex networks of seen and unseen interactions, then the ideological emphasis on individual bodies disconnected from space can be unraveled in generative ways.[37]

Moreover, the ethical implications of the kinds of connections we allow and disallow become clearer, which is part of why FC is so controversial; biases against certain kinds of persons lead to biases against certain forms of communication and the connections they index and create. As I discuss in chapter 2, the denial of connection is especially pernicious in the care for individuals who seem to be unable to express culturally scripted forms of connection and intimacy. What is required to overcome this bias is an animating medium that allows for interactions that are based on shared interests and experiences.

Drawing on the experiences of two families, the Suskinds and the Karasiks, I discuss animation as a way that connections between persons are made lively and that becomes the basis for the development of subjectivity.[38] What this means in practice is that individuals are interacted with as persons—by family members, physicians, psychiatrists, and institutions—through a medium, and this interaction allows for the flourishing of nonnormative subjective forms. This is the case especially for the Suskinds, who treat their son, Owen, as a person with desires of his own (in his case Disney animated films) and who use this shared basis for interaction as the grounds upon which to facilitate Owen's maturation and socialization. This developmental experience for the Suskinds shapes the whole family over time through their shared interactions mediated by the Disney films and through Owen's media consumption and production. Animation serves as a way to conceptualize the necessary bases of interactions in media. This can include media such as language, storytelling, and institutions that make demands on the performance of particular forms of subjectivity. In making this argument, I am interested, like Mel Chen, in destabilizing our conceptions of what is animate and inanimate, and in what kinds of impacts the animate and inanimate have on the experience of life.[39] Animation can exist wherever shared bases for interaction are found; animation and subjectivity are shaped by the mediums through which they occur.

Undergirding this need for animation is a capacity for mimicry, which is most obvious in the mimicry at the heart of socialization and enculturation that "normal" children seem to evidence but that children with neurological disorders seem to upset. Mimicry can be seen in the calls for children to parrot language and behaviors, to become civilized in their culture-bound interactions with others in their worlds as well as with their own body.[40] Mimicry can also be seen in the practices that individuals use to interpret the actions of others. Through replication or deduction—as in the case of Henry Kisor's lipreading, which I discuss in chapter 2—the capacity for mimicry serves as a mechanism to bring bodies together in their intentions and experiences. Like connectivity, a misunderstanding of mimicry as mere imitation can frustrate the actions of parents, caregivers, and physicians. In chapter 2, Noah Greenfeld's seeming refusal of behavioral modification indicates to his parents that he is unable to mimic in fully human ways. Instead, we might consider what needs to occur—what changes in the animating basis of facilitation—to make Noah's mimetic abilities as patterns of pattern making more apparent and serve as the basis for his and his family's shared desires. Mimicry is thus a language unto itself, which differentiates it from imitation as the rote reproduction of actions. Accepting mimicry as principally a form of communication moves the expectations of communication away from an imitative act that comes from within an individual and replaces it with an interaction between bodies.

Against the normative demands of many American institutions, I argue for modularity—that is, the need to conceptualize capacities for interaction as shaped by the institutions that individuals interact with and which provide the interpretive basis for conceptualizing behaviors and capacities. Against disciplinary forms of power, modularity points to the importance of reconfiguring institutions to allow for a broader expression of human capacities. The politics of recognition central to the liberal subject demand that individuals be recognizable in particular ways; such a politics depends on the coercive performance of self that make individual lives legible.[41] In this way, the performance of subjectivity is fundamentally shaped by the institutions that compose our everyday lives; subjectivity follows the demands of the institutions that individuals interact with. Institutions can change, but the dynamic process of subject formation and institutional reform is slow and shaped by those in power more than social movements.[42] But as I discuss in chapter 2, experiments with social forms that unravel institutional demands help to expose how institutions might be organized to allow for nonnormative subjectivities and new possibilities for interaction. Modularity inverts Gilles Deleuze's control societies, his shift away from Michel Foucault's disciplinary institutions. It suggests that if norms are proliferating in our current moment of discrete and disconnected institutions, then there is an opening to consider how institutions and interactions between persons might be generatively refashioned to allow for new connections, facilitation, and animation.[43] This is to take seriously experiments like Jean Vanier's L'Arche homes and Jean Oury and Félix Guattari's La Borde, both of which seek to carve out spaces for allowing persons to exist in nonpathologized yet facilitated ways.[44] In disrupting the impulse to pathologize particular forms of life, there are spaces for care without the need to impose normative demands on the articulation of subjectivity.[45]

Disliberalism and the Rejection of Value

Over the course of the last two hundred years, liberalism has led to its intensification in the form of neoliberalism. Neoliberalism occurs at the level of the economy, property, and individual lives. At the level of the economy, neoliberalism embraces the financialization of the economy, moving away from the material basis of currency in industrial production and gold standards.[46] At the level of property, neoliberalism moves away from state control and ownership of public goods and toward models of privatization. And at the level of individual lives, neoliberalism intensifies focus on self-determination and individual rights.[47] As a unified cultural logic, neoliberalism tends to emphasize individuality. In the sciences, this emphasis on individuality is especially clear in genomics and neuroscience, which posit that disorders arise in the individual based on one's genes or one's brain—not that they are effects of social determinants or cultural expectations of "normal" behavior, growth, and development.[48]

Two alternatives to neoliberalism are communitarianism and collectivism, moving the focus away from the individual and toward the community. Collectivism tends to be ascribed to cultural norms, suggesting that a collective interest in the social good serves as the basis to critique the actions of others and make decisions that favor collectives—the family, the community, society—over the individual.[49] Communitarian critiques are based on a conception of the economy driving cultural forms and that a more community-focused approach to understanding the responsibilities we share to one another necessarily challenges the structure of capitalism.[50] Both of these models share a focus on how the individual and individual rights obscure the relational forms that enable the individual to appear free and self-determining. Communitarianism and collectivism share an interest in arguing against the perceived naturalness of the individual as the base unit of ethical concern.

All of these traditions are deeply humanist. In each case, they conceive of human worlds wherein nonhuman animals, inorganic matter, and environments are the milieu that humans exist within, which may or may not have the capacity to shape human lives and actions. Across humanistic traditions, humans are seen as not merely different in qualities but in kind, and discourses about human rights take as their argumentative basis the need to recognize this inherent difference between humans and nonhuman animals.[51] This inaugural difference, which is shared across philosophical and scientific traditions that see the human as fundamentally different than nonhuman animals, coevolved with ways of thinking that separated humans from other humans on the basis of perceived animal characteristics or lack of access to specific, human capacities. This has been most evident in the history of racism and sexism in the North Atlantic, with nonwhites being associated with animal instincts and capacities compared to their colonial, white counterparts, and women being associated with nature.[52] Children have also been subject to this kind of thinking, but children are accepted as changing as a function of the civilizing process, which makes of them adults with full capacities.[53] The same logic of differentiation has undergirded thinking about disability, with individuals seen as having impairments being accorded lower, not-quite-human status compared to able-bodied individuals.[54] Over the course of the late twentieth century, disability rights activists have struggled to assert the full personhood of individuals associated with a variety of disability categories. In its earliest phases, these movements focused on individuals with mobility and sensory impairments, which led to the adoption of accessible designs in urban and built environments. Over time, disability rights advocacy sought to also include nonnormative intellectual and cognitive styles, most famously enshrined in calls for neurodiversity: the view that, while different, nonnormative cognitive styles and capacities are worthy of social acceptance and are nonpathological.[55]

Lennard Davis has suggested that we are currently in a period of dismodernism.[56] Davis argues that North Atlantic societies have entered a period of intense interest in the body, notable for its focus on care of, for, and about the body. In its intensification of focus on the body—which Davis characterizes as a form of oppression—the disabled body serves as a model for subject formation. Everyone, both able-bodied and disabled, is entreated to think of him- or herself as lacking characteristics or capacities that self-care, prosthetics, and pharmaceuticals might provide.[57] Disability serves as a mechanism to destabilize the category of the human, which Davis suggests is an antihumanist position, replacing the normative body with a more unstable, less unitary body. In his argument, Davis is contributing to a larger trend in disability studies to articulate a posthumanist conception of disability.[58] Such a view does away with the distinction making between humans and nonhumans—and, more radically, between the organic and inorganic.[59] This more extreme position is the one I adhere to here. This erasure of distinctions between human and nonhuman, organic and inorganic, provides a foundation for a cybernetic, affective conception of the human, with distinctions that we make between human and nonhuman, organic and inorganic, as ideological and as indebted to an impoverished, humanist tradition in Western thought that has long sought to position the human—and by extension particular kinds of humans—as fundamentally different from our worldly cohabitants.[60]

Because of their focus on the individual, liberal and neoliberal social formations compel the tactical use of identity for individuals to be recognized by institutions as persons and subjects. When individuals are compelled to claim a normative disability identity in order to receive this recognition, this is a form of disliberalism. Dismodernism has been criticized for potentially weakening the claims made by individuals who seek recognition for their status, both as clients of institutions and as persons.[61] Dismodernism, as Davis's critics suggest, threatens to make all disabilities mere performances for the sake of recognition; yet liberalism depends on the performance of identity across categories that are recognized by dominant institutions. When individuals—or families on behalf of family members—make entreaties for recognition, they are enacting a disliberal subjectivity.[62] Disliberal subjects are compelled to perform their deservingness of recognition by demonstrating their nonnormative capacities within the context of normative identity categories. In the case of individuals with neurological disorders, this has developed into an appeal made through neurodiversity, which argues that nonnormative cognitive styles are nonetheless valuable.

Any recourse to the value of difference faces two challenges. The first is the slippery slope of value, which can lead to some lives being valued while others are not.[63] This is most apparent in "quality of life" as a medical and bioethical decision-making concern. Individuals who are judged as having a low quality of life are often seen as requiring more resources to support them than they are able to return, or whose lives are severely impaired, requiring life support and constant care with minimal signs of consciousness or interactions with their worlds.[64] The second challenge is the differential subtext of such claims to liberal subjectivity. By making claims on behalf of an individual or an identified group, an inherent difference is made between those inside and those outside of the group.[65] This has been the case with the differences made between so-called high-functioning and low-functioning people diagnosed with autism. The words "high" and "low" tend to correspond to verbal capacities as well as to the ability to labor in socially valued ways.[66] This kind of distinction making has been central to liberalism throughout its history, and it has motivated claims to full personhood and subjectivity for individuals and communities seeking recognition, who rely on differentiating themselves from those who are seen as lesser along a human–animal spectrum. Wherever the discourse of value rears its head, it should be destroyed.[67] The more radical position is to claim personhood for everyone, regardless of putative status as disabled or able-bodied, abnormal or normal, human or nonhuman. If life is judged not by what it produces but by the facilitations it enables, then claims to value and recognition can be discarded in favor of a more inclusive politics of facilitation and interdependence.

This disliberalism is another reason why I have trepidations about writing about my son, my father, and my life more generally. If liberalism requires of us a performance of the self to garner recognition by institutions and their actors, then we have also accepted this performance of the self as a way to judge the value of individual claims to participation in society and its communities. After giving a talk from this book entitled "Neurodiversity Is Not Enough," an audience member challenged me during the question-and-answer period as to what right I had to critique the concept of neurodiversity. The audience member seemed to be suggesting that only those with a legitimate claim to the community—as autistic, or as a family member of an individual with autism—could critique the concept. This performance of the self is precisely the kind of essentialization of identity that liberalism requires, and in so doing, it takes what is socially constructed (e.g., a diagnosis like autism) and makes it natural and seemingly self-evident. At the time, I'm sure I dissimulated my way through an answer. Now I would be clear that my problem with neurodiversity is that it is not capacious enough to fully unsettle the disliberalism at the heart of liberalism and its politics of recognition. This is in part due to neurodiversity's liberal differentiation of kinds of persons, but it is also in part due to its reliance on a pernicious form of neuroreductionism.

Neuroreductionism versus the Nervous System

Neuroreductionism posits that we are reducible to our brains.[68] In neuroreductive approaches to thinking about human life, the capacities we exhibit are extensions of our brains, meaning that if a part of our brain is damaged or different in some fundamental way, so too will our capacities differ from the norm. Moreover, evolutionary understandings of the brain and its parts are used to explain not only human differences from other animals but also instinctual human behaviors. Recourse to the lizard brain and prefrontal cortex do the same thing: they associate a perceived behavior or its lack with an underlying material part of the brain. Such rhetorical work reduces complex social phenomena to a perceived function of the brain.[69] Neuroreductionism misses two important things. First, the human brain has continued to evolve from its earlier forms, and although parts of the brain can be associated with earlier forms of life and nonhuman contemporaries, the functions they serve in the modern human brain are not reducible to what the brain did in its earlier form.[70] Second, the brain is a node within a complex world.[71] Even claiming that a behavior originates in the brain ignores that behaviors are reactions to stimuli in and outside of the body, and that behaviors are only behaviors to the extent that they are interpreted as behaviors in a given cultural context. Additionally, the sciences that associate parts of the brain and the brain's evolutionary changes to behaviors are themselves subject to cultural influences that shape the practice and beliefs associated with the science.[72] Brains are important, but they do not act alone. Behaviors are important, but they do not exist outside of their interpretation. The association between behaviors and brains is more complex than neuroreductive approaches allow.

The alternative to neuroreductionism is to reinvigorate our conception of the nervous system. I use the term "nervous system" metaphorically in an effort to unsettle how we conceptualize the nervous system as a material, bounded thing, resident in animal bodies and disconnected from its environment. As popularly understood, the nervous system comprises the network of cells and fibers that transmit signals throughout the body, responding to internal and external stimuli. As a response system in this way, the nervous system brings the outside world into the individual—or, in a cybernetic framework, mediates the experience of what is categorized as inside and outside.[73] This experience of the inside and outside is a specious one. It depends on phenomenological models that see the individual as irrevocably divorced from its environment, producing bodily boundaries as well as discrete objects in the environment.[74] Spinozist approaches to embodiment seek to establish a conception of the world and its inhabitants as irreducible to isolatable objects. Instead, bodies are expressions of an underlying shared substance. Such an ontological position can be difficult to make intuitive sense of, but it is useful for the purpose of critiquing the inherent individualism of dominant models of personhood that depend on a foundational assumption of isolated bodies, brains, and experiences.

Nervous systems comprise the animating environments that individuals are a part of, eroding the boundary between the internal and the external. It is not that bodies exist in environments but rather that bodies and environments are made possible through immanent interactions between forces. These forces create the capacities that are ascribed to specific bodies, making individuals able to act and react in accordance with the capacities that bodies are produced to have. The implication of this way of conceiving the world is that there is a network of connections that compose an individual and his or her environment, and this network is both visible and invisible. Moreover, the network both facilitates some capacities and impairs others. Facilitating personhood and subjectivity in such a schema is not simply a matter of interpersonal interactions; rather, it is based on a diverse set of connections made possible by one's environment that rely in no small part on conceptions of which connections are important and what constitutes a connection at all.

Recent turns in the humanities, social sciences, and laboratory sciences have pointed toward the importance of taking into account the more-than-human worlds that we live within. Unraveling the human and nonhuman distinctions that lie at the heart of liberalism and its institutional forms requires adopting a more inclusive, less anthropocentric conception of interrelatedness and dependency. This includes moving beyond anthropocentric conceptions of kinship that see kin as only human, and only humans that are recognized as kin through traditions of law and biological reckoning.[75] Instead, kin might be more generatively extended to the human and nonhuman, organic and inorganic bodies that comprise the nervous system that individuals are facilitated by and animated through. Such a view moves subjectivity out of human-centric biases and toward a more affective conception of facilitation and animation. The roles of technology in shaping subjectivity are often denied to the detriment of recognizing how vital technology is in making lives livable. Moreover, a lack of attention to technology serves to focus on the individual and his or her perceived disorders as naturally occurring. A more capacious conception of the world helps bring together the many human and nonhuman factors that make lives livable; it recognizes how power manifests itself across a social field of interactions between humans and their environments. The animal/human and inanimate/animate distinctions that undergird humanism help to inaugurate the human as the foundation for exclusionary and inhumane practices that target those who are seen as less than full humans or less than fully agentive. I follow Sunaura Taylor and Mel Chen in making this argument,[76] but I draw on my philosophical interests in Spinozist monism to ground it. Making distinctions such as between the animal and human and inanimate and animate serves those who make the distinctions, often at the detriment of those who are being distinguished as less than full humans or full agents. Such distinctions also serve to obscure the interdependencies and interconnections between individuals and their more-than-human worlds.[77] Animal/human distinctions are especially important—and important to subvert—in the context of the animal model research that is conducted by scientists who simultaneously seek to establish the likeness between animal models and humans and to conduct their research on animals precisely because they are not humans and do not have the rights accorded to human beings.[78] Two scientists I discuss— José Delgado and Harry Harlow—are especially interested in working with nonhumans to understand human brains and social worlds. My engagement with their work is in an effort to think through the violences that the animal/human distinction have enabled, but also how eradicating such a distinction can become the basis for a more inclusive ethics. Inhabiting a world with nonhuman actors demands what Donna Haraway refers to as an ethics of touch—the recognition that life is materially interdependent and interconnected. Rejecting the logics of animal/human and inanimate/animate distinctions that insist that particular kinds of connections are more meaningful, valuable, or important helps us recognize the more-than-human determinants of making lives possible.

Focusing on facilitation, animation, and modularity moves toward a view of the individual as a node in a cybernetic network of relations and connections. If there is a single thinker who motivates the whole of this book, it is Gregory Bateson. Bateson was an irregular anthropologist who started his career doing ethnographic fieldwork in Melanesia on socialization and its effects on individuals.[79] Over time, out of curiosity and geography, he became involved with a series of interdisciplinary interlocutors, which led him through animal studies of communication, family dynamics, and eventually theories of consciousness. Bateson was central in the development of cybernetics in the middle twentieth century, but whereas cybernetics eventually became synonymous with information theory, Bateson saw it as a way to conceptualize the dynamic relationships between individuals and their environments.[80] Over time, he came to see this relationship as tautological: not merely socially constructed, a tautological conception of the world shapes the world through its understanding.[81] As we change, our world changes apace, and as our world changes, so do we. This immanent way of seeing the world attempts to move beyond the strictures that we find ourselves in so we can work toward new possibilities. Importantly, it attempts to reconcile our material worlds with our personal ones, moving away from naive idealism and toward an understanding that our ideational capacities fundamentally shape our material experiences of ourselves and our worlds.

What does this all add up to? Distinctions should not be made between kinds of persons. If a thing—human or not—is considered a person, then it ought to be afforded unconditional personhood and the facilitating care that sustenance requires. Personhood and subjectivity do not exist outside of their animation; there is no innate personhood or subjectivity. Static institutions demand the performance of particular forms of subjectivity to recognize persons; modularity seeks to carve out spaces and forms of interaction that allow for different forms of subjectivity to flourish. Accepting the connectedness and interdependence of the living and the unliving is not necessarily an uncomplicated pro-life position. Instead, it demands an ethics that derives its obligations from the recognition that there are affective repercussions for any decision about connection, life, and death. Those repercussions are not limited to the immediate world of a person, but there is a priority to those who animate and are animated by a person. Ethical decisions should not be made on the basis of value or on ideals but on the affective connections that are affected by a particular decision. In the final pages of this book, I turn back to this question and play with the idea of subjunctive grief as a way to think about the effects of affective loss. I use subjunctive grief as a way to think about loss in the future tense—not as something that has been lost, but for something that will be. In this way, subjunctive grief compels future thinking, demanding that an anticipation of loss motivate action in the present.

Methodology and the Content of the Book

As I have been writing this book, I tell friends that it is a perverse Oliver Sacks book. Sacks, like me, was trained in the case study method of analysis, a tradition in medical thought that extends to early modern medicine.[82] In the case study method, individuals are taken as representative of a diagnostic category; individuals are presented to demonstrate what the actualization of a medical category looks like. At times the case study method is also used to present medical mysteries: given a set of symptoms that seem inscrutable, can a canny doctor figure out what's really going on? Individual lives are set against scientific knowledge that provides an explanation for what is being observed, as if a diagnosis can cure the problems at hand. Individual lives are curiosities, ways into thinking about phenomena that might otherwise be mysterious. In the case study method, medical science can be rather imperial, taking without giving much back.[83] Medical practitioners position themselves as objective, as having the answers. Here I subject scientists, psychiatrists, and neuroscientists to the same kind of case study method, seeking to put them on equal footing with the people they would seek to treat as cases. I invert the relationship between patients and physicians, drawing explanatory power from the experiences of families and individuals who challenge the strictures that neurological disorder places on them and who develop alternative ways to conceptualize interactions, facilitation, and the animating bases of subjectivity. Likewise, methodologically, I attempt to pervert the history of neuroscience and liberal thought about persons and subjects.

This book is the result of a project on noncommunicative individuals that I have been working on since 2006, specifically focused on how the capacity for communication is accepted within American neuroscience and society as an indication of normalcy[84]—or at least normal neurological development. As a means to account for the experiences of a diverse group of individuals and families who experience challenges with communication, I turned to memoirs.[85] The sample of memoirs totaled sixty and was constrained by their publication dates' being limited to the twentieth and early twenty-first centuries to align with the development of neuroscience as a discipline.[86] They were further limited by diagnostic category: autism, stroke, and meningitis-caused deafness,[87] as well as several memoirs written by the parents of idiopathic deaf-mute individuals and some about children who were never officially diagnosed yet who experienced symptoms that accord with contemporary understandings of autism. Alongside the textual analysis of these memoirs, I conducted fieldwork with neuroscientists, psychiatrists, clinical neurologists, and psychoanalysts, motivated to understand how they conceptualized communication and its relationship to neurological development and normalcy.[88] I also attended public events for parents and caregivers of nonverbal individuals diagnosed with autism. These two more traditionally ethnographic approaches motivated my interests in archival research of neuroscientific experiments in the twentieth century focused on communication and its relationship to sociality. Taken together, this diverse body of data helped me build a history of American conceptions of communication disorders over the course of the twentieth and early twenty-first centuries, as well as the various interpersonal, institutional, and technological efforts to make "normal" communicators of nonverbal individuals.

Throughout this book, I engage with a series of experiments in conceptualizing and actualizing personhood and subjectivity. These include the laboratory experiments of Harry Harlow and José Delgado, two twentieth-century scientists interested in the relationship between the brain, behavior, and society; Sigmund Freud and Antonio Damasio, two scholars interested in how meaning shapes the experiences of the self and others; and Félix Guattari and Mony Elkaïm, two therapists interested in novel approaches to the treatment of individual and social disorders. My purpose is not to judge them for their acts but to use their work to conceptualize what capacities are seen as fundamental to being human and what the absence of these capacities means for conceptualizing neurological disorders. In parallel to these practitioners, I take the families at the center of this book as experimentalists in their own right, as each family works in its way to modify expectations and environments to meet the needs of family members categorized as disorderly. These families also work with a wide variety of technologies to attempt to bridge communicative divides between individuals. I am interested in what experiments make possible, specifically in how personhood and subjectivity can be unraveled and reconceptualized through experimental practice.[89]

In each case—and this is sometimes challenging—I accept the intentions of the experiments to be not the revelation or discovery of something but rather the invention of its object.[90] The experiments provide new ways to think about behaviors and relationships, and in so doing help to make new forms of facilitation and connection possible. In these ways, there are embedded—and sometimes explicit—ethical considerations in the experiments: What kinds of persons are they making? What kinds of capacities are they shaping? What kinds of normative and antinormative subjectivities do they engender? At their best, these experiments make new forms of personhood and subjectivity available, and at their worst, they foreclose possibilities for individuals to inhabit and make worlds smaller and less hospitable. Recognizing that understandings of communication, the individual, and disorder work together to marginalize a wide variety of individuals and families is one step toward a reparative stance that might work to create new institutions and modes of social engagement. Working toward those modular institutions and engagements will require invention—experiments that make new persons and subjects possible and that reconfigure the world in emergent ways.

Over the course of the families and scientists I follow, I attend to how subjectivity is differentially produced with competing conceptions of personhood. In chapter 1, I focus on neurological subjectivity as developed in neuroscience, particularly in the work of Antonio Damasio. For Damasio and others who follow in his wake, the material stuff of the brain is paramount in conceptualizing how an individual's subjectivity develops. If a brain is injured, damaged, or otherwise abnormal, then subjectivity is shaped by this difference. What results is the view that behavior is an index of interior processes, and also a window into what might be abnormal in the brain, which is upheld by theories of localization of brain capacities. The problems with this view of subjectivity are twofold: first, all social phenomena are reduced to material structures in the brain and its noncognitive processes; and second, material differences in the brain mean that some individuals are foreclosed from normative forms of subjectivity and personhood because of the understanding of their brain as being fundamentally, materially "abnormal."

In chapter 2, I turn to the opposite extreme and focus on symbolic subjectivity as elaborated in Freudian and Lacanian psychoanalysis, and as embraced by a variety of contemporary scholars who are influenced by the idea of recognition as the basis of subjectivity.[91] In looking at how individuals are foreclosed from participation in symbolic registers of communication because of neurological differences, it becomes clear that symbolic conceptions of subjectivity foreclose a variety of individuals from normative forms of personhood and subjectivity on the basis of assumptions about communication as an expression of the self and means of self-conception.

Chapter 3 turns to the idea of materialist subjectivity, or the understanding that subjectivity is the product of an individual's material environment and its impact on his or her body, especially the brain. In focusing on mid-twentieth-century experiments with material operations on the brain and how individuals with neurological disorders use technology to facilitate their communication with those around them, I show how attention to the material conditions of subjectivity is useful in conceptualizing how human and nonhuman elements in an environment can make subjectivity possible, but I also raise questions about how individuals can control the outcomes of their exposures to environmental forces that shape subjectivity in determinative ways.

Each of these approaches—neurological, symbolic, material— has merits, but each renders some individuals as nonsubjects and nonpersons as a result of their reduction to "normal" brains, modes of communication, and material environments. Cybernetic subjectivity brings these approaches together and is the basis of chapter 4. By focusing on animation and how individuals and their environments exist in mutually supporting and determining fashion, I bring together the strengths of each of the preceding models of subjectivity in an attempt to overcome the normative impulses undergirding emphasis on the brain, symbols, and material environment alone. A cybernetic approach accepts that bodies, the symbolic, and our material environments all equally affect the development of subjectivity, and that by embracing emergent forms of facilitation, specific forms of subjectivity can be developed. In chapter 5, I consider the ethical consequences of cybernetic subjectivity and how it might affect the care we afford one another through interpersonal and institutional facilitation.

As theory producers, the scientists, theorists, practitioners, individuals, and families in each of the chapters point toward a set of features that might be taken as fundamental capacities of human beings, particularly mimicry and connectivity. Inseparable from the facilitating networks that make these capacities possible, these are not inalienable features of some primordial human nature that science, medicine, and experience reveal but rather capacities that are produced as fundamentally human and are the basis for knowing orderly and disorderly bodies.

Rather than assume that the ability to recognizably communicate is inborn, in chapter 2 the experiences of the Greenfelds and Kisors point to the necessity of conceptualizing mimicry—the ability to recognize and repeat patterns—as a fundamental capacity of human personhood that needs to be facilitated and that is fundamentally a form of communication and a language unto itself. Henry Kisor's learning to lip-read and Noah Greenfeld's apparent inability to acquire language point to the necessity of communication as fundamental to the facilitating networks humans find themselves parts of, but in ways that break significantly from symbolic forms of communication catalyzed in twentieth-century psychoanalysis. Focusing on mimicry moves communication away from a purposeful behavior of individuals and toward a conception of communication as always necessarily an interaction, a connection, and means of facilitation. Attending to a more expansive conception of communicative acts also suggests that building modular worlds, ones that move toward more open systems, might facilitate nonnormative ways of communicating.

In chapter 3, CeCe Bell's experiences with her hearing aids and Peyton Goddard's use of FC both make evident how the technologies that make up sociotechnical environments are integral to facilitating relationships between persons but also between individuals and their environments. Connectivity depends on the capacities that our organs, inborn or prosthetic, allow. From Goddard and Bell, I turn in chapter 4 to the Suskind and Karasik families, both of whom have a child diagnosed with autism but are separated by forty years. However different their experiences of the medical–industrial complex are, Owen Suskind and David Karasik share an intense interest in media. I draw on their experiences with their families and the media they love to conceptualize the role of animation, of making something lively through media. I develop a way to think about the family as a particular kind of network that enables animation through reciprocal facilitation by drawing on the Suskinds' and Karasiks' experiences, the work of experimental psychologist Harry Harlow, and cyberneticists inspired by Gregory Bateson.

In chapter 5, I attend to two families, the Schiavos and the Ackerman–Wests, as they confront the inability of an individual in the family to communicate as a result of perceived damage to the brain resulting in severe neurological disorders. In the case of the Schiavos, lack of oxygen results in Terri's persistent vegetative state, which she never recovers from, and which her husband, Michael, and a team of caregivers support her through. In Paul West's case, a stroke leaves him aphasic, struggling to return to language. His wife, Diane Ackerman, and a variety of caregivers aid him in reacquiring his communicating capacities. In the end, I argue that a bioethics that focuses on the capacities produced through connections and guided by subjunctive grief is vital to displace contemporary neoliberal concerns with meaning, communication, and the speaking subject.

But before those chapters, in chapter 1 I turn to a partial history of neuroscience, psychiatry, and cognition in an effort to unravel the place of the individual as the basis for institutional intervention. In so doing, I attend to debates on the relationship between sensation and cognition through an originary and exemplary case, Phineas Gage—a favorite of neuroscientists. From there, the questions of facilitation, connectivity, modularity, and animation motivate my readings of the succeeding cases. Each of these ideas derives from the cases discussed, usually using the same language as that used by the memoirists. The effect of this inclusive approach of a wide variety of memoirs and monographs is to create a countergenealogy of the brain, neuroscience, and neurological disorder. If the story that is accepted about these objects, practices, and ways of knowing and being in the world is one of linear progress toward greater objectivity in scientific practice and medical diagnosis and the material reality that disorder lies in the brain,[92] then the countergenealogy I knit together here is an attempt to intensify resonances across time—ways of thinking that haunt us still and might provide ways of conceptualizing human capacities and how they might be facilitated differently to be more inclusive.[93] Where the limited materialist reductivism of neuroscience would seek to vacate the social from conceptions of disorder by displacing causation into the brain's matter and the inevitable forces of nature, this countergenealogical approach puts the social back into the material by focusing on how interpretations of the causes of disorder resonate over time and destabilize perceived objectivity by making evident the long history of liberalism in neuroscientific conceptions of the individual. Reading history in the way I do shows how the material is always animated by the social; neurological reductivism is only made possible because of its appeal to liberal humanist conceptions of the individual. A cybernetic approach offers a way to displace the reductivism of neuroscientific materialism and replace it with an understanding of disorder as an interpretation of the combined material relations between the body and its environment. With this cybernetic conception of personhood and subjectivity, we might work toward more modular institutions that facilitate inclusive ways of being in the world.

Coda: Temporality and Disorder

Disability studies scholars have long made recourse to the inevitability and contingency of impairment.[94] We will all become impaired at some point through the process of aging. Our memories will fail us, our bodies will move more slowly and less gracefully, we may lose the senses of hearing, sight, taste, and smell. Our able-bodiness—if we are able-bodied—is a temporary condition, and it is only a matter of time before these taken-for-granted capacities begin to shift and require social or medical support. Able-bodiness is also contingent on a vast array of circumstances: exposure to dangerous conditions, being in a severe accident, or becoming ill can all render the body impaired in chronic ways.[95] Conceptualizing able-bodiness as temporary and contingent points to the temporal nature of embodied experience and how the subjunctive, the anticipatory future tense, infuses relations with one's body and with the bodies of others.[96] Such a view helps move away from the idea that disabled bodies have lost something and are in need of prosthetic remediation to become normal bodies; bodies do not proceed from loss, they approach it.[97] The possibility and inevitability of loss motivates care for the self and others. This anticipation of future loss, this subjunctive grief, provides a way to ground practices of facilitation, animation, and modularity. Anticipation rather than compensation might help us move away from conceptualizing individual bodies as not having particular capacities and instead move us toward working on the reorganization of society and implementation of technologies that make varieties of life livable.

If I have trepidations about writing about my son, my father, and our family, they are eased by my ethical commitments to reconceptualizing personhood and subjectivity in this moment of intensified emphasis on the brain as their basis and the possibility that emergent futures can be wrought into being. My enactment of disliberalism extends beyond the invocation of my relationships and my care for others to the whole of *Unraveling*: these lives, these experiments, help disrupt the normative demands of liberalism and its reliance on particular forms of communicating selves, persons, and subjects. If disliberalism can often be coercive and reinforce liberalism's tendencies to demand particular performances to garner recognition of personhood, then its use can also be intensified and used as a tool to dismantle liberalism's biases and their enshrinement in scientific and medical models and practice.[98] If my life has predisposed me to an awareness of facilitation, animation, and modularity—which has become refined between the first version of this book and this final version, as Iggy has grown over the last year and our family has changed apace—it was first the families I encountered through memoir that suggested how liberalism might be dismantled through the careful deployment of neurological disorder to undo liberalism's normative impulses and the exclusions they produce for individuals, families, and communities, all based on a reductive view of human biology. Reconceptualizing a modular, worldly nervous system and the facilitations and animations it can produce makes new kinds of persons, subjects, and connections possible.

ONE

Neurological Subjectivity

How Neuroscience Makes and Unmakes
People through Neurological Disorder

Neurological subjectivity holds that the ability of an individual to conceptualize him- or herself is wholly dependent on the material stuff of the brain. In this model of subjectivity, an "abnormal" brain will result in abnormal forms of subjectivity. An individual with damage to a particular part of the brain will exhibit—or be unable to exhibit—specific behaviors associated with that localized area of the brain. For individuals whose brains are seen as materially different in some way, this helps to account for their abnormal behaviors. This can range from views about chemical balance, as in the case of depression,[1] or discussions of wiring or programming in relation to autism, dementia, or aphasia.[2] In all of these cases, the material organization of the brain is seen as determining what kind of subject a person can become. In its most dogmatic iterations, such neurological reductionism also makes distinctions between who counts as a person and who does not. This approach to subjectivity and personhood is synonymous with the rise of the neurosciences and is emblematized in the work of neuroscientist Antonio Damasio. At the start of his career in the 1980s, Damasio evidenced a nuanced understanding of how the brain works as a mediating organ between individual bodies and their environments. Damasio's earliest work exhibited a humanist tendency that advocates for more nuanced and less reductionist approaches to individuals with abnormal brains.[3] But over time, his work has led him to develop a notion of biological value that epitomizes neurological reductionism.[4] Biological value takes the motive powers of the brain and its component parts to their extreme, seeing in the brain all the determinative features of neoliberal capitalism but rooted in natural processes. Where once his emphasis on the "body-minded brain" was deeply humane,[5] his pivot toward ideas of value makes evident the pernicious and dehumanizing effects of neoliberal conceptions of the person and subject.

The earliest iterations of neurological subjectivity posited that behavior is shaped by the brain. This was rooted in Damasio's reading of cases such as that of Phineas Gage, who was seen as exhibiting abnormal behaviors that resulted from damage to a specific part of his brain. Rather than see behaviors as willful, as emanating from some intent of the individual that seeks to establish his or her status as a particular kind of subject, it is useful to invert this dynamic, emphasizing the interpretation of an action as a meaningful behavior. The structures of meaning lie outside of an individual's intent, and actions are sorted into recognizable behaviors by others only through interpretive acts that make them recognizable as kinds of behaviors. This epiphenomenal approach to subjectivity suggests that rather than dialectically resolving interior intentions with exterior interpretations, exterior interpretations determine interior intentions after the fact. First there is the action, then the interpretation, and then the process of subjection resulting in an interiorized subjectivity. This accords with anthropological theories of personhood that see the recognition of persons as existing within cultural matrices of meaning, separating some kinds of individuals—nonhuman animals, babies, ancestral spirits—from others, with attendant ethical obligations to those considered persons and other ethical regimes applying to nonpersons. An epiphenomenal approach to subjectivity seeks to reconcile the externalization of personhood with the interpretive nature of behavior, which works against neurological reductionism through attention to the modular interactions between individuals, and between individuals and their environments.

In the following, I focus on Phineas Gage, who in the nineteenth century helped physicians and scientists think about the relationships among the brain, behavior, personhood, and subjectivity. In assessing Gage, experts confronted their conceptions of the human/nonhuman divide; what kinds of behaviors are only possible for humans as humans? The inheritors of these traditions in the twentieth century—neuroscientists interested in Gage's brain injury and his resultant behaviors—use Gage's case to confront the relationship between the material stuff of the body, especially the brain and the nervous system, as they consider what the relationship between personhood, particular kinds of capacities, and their material foundations are. I turn next to the question of behavior and how it plays a central role in Damasio's understanding of biological value. For Damasio, behavior and the production of value depend on an understanding of intention as arising in the brain. Such an understanding draws a bright line between those he can consider human and those who are not quite human, thereby rendering individuals with particular kinds of neurological disorders as less than fully human; biological value and neurological models of subjectivity do not just render individuals as disabled but as inhuman. In the final section in this chapter, I turn to my ethnographic work in educational settings to argue that behavior needs to be reconceptualized as existing outside of the individual, thereby moving personhood and subjectivity away from an inborn capacity to one that is facilitated by the connections made possible in a social world.

The Man with a Hole in His Head

NEUROLOGICAL SUBJECTIVITY AND THE
IMPORTANCE OF BEHAVIOR

In rural Vermont in 1848, while working on the installation of railroad ties, Phineas Gage had an iron rod propelled by an explosive charge pass through his left cheek, through the base of the skull, against the front of his brain, and out through the top of his skull. Gage sustained damage to his brain as well as extensive damage to his skull. Gage began to exhibit behavioral changes—changes that in the twentieth century came to be associated with this brain damage. Where once he was polite and followed social norms of address and conversation, he began to behave in crass and disruptive ways, often swearing in public. Where once he behaved in a thoughtful and responsible manner, he began to often miss work deadlines, behaved disrespectfully to his coworkers, and was unable to meet workplace expectations of his performance. There was no way to restore his brain to its previous state, and no amount of social correction would lead him to change his behaviors. He became listless, unable to hold down a job, and traveled frequently, working odd jobs, relatively estranged from his family. All of this, it seems, was due to the damage to his brain, which marked a fundamental shift in his behavioral capacities. At least, this is the story as it is popularly told in neuroscience and psychiatry, a seemingly clear case of localization—that specific parts of the brain are associated with particular capacities and their injury results in socially apparent disorder. As his case is interpreted by contemporary neuroscientists, Gage's frontal lobe—often associated with the regulation of behaviors related to the maintenance of social norms, like monitoring interactions and anticipating the future—was damaged enough to alter his sense of social propriety but not so damaged as to be life threatening.

Gage was the focus of intense scrutiny at the time of his accident and shortly thereafter, but once the novelty of his case wore off, he was largely forgotten. Gage went on to live thirteen years after his accident—no small feat for nineteenth-century medicine, as he experienced infections after the injury and an open wound in his skull for the rest of his life, although the skin apparently grew to cover the exit wound and sealed the wound on his face. Gage was estranged from his family for a long period of time, having spent years traveling and moving from one job to another; eventually he returned to his family shortly before his death. Only after his death did his case begin to elicit interest again, and especially only in the late twentieth century did Gage become a medical celebrity, which has largely been the result of neuroscientists constructing a genealogy for their practice, focusing in no small part on localization.

Gage's story has been told many times before, and my purpose for retelling it here is twofold. First, it is an important case in the context of neuroscience, and neuroscientists often refer to Gage's case as proof of the neurological basis of personhood and subjectivity—as exemplified by Antonio Damasio, who begins *Descartes' Error* with the story.[6] Second, Gage shows how emphasis on meaning and value are misguided in a neurological framework, which often conceptualizes meaning to be immaterial in some fundamental way. For neurological reductionists, in its materiality, the brain can be acted on in direct ways to produce results through particular forms of intervention, particularly through pharmaceuticals and surgery. For Damasio and others who follow in his way of conceptualizing the brain, Gage provides evidence for a neuroreductive genealogy of neuroscience. Contrary to those who might see the mind or consciousness as existing outside of or as superadded to the brain, for neuroreductionists, Gage makes it clear that fundamental components of what we take to be our individual identities—like our interpersonal behaviors—and our social interactions are rooted in the material structure of the brain. And importantly, there are material limits to behavior, as seen in theories of localization. Whereas some might argue that it is possible to instill in an individual a better adherence to social norms through discipline, Damasio uses Gage to make it clear that some brains are structured—through injury or inheritance—in ways that limit the social corrections they can receive; some brains are neurologically disordered. No amount of attention to meaning will correct this, nor, seemingly, can any operation fix this, making individuals doubly disabled, first by the material stuff of the brain, and second through the lack of social affordances for cognitive differences. For neuroreductionists, when material damage occurs to a brain, it fundamentally alters the capacities of that brain, and the preservation of meaning, memory, and selfhood are secondary to the preservation of life itself. This assumption has led in some cases to operations like leucotomy and lobotomy,[7] which are attempts to change the physical structure of the brain to achieve particular therapeutic effects. But a materialist assumption also underlies the conception of the individual as innately connected with his or her own environment in deeply material—as opposed to wholly symbolic—ways. What the neurological model of subjectivity gets wrong through its reliance on localization of disorder in the brain of the individual is that symbolic and environmental forces are material too, and have profound effects on the brain.

Localization is the understanding that specific areas of the brain are responsible for particular capacities. In the case of Gage, planning and anticipation are seen as governed by the prefrontal cortex, a part of the brain than many see as being uniquely human. His brain damage meant that Gage's prefrontal cortex was significantly reshaped, as were his capacities for planning and anticipation. There are two problems here. First, localization is largely theoretical. Outside of specific, often named areas—the Broca area, the Wernicke area—the proof that any particular area of the brain governs a specific capacity for any specific individual is largely only known through pathology; that is, only through injury, disease, or damage and the loss of a particular area of the brain does it become clear that it was associated with a specific capacity for an individual. Second, the damage to Gage's brain has been reconstructed by contemporary scientists, including Damasio, and there is evidence that the damage to Gage's brain was quite different than the modeling that Damasio conducted. In a thorough study of Gage and the early origins of neuroscience and theories of localization, Malcolm Macmillan has shown that Gage was not the person whom contemporary scientists have made him out to be; nor was the damage itself what Damasio would make of it.[8] To say that Gage is proof that the prefrontal cortex governs specific capacities is difficult to definitively claim, yet neuroscientists have done so since the early twentieth century. This neuroreductionism puts the problem of neurological disorders into the individual rather than as an effect of society.

Damasio relies on John Martyn Harlow's initial report of Gage's injury as well as a later report he provided after Gage's death in 1860. On the basis of these reports about the nature of the injury and the changes perceived in Gage, Damasio and his laboratory set about reconstructing Gage's injury and the damage that it seemed to do to his brain. But Damasio and his colleagues worked from the present understandings of localization backward to Gage, finding reference to a change in his temperament as evidence of damage to specific parts of his brain. In Harlow's second report, he writes that after his injury, Gage

> applied for his situation as foreman, but is undecided whether to work or travel. His contractors, who regarded him as the most

efficient and capable of foreman in their employ previous to his injury, considered the change in his mind so marked that they could not give him his place again. The equilibrium or balance, so to speak, between his intellectual faculties and animal propensities, seems to have been destroyed. He is fitful, irreverent, indulging at times in the grossest profanity (which was previously not his custom), manifesting but little deference for his fellows, impatient of restraint or advice when it conflicts with his desires, at times pertinaciously obstinate, yet capricious and vacillating, devising many plans of future operation, which are no sooner arranged than they are abandoned in turn for others appearing more feasible. . . . his mind was radically changed, so decidedly that his friends and acquaintances said he was "no longer Gage."[9]

Harlow seems to have kept track of Gage for a number of years after his accident, corresponding with him and his family, but these notes and letters were eventually lost. Gage spent nearly a decade in Chile as a coach driver, and he returned to the United States to spend his last months with his family, during which time he experienced a series of epileptic seizures and was unable to hold down a job. Upon Gage's death, his family contacted Harlow again to let him know of Gage's passing, at which point Harlow asked for an autopsy that it was already too late to have conducted; instead, Gage's family sent Harlow Gage's skull. Harlow's accounting of Gage's life indicates that Gage seemed to have largely recovered—in the behavioral sense—from his injury, but Damasio and others who mobilize Gage's story elide this, in some cases making up details about Gage's biography that have no basis in any of the contemporary reporting of Gage's life; nor can they be corroborated in the historical record.[10] Moreover, many of these interpretations of Gage miss two things: first, all of the reporting about the changes in Gage came only after his injury; there is no baseline to compare his later behavior to in order to draw significant conclusions about long-lasting change. And second, the damage to Gage's brain was far more extensive than any interpretation based on localization would suggest. The iron rod was hardly a precise instrument, and shrapnel of the skull punctured the brain, leading to damage in other parts of the brain that could not be accounted for without an autopsy. Did Gage change as a result of his accident? Yes, but to say that it was due to a highly localized effect is to misread his injury and to impute changes that may not have been changes, nor were permanent. This misreading of the evidence is possible because neurological subjectivity relies on reducing all social effects to the brain of the individual and renders him or her impaired through this interpretation.

HOW GAGE ANIMATES NEUROLOGICAL SUBJECTIVITY

Despite these problems with Gage's case, Damasio's reconstruction and retelling of Gage's injury and social experiences has led to Gage's case being frequently used as an example in neuroscience textbooks as an example of localization and the material explanation for what brain damage can do to an individual. In *Neuroscience: Exploring the Brain*, Mark Bear, Barry Conners, and Michael Paradiso follow Damasio in suggesting that Gage's change in personality is entirely based on the damage to his brain. Following a discussion of Harlow's later article, the authors write, "The iron rod severely damaged the cerebral cortex in both hemispheres, particularly the frontal lobes. It was presumably this damage that led to Gage's emotional outbursts and the drastic changes in his personality."[11] Or, more reductively, in *Basic Clinical Neuroscience*, Gage's story is summarized in the following way:

> Insight into the functions of the prefrontal cortex was first reported in the middle of the 19th century when a railroad construction foreman, Phineas Gage, suffered prefrontal lobotomy when a dynamite tamping rod was accidentally blown through the front of his head. Prior to the accident, Gage was a model employee—punctual, hardworking, gentlemanly, and highly respectable. Following recovery from the accident, Gage lost all sense of responsibility; became impulsive, irascible, and profane; and drifted aimlessly the rest of his life.[12]

Following a discussion of Gage's injury, Neil Carlson writes in *Foundations of Behavioral Neuroscience:*

He survived, but he was a different man. Before his injury he was serious, industrious, and energetic. Afterward, he became childish, irresponsible, and thoughtless of others. His outbursts of temper led some people to remark that it looked as if Dr. Jekyll had become Mr. Hyde. He was unable to make or carry out plans, and his actions appeared to be capricious and whimsical. His accident had largely destroyed the orbitofrontal cortex.[13]

(Incidentally, Robert Louis Stevenson published *The Strange Case of Dr. Jekyll and Mr. Hyde* twenty-six years after Gage's death, so no one in Gage's social circle was calling him Mr. Hyde.[14]) This is by no means an exhaustive study of the occurrence of Gage in neuroscience textbooks, but it is representative of how Damasio has been successful in animating Gage as an originary case for neuroscience to conceptualize the relationship between behaviors, their interpretation, and the material conditions of the brain. With a case like Gage in hand, neuroscientists have been able to argue for a particular understanding of localization based on associations between parts of the brain and specific capacities, particularly the social ones that Gage seemed to lose after his injury. Neurological subjectivity holds that behaviors originate in the brain and that material disorder of the brain limits capacities. Gage demonstrates this elegantly—at least as he has been reconstructed in the twentieth century.

Throughout his work, Damasio establishes the relationship between changes in the physical structure of the brain with changes in behavior and individual patients' sense of self, showing how injury to the brain often results in unpredictable or unprecedented reactions on the part of damaged individuals despite an environment that is unchanged. In each case, Damasio stresses the profound social impacts these changes in the brain entail, often disrupting marriages, ending careers, and leading to ongoing secondary medical and psychiatric issues. For Damasio, consciousness arises in the interaction between the individual and his or her environment, a by-product of the chemical and electrical reactions of the brain. Personhood is tertiary, accumulating through the repetition of responses to stimuli. When the material structure of the brain changes so that reactions are not the same as they were, an individual's personality is seen as changing. That is, in individuals who experience some kind of brain damage, what used to enthrall or anger them now may only elicit mild interest; or what was once beneath notice is now compulsively focused on. Such people change, yet those around them expect that the brain-damaged individuals will continue to act as they did previously. On the basis of neuroreductive localization, it is assumed that when specific parts of the brain are damaged, particular capacities are diminished—as Gage seems to show with his imputed loss of his ability for forethought and social awareness—leading to individuals who stop being themselves or the selves that they were.

This is critical for reductive neuroscience: the physical structure of brains determines an individual's capacities. By extension, the material structure of the brain makes certain kinds of personhood and subjectivity possible. How a person acts is an indication of the material structure of the brain. Taken together with ideas about localization, these assumptions allow for the possibility to see an individual's aphasia as being related to damage to a specific area of the brain; or, more generally, that an experience like depression is based not on social factors but on chemical conditions within the brain. This reductionism—that everything is reducible to the material structure and processes of the brain—provides neuroscience with a powerful ability to explain behaviors of individuals and leads to the erosion of conceptualizing individual experiences of the world as being meaningful. In this materialist frame, humans are biological computers, taking in stimuli, collating it with experience, and outputting behavior that is taken as meaningful by others. When these behaviors are disruptive or seemingly meaningless, it is clear to neuroreductionists that the aberrant individual has some mechanistic problem that can be intervened upon through surgery or pharmaceuticals. Gage is important because he makes this clear; as an originary case in neuroscience, it is precisely because of his material situation that he is disabled in the eyes of those around him. This is not his choice. Medicine at the time was unable to do anything other than attempt to keep him alive; there were no available surgeries or medications he might take. Neuroscience can excuse the behavior of individuals like Gage and draw sympathies toward their experience of the world, but unless it has remedies to surmount specific material conditions, it is powerless to effect change. In deploying Gage's story as a founding myth in neuroscience, Damasio and other neuroscientists simultaneously make an argument for neurological reductionism in understanding the plights of individuals and for the vexed abilities for neuroscience to do anything about it—other than explain that a mechanical malfunction is to blame, not society or the environment.

But Gage also appeals to Damasio's humanism, as well as the dormant humanism in psychology and neuroscience more generally: Gage's story is more than an exceptional injury and concomitant recovery that defies all odds. It is, more important, a moral tale about the brain, its capacities, and neuroscience. The physical damage that Gage experienced is incidental to the social damages that his injuries led to; Gage helps to show how intolerant society can be toward an individual with a neurological disorder beyond his control. Gage, like many of Damasio's own patients, is portrayed as experiencing a cascading set of social failures that are brought on by his injury, and for which medicine and science have no immediate answer. Individual bodies can be acted upon, but the damaged social lives of those with brain injuries cannot be easily repaired, and this is what Damasio hopes to change. By drawing attention to the uncontrollable effects of brain damage, Damasio points to the limited social capacities of individuals who have experienced such trauma. Social allowances, he suggests, need to be made for these individuals. Science and medicine, he argues, are increasingly able to diagnose physiological problems and to impute their potential effects, but they are unable to address the social damages experienced by those with diminished capacities. In animating a figure like Phineas Gage, Damasio is able to create a character who explains why the material conditions of the brain are important to take seriously—and why neuroscience needs to look outside of itself for solutions to the problems that individuals with brain damage experience. The brain may determine behavior, but it does not determine interpretation.

Antonio Damasio and the Neurological Subject

THE REDUCTIONISM OF NEUROLOGICAL SUBJECTIVITY

The use of Phineas Gage as an exemplar points to a set of assumptions about the relationship of the brain to personhood: namely, that the brain determines the self in a fundamentally material way. This is the neurological subject imagined by Antonio Damasio and other neuroreductionists. Gage's damaged brain means that his self is damaged as well—he becomes rude, insensitive, and lacks forethought. Gage has facilitators, but, as far as history is able to recount, in his lifetime, they were the people who made up his everyday life, and to a degree the doctors who attended to him after his accident. Gage was facilitated by others, but based on the historical evidence, it may not have been enough to enable him to return to his everyday life, even with the support of his family and doctor. After his death, Gage is animated in yet other ways, being written about, reconstructed, and reinterpreted to show how critical the prefrontal cortex is to human sociality. Gage's case depends on a categorical distinction: what it means to be human, where the threshold exists to differentiate the nonhuman from the human, and how this exists along an axis of ability and disability. Central to humanity in this neuroreductionist paradigm is the difference between sentience and consciousness.[15] Nonhuman animals are sentient, and they may be conscious of themselves as individuals and as part of a community in a limited way, but humans, or so the assumption goes, are fully conscious, resulting in a subjective sense of self, of relationality, and of purpose, futurity, and history, all of which are based in the brain. To be less than fully conscious is to be less than a full subject, which Gage makes clear: by appearance, he is like people around him, but his damaged brain limits him in a fundamental way, making him unable to meet the social demands expected of an adult man of his era. The conclusion to draw from this distinction between sentience and consciousness is that the brain makes the person—and that damage to the brain results in limits to the subject. This is the neurological subject, determined entirely by the capacities of the brain and contained in the individual body. In this view of the individual, those with severe neurological disorders are in danger of being treated as nonpersons and nonsubjects, more animal than human, which comes to be justified through recourse to neuroscientific explanations of the lack of key cognitive capacities.

The distinction between sentience and consciousness is one that relies on a difference between feeling and cognition, between sensation and thought.[16] In making this kind of distinction, the physical is divided from the mental; feeling and sensation are assigned to lower-order life-forms like amoebas and paramecia, whereas cognition and full consciousness are granted to higher-order life—creatures like dogs, monkeys, and humans. All life feels, but only some kinds of life can think about feeling, or so neurological subjectivity holds. All humans are sentient, and most humans are conscious, but there are those who may only be the former and not the latter: people who are in persistent vegetative states, people with extensive brain damage or who are experiencing neural deterioration, and fetuses—and Phineas Gage, who reacts in a sentient way but who seems to lack fundamental aspects of consciousness that would make him a full subject. The construction of Gage as a case of neurological subjectivity is intended to show that he loses something fundamentally human in his brain injury. In losing part of his brain, he loses part of his humanity—specifically his abilities for full cognition related to planning and social norms—which make him less of a subject. This way of conceptualizing humans is deeply troubling. It depends on a conception of the liberal subject that relies on assumptions about the individual as an autonomous, self-motivating, self-directing, fully cognizant actor.[17] In so doing, it is fundamentally ableist; anyone who varies from this baseline is labeled as disabled by this standard.[18] It also depends on the ability of individuals to make themselves known as subjects; it depends on communication in an untroubled way and assumes that the communicative acts individuals participate in are transparent indexes of intent. I know who I am, I know what I want and need, and I am able to make those concerns known to others in my world. In the context of neurological subjectivity, being unable to access one's subjectivity in this way marks variance from the norm; being unable to communicate in a transparent way marks one as disabled. In neurological subjectivity, consciousness makes subjectivity possible, and subjectivity is required for personhood.

These assumptions are the basis for categories of neurological disorder. In this respect, consider how Damasio conceptualizes the relationship between subjectivity, consciousness, and what he refers to as biological value:

> The history of consciousness cannot be told in the conventional way. Consciousness came into being because of biological value, as a contributor to more effective value management. But consciousness did not *invent* biological value or the process of valuation. Eventually, in human minds, consciousness revealed biological value and allowed the development of new ways and means of managing it. . . . The emergence of consciousness opened the way to a life worth living. Understanding how [consciousness] comes about can only strengthen that worth.[19]

For Damasio, biological value makes life possible, but consciousness makes life worth living. Such a claim draws a distinction between sentient, feeling creatures and those who are able to recognize their own biological processes and needs, with humans at the top of that list. In this view, other creatures have some access to consciousness, particularly higher primates, but humans stand out as the species that has come to recognize how biological value operates, and how it might be made central to a conception of life itself. Biological value derives from the operation of the brain stem, what Damasio sees as the most basic part of the human—and animal—nervous system.[20] Damasio then asks, "Why do we take virtually everything that surrounds us—food, houses, gold, jewelry, paintings, stocks, services, even other people—and assign a value to it? Why does everyone spend so much time calculating gains and losses related to those items? Why do items carry a price tag?"[21] Ignoring the cross-cultural record regarding value accumulated by anthropologists and historians,[22] he explains, "Value [is] indelibly tied to need, and need [is] tied to life. The valuations we establish in everyday social and cultural activities have a direct or indirect connection with homeostasis. . . . Value relates directly or indirectly to survival. In the case of humans in particular, value also relates to the *quality* of that survival in the form of *well-being*."[23] Damasio goes so far as to explain that all notions of value derive from this basic biological function, imputing all aesthetic, ethical, and social values as derived from the fundamental biological drive toward life's continuance and homeostasis.[24] This is biological reductionism at its most sweeping, and despite Damasio's claims that he values culture as a driver in human society and the possibilities it provides for new steps in human evolution, at its base, Damasio argues for a conception of life that is intrinsically tied to the pursuit of its continuation. On its face, such a claim is relatively benign, if too simple. But Damasio's linkage of biological value with worth and quality implicitly suggests that some lives are more worthy than others and that some individuals implicitly have a higher quality of life than others. In creating this spectrum, the danger becomes justifying the treatment of specific individuals in dehumanizing ways based on their inability to attain or sustain a quality of life that is seen as desirable.

In a discussion of the beginnings of mind, which Damasio sees as a precursor to consciousness, subjectivity, and therefore personhood, he introduces the case of hydranencephaly, a condition wherein a child in utero experiences a stroke and as a result is born with a brain stem intact but lacking the cerebral cortex, thalamus, and basal ganglia.[25] These children are born with a skull full of cerebrospinal fluid, which gives them the appearance of normality. In Damasio's estimation, without most of a human brain, these children lack the ability to conceptualize what is happening and are instead merely feeling, reactive beings. As Damasio explains, "They have expressions of emotions in their faces, they can smile at stimuli that one would expect a normal child to smile at—a toy, a certain sound—and they can even laugh and express normal joy when they are tickled."[26] They exhibit "real *felt* delight, even if they cannot report it in so many words."[27] Damasio concludes, "The degree of sentience, feeling, and emotion that is possible in these cases is quite limited, of course, and, most important, disconnected from the wider world of mind that, indeed, only a cerebral cortex can provide."[28] People diagnosed with hydranencephaly are important to Damasio because they only have access to human feeling, lacking human cognitive capacities altogether. They can experience joy or humor in an immediate way, reacting as they do to sound and touch, but they are unable to attach meaning to interactions. For Damasio, they are unable to do the basic human work of creating a conscious understanding of themselves. Like Gage, people diagnosed with hydranencephaly are brain damaged in Damasio's understanding, but whereas Gage was damaged in an accident of human industry, people diagnosed with hydranencephaly are damaged through a random occurrence of physiological processes. Where Gage is construed by Damasio as having impaired cognitive functioning that limits his consciousness, people diagnosed with hydranencephaly are understood by Damasio as exhibiting the basest functioning of human life—pure feeling unmediated by consciousness. True human beings, for Damasio and others who would see human life in such starkly neurologically reductive terms, are those who are able to move beyond pure feeling and to use feeling as the basis for cognition and the elaboration of a sense of self.

This imagined status of conscious subjects being aware of their own cognitive and sensorial functioning is how neurological subjectivity moves from the material to the social. Neurological subjects are more than sentient; they are not only aware of their consciousness but also that consciousness derives from the operations of the brain. This conception of the self is both historically new (only possible since the invention of psychology and neuroanatomy at the end of the nineteenth century) and geographically specific: one has to accept that the self and consciousness derive from the brain and its functions.[29] Moreover, neurologic subjects are potentially divorced from their environment. One might come to the realization of subjectivity through only internal processes rather than in dialogue with and in response to environmental and social forces. This view of the fundamental self-sufficiency of individuals to realize their own subjectivity is contrary to what subjectivity is generally accepted to be: an effect of interpersonal, historical, and interactional processes. But what does it matter what a person thinks or feels unless it is in response to stimuli? The brain may be reactive, and it may inspire new actions and thoughts in response to its world, but neurological subjects exist before or beyond responsiveness; the state of the brain, its pristine or injured state, make subjectivity possible in reductive and materially constrained ways. In the context of neurological subjectivity, biology is destiny, again, and if one's brain is abnormal, only disorderly forms of subjectivity are possible. The subject is merely an extension of the material functioning—or malfunctioning—of the brain.

THE SHORTFALLS OF NEUROLOGICAL SUBJECTIVITY

There are two complications to this conception of the neurological subject, which finds much of its strength in liberal appeals to individual personhood. The first is the cross-cultural record, in which ideas about personhood, subjectivity, and agency vary widely. The second derives from an increasing attention to nonhuman agency. In the case of the cross-cultural record, what counts as personhood can be widely different given historical and social conditions. It can include humans and nonhuman animals, but also inanimate objects, gods, plants, spirits, and a long list of visible and invisible actors, including, in the United States, corporations.[30] More important, which individuals count as persons can vary widely across societies as well, with many societies not recognizing infants as people until they reach a critical developmental stage, often marked by a naming ceremony in which the child is officially recognized as a person in the community.[31] In a more subtle way, claims to personhood can vary in a society across time, with the claims individuals have to social recognition changing as they mature, earning rights and responsibilities as laid out in social contracts, and losing those rights and responsibilities through crime, age, or impairment. Moreover, in reading through the cross-cultural record, the very assumption that the individual is the base unit of personhood is frequently unsettled, as many societies start with the assumption of the "dividual," the necessary comingling of individual bodies that over time resolves into individuated subjects. The connection between infant and mother might be accepted as a given in North Atlantic societies, where the individual is a discrete entity, but for societies where the dividual is the foundation of personhood, the baby–mother dyad is not so clearly demarcated; where does the suckling mouth end and the nutrient-giving nipple begin? This view of interconnection is one that is embraced in the North Atlantic as well, albeit in the context of romantic love, wherein two lovers' lives ideally intermingle to the point of indeterminacy.[32] The conclusion we might draw from this is that personhood, subjectivity, and agency are attributed, not intrinsic.

That is, rather than being qualities that naturally arise in an individual as an effect of the biological processes that Damasio outlines, which some people exhibit and others do not, these qualities and powers of personhood, subjectivity, and agency are attributed to individuals by others as a result of what is accepted as individual behavior. Persons are made out of individuals; subjectivity is imputed to persons; and agency is a causal explanation provided by observers. Damasio might contend that these phenomena only become possible because of the underlying biological conditions that allow them to exist, and that the division between intrinsic qualities and attributed ones is relatively insubstantial. But personhood and subjectivity are social effects, and the demarcation of a behavior as meaningful exists only as an effect of social regimes of interpretation.

Nonhuman agency has become a way to conceptualize how nonintentional actors shape the worlds they inhabit. These actors are a diverse lot, including anything that can be shown to affect a situation, from geological structures to pharmaceutical chemicals, from nonhuman animals to the material capacities of technologies.[33] In terms of the brain, part of what Damasio is working to conceptualize is the agency of cells, including, importantly, neurons. Damasio understands cells to be agents that seek their own prolongation of life, which in turn extends the life of the thing they make up. Pushing a conception of nonhuman agency into human physiology, as Damasio does, suggests that the various agents that make up an individual's body might be working at cross-purposes, and such a conception of life accounts for diseases like cancer, where cells have the wrong programming and proliferate in adverse fashion. Or, more to Damasio's point, the neurons at work in one's brain can send the wrong messages or inhibit the right messages from being relayed, resulting in the experience of a neurological disorder. Such a conception of life is accidentally Cartesian, splitting the individual between the material functioning of the body and the subjective sense of one's self that is produced as an effect of these interior physiological processes. Additionally, such a conception of life is strangely monadic; it conceptualizes an individual as primarily, if not only, the product of internal forces rather than the creation of internal and external relations. Damasio backs away from materialism by creating a new spiritualism that finds its roots in the brain's capacities for self-conception and reflexivity without an awareness that these capacities are only made possible through relations that exceed the individual brain.

Contrary to this model of neurological subjectivity, personhood, subjectivity, and agency are made possible through connectivity. As individuals, we only have these capacities of personhood, subjectivity, and agency in a world of connections. Our bodies make connection possible, but how we categorize those connections and the motives that make them desirable, normal, and actionable are subject to the constraints and ideologies of dominant institutions in a society that facilitate some forms of personhood and subjectivity but not others. That Damasio sees these qualities as arising in the individual is an effect of liberalism, which posits the individual as the foundational unit of social relations. That Damasio sees all value systems as derived from biological value reads the effects of capitalism backward. It is not that we see value in economic systems, aesthetic works, and particular activities and foodstuff as a result of our biological drives ascertaining value in our physiological functioning, but that capitalist theories of valuation color the way that biological activity comes to be conceptualized by scientists and their publics. In forwarding the framework that he has put together, Damasio is crafting neuroscience as a neoliberal science, if not *the* neoliberal science: all activity, from evolution through everyday interactions, can be understood as the search for maximizing individual value. Damasio has a theory of everything that results in the neuron's being the most valuable of cellular structures, and he sees the evolution of life toward humans as enabled by these tiny agents; humans are the inevitable outcome of the search for value.

Gage's case is compelling to Damasio in no small part because it makes evident that the normal operation of the brain leads to the production of value. Gage was a good worker and a respected member of his community. Then the accident occurred. Gage's ability to self-monitor was damaged, resulting in his inability to ascertain social values and his lack of desire to produce labor value. For Damasio, the explanation is in Gage's brain damage: the material disruption of Gage's brain leads to his social disorders. It is not that Gage is unwilling to control his behaviors; rather, it is that the underlying material capacities for doing so have been destroyed. Gage's impairment, derived from his brain's damage, is a disability in the sense that it disables him from being able to recognize value and participate in a capitalist society. Damasio's use of Gage—and Gage's use as a case in neuroscience more broadly—is caught up in neoliberal conceptions of the individual and the production of value that find justifications of personhood and subjectivity in the capacities of individuals to produce and recognize value.

In this neoliberal view of consciousness as an outcome of cognition, and true self-expression as possible through normative forms of consciousness, Gage is neurologically disordered. Gage is an exemplary case of neurological disorder because his access to full consciousness and self-expression has been diminished by his injury. Gage becomes too close to sensation, too close to feeling, and in so doing too far removed from cognition and consciousness. He becomes too animal. For his neuroscientific interpreters, through his accident, Gage becomes less than human because he lacks full personhood and subjectivity arising from a "normal" functioning brain. This is important because he once had full human capacities—or at least that is how Damasio and others read the historical record—and the injury removes these capacities. Gage might look human, but his behaviors index something else, at least by any normative standard. At the least, they index that he lacks full, human cognitive capacities. When behavior is taken as indexing an interior world, individuals like Gage are interpreted as either making bad decisions or lacking the material basis for making the right decisions. For those who would reduce everything to the brain, in this model of neurological subjectivity, Gage—and by extension other people who make similar bad decisions and who lack the ability to ascertain value—must have something wrong with the functioning of his brain. There must be a material cause and a material solution.

How to Have Behavior without Intent

INDIVIDUAL BEHAVIOR AS SYMPTOM OF DISEASE

Behavior has long served as a means to conceptualize an individual's social conduct and personal comportment, but in the nineteenth and early twentieth centuries, it became paired with the rise in Taylorist and Fordist conceptions of labor.[34] The shaping of the behavior of others—children being trained by their parents, students being educated by their teachers, workers being coordinated by their managers—became a way to create the modern subject.[35] Individuals who failed to meet the behavioral standards embedded in dominant institutions—bad parents, bad students, bad workers—became subject to interventions, often in the form of state-based institutions. In the context of disciplinary institutions, abnormalities could be expressed through behavior, and these behaviors came to be read as symptoms of increasingly categorized ideas about human disorders, whether of criminal types, physiological abnormality, or mental illness. Where once behavior seemed to index a relationship between an individual and society in the broad sense, it increasingly came to be seen as a way to conceptualize the relationship between an individual and a specific kind of institution or set of institutional demands. It is as a result of this changing landscape that Gage's behaviors come to be diagnosable as abnormal by Damasio and other thinkers, even when his attending doctor does not see Gage as socially disruptive to the same extent. In the hands of Damasio, Gage becomes a representative of this mode of conceptualizing individual behavior, but it depends on his case being written in such a way that his experiences and actions can be translated into symptoms of a neurological disorder—and a disorder that is understood as rooted in the material condition of Gage's brain, making his behaviors simultaneously unintentional by him and meaningful to others.

In the context of disciplinary institutions and control societies, disorder becomes obvious through behavior. As a way to think about the actions of individuals, the language of behavior assumes intent; behavior reflects the intentions of the individual who is enacting a particular behavior or set of behaviors. Alongside this assumption of intent is the belief that behavior can be controlled. This control might be through the shaping of the individual, which occurs for most individuals through their participation in the institutions that make up a society, especially the family, school, and work. When these primary institutions fail, therapeutic and juridical institutions attempt to shape behaviors, either by medical or psychiatric treatment or through legal proceedings. The histories of medicine, psychiatry, and law weave around these questions of behavior, and their practices as disciplines are mutually indebted to one another, as disorderly individuals who are seen as criminal in their behavior are normalized through the use of medical or psychiatric treatments.[36] When this occurs, it is because the brain is identified as the motor in an individual's actions; through pharmaceutical or therapeutic intervention, the material functioning of the brain can be modified to produce the right, orderly behaviors. When efficacious, these interventions help to establish that disorderly behavior can exist without intent; such behavior is merely an unintended effect of a disordered brain.

Phineas Gage's behaviors are important to Antonio Damasio not because of the actions themselves but because of what they index about Gage's interior material workings. In effect, Damasio seeks to reduce Gage's social behaviors to symptoms of a material condition that is otherwise invisible. In so doing, Damasio implies that behaviors are meaningful to the extent that they index an interior state or condition; they are not especially important for the social work they do outside of medical semiotics.[37] Erasing the immediate social context of Gage's behaviors evacuates his behaviors of their meaning-making potential and installs them as symptoms of an underlying brain state. In effect, Damasio removes the symbolic content of Gage's behaviors and renders them instinctual. Gage becomes more animal, emotional, and feeling, and less intentional and cognizing. But Gage's actions depend on a social context to permit inference of their status as symptoms. Gage's brusqueness and lack of forethought can only be known as symptoms of neurological disorder because he fails to behave in ways that people expect him to as a respectable member of society, which indicate that something about Gage has changed.

Behavior is popularly thought about as deriving from either instinct or intent, from some base biological drive or from some higher cognitive functioning.[38] In making this distinction, behaviors are aligned with two regimes of agency, the first symbolically meaningless and the second symbolically meaningful. Symbolic meanings can become attached to biologically derived instinct, which is what Damasio does in diagnosing Gage's neurological disorder through his behavior. This kind of symbolic recoding occurs at multiple scales, including the imputation of motives to cellular agents in the neurological model of subjectivity, the social interactions between individuals, and the cultural workings of whole populations. In Damasio's view, biological instinct is always focused on the prolongation of life. The intentional production of meaning, however, can be much more complex. As psychoanalytic approaches to subjectivity emphasize, the conscious production of meaning can be influenced by unconscious forces that, at their most benign, can traffic in shared interpretation of symbols; at their most pernicious, they can be determined by deep species drives toward death, violence, and sex, and may be the expression of pathological psychiatric conditions.[39] Moreover, the intentional production of meaning can work against what are perceived as instinctual drives toward preservation and reproduction, as individuals, institutions, and whole societies can be invested in self-destructive behaviors and practices.[40] Most important, humans are not alone in being able to create meaningful communication. There is increasing evidence that a variety of animals have the ability to perceive the existence of threats, which preserves individual and community lives, but also that animals experience a desire for play.[41] The reduction of meaning to only a biological phenomenon ignores the complex variety of signaling that animals engage in, and it also ignores how all interpretations of behavior are always social.

The assumption underlying Damasio's conception of behavior is that behavior is meaningful only in that it is goal oriented. I reach for a glass of water because I am thirsty. The exterior state indexes an interior drive. I write a book to express a set of thoughts. The material product is reflective of interior action. I have a conversation with a friend. Our communicative acts serve to bind us together as a social unit. I marry my partner to ensure my reproductive fitness and the well-being of my children. I have children because of some deeply instinctual drive to the prolongation of our species, facilitated by some investment in fostering my own lineage. One of the challenges that begins to arise in thinking through this list of actions is the deferral involved between the biological instinct initiating a behavior and that behavior's coming to fruition. I am thirsty, I drink, my thirst is gone. I am instinctually interested in prolonging our species's life span. The chain of events that leads to having children is far more complex than taking a drink of water—although one might argue that modern society is the problem here, distancing us from our biological drives. But modern society also provides the infrastructure for clean, widely available drinking water, making it apparent that at the individual and social level, deferral is an important aspect of desire, requiring individuals and communities to invest in future-oriented projects for individual and collective benefit. In Damasio's reductive reading, we take the good with the bad in accepting cultural advancements, knowing that overall, they add to our species's life span and the production of biological value. The form of investment that Damasio imagines motivates individuals and societies is deeply neoliberal, depending on the deferral of value through the strategic investment of individuals in their everyday lives.

Philosophers, psychologists, and zoologists have long made distinctions between instincts, drives, impulses, behavior, and action, all in an effort to clarify the role of intention in the interactions of individuals. Humans, being a higher order of life, would seem to benefit from the capacities of forethought, which can come to shape their behaviors. In neoliberal conceptions of the subject, if our behaviors benefit from our capacities to meditate on their perception by others, surely they carry meaning; if individuals actively shape their behaviors, then those behaviors by extension indicate something about the individual enacting them. However, take, for example, individuals with Tourette syndrome, a nervous disorder that results in the exhibition of frequent tics, including verbal outbursts and body movements. Often these tics are repetitive, with individuals saying the same word or phrase repeatedly or enacting the same movement over and over again. Others might see these speech acts or movements as exhibiting some kind of intent or meaning—individuals with Tourette syndrome speak and act normally when not experiencing a nervous tic—but in the context of neurological subjectivity, these speech acts or movements are expressly divorced from the intent of the individual.

Similarly, avoidance of eye contact is common among individuals with autism, social anxiety disorder, and introversion. But when is avoidance of eye contact purposeful, meaningful, or inadvertent? Upon entering a room, I might look around, fleetingly engaging others with my eyes. When I look at them, they look back, but my gaze continues to move so as not to make direct, lingering contact with anyone. In meeting someone, I make direct eye contact to let her know that she has my full attention. But when I take a turn to speak, my eyes might wander, scanning the room for other people I know or fixing on an object or feature of the space. When asked to address the whole room, my eyes wander, not making too direct contact with any one person; I'm aware that locking eyes with someone will be uncomfortable for that person, and might indicate to the rest of the audience something about me as a person. All of these eye movements and interactions might be interpreted as my obeying normative expectations of behavior—the right thing to do in these social contexts. But at no point do I consciously decide what I do with my eyes. Only when whomever I am interacting with breaks these unwritten rules do I become aware that something is going wrong in an interaction: when someone locks eyes with me during an interaction, making it difficult to look away; when someone intently stares at me during a lecture; when someone averts his eyes throughout an interaction. These behaviors all defy my expectations for social interaction, just as an audience would likely be unsettled if I spent the entire time giving a speech with my eyes locked on one audience member.[42]

Improper eye contact can be read as a symptom of a neurological disorder, and this is particularly the case in affect disorders like autism and schizophrenia. Improper eye contact can also be read as an individual defying social conventions—or being unaware of them. In the context of neurological subjectivity, there is an underlying organic conception of why the individual behaves so; there is something beyond the individual's control that initiates particular behaviors. When this is the case, it is erroneous to assume that there is any meaning inherent in the actions undertaken; the actions are initiated beyond conscious choice. When foreigners come to visit a new community, they may similarly defy social expectations among their host society: too long of an interactional gaze might be seen as rude or might be experienced as uncomfortable, but assuming that they are intentional in their defiance of local social norms depends on the assumption that these interactional codes are the same everywhere. Doing so would falsely impute intent where there is none. In both cases, social actions are read as if they are intentional, as if individuals whose behaviors are irregular are willfully choosing to act in an antisocial or asocial way. Assuming that an action is intentional in this way imputes meaning to it; the antisocial or asocial act indicates something about the individuals who choose to act in a specific way. But in both of these cases, there is no meaning to be found in these antisocial or asocial actions, grounded as they are in material and social difference.

This is not to say that all actions are not intentional. Rather, associating behavior with meaning is misleading. Consider this example, from the School of the Redwoods, which is dedicated to education for children and young adults diagnosed with autism. Jason, one of the teachers, tells an audience of parents and caregivers about the difficulties of parenting an adolescent and then young adult child diagnosed with autism. Jason is young—in his late twenties—and has been teaching at the School of the Redwoods for eight years, since he graduated from college. Jason hadn't planned to go into special education, but his philosophy degree wasn't about to get him a better-paying job. As he talks, he seems like a thoroughly philosophical teacher—patient, pragmatic, compassionate, and insightful. His presentation is long—nearly three hours—and filled with PowerPoint slides recycled from other presentations he has given, as well as slides borrowed from colleagues. No one takes notes except me; most of the information appears to be old for the other attendees. What people pay the most attention to are the cases that Jason presents, as he details the strategies he uses in dealing with complex and sometimes inscrutable situations. He talks his way through a few slides, unpacking bullet-pointed information, and no one asks any questions. But after an illustrative case, the audience opens up. He tells us about Bluetooth therapy, which is a technique for social integration, and which the caregivers around me find compelling.

In Bluetooth therapy, a client diagnosed with autism wears a Bluetooth headset while the coach sits nearby on a telephone through which they communicate. The client then goes about a set social interaction—going into a grocery store to buy a drink, going into a fast food restaurant to order lunch. This mission is determined by the coach, who sees it in an opportunity to rehearse a set of actions. Although the client can fulfill the components of the mission that do not involve direct social interaction with another person, the coach is on hand to help the client through any social interactions that might arise. But rather than give directions, the coach voices for the client what the latter should say to anyone who inquires if he or she needs help or who greets them. The client is there to parrot whatever the coach says; the client is not meant to communicate in a way that is meaningful to him or her, but meaningful to the person he or she is interacting with. The therapeutic goal in this practice is for the client to recognize the social cues and to respond accordingly. The person diagnosed with autism is meant to learn how to mimic socially meaningful interactions. As I sit in the audience jotting notes, I wonder whom this therapy is for. If the therapeutic process is intended to instill a behavioral response without an understanding of meaning, is it for the benefit of the client undergoing the therapy? Or is it for those that interact with the client?

Answering these questions leads to conceptualizing behavior as an epiphenomenon. Rather than conceptualize behavior as an extension of the intents of the actor, consider what happens when behavior is understood as being primarily meaningless. First, it vacates the assumption that any specific action is inherently meaningful, and by extension that it has a set meaning, either within a given society or across societies. It follows that any action is not reflective of the attempts of individuals to convey a particular meaning to their social others. Instead, meaning is something produced in a specific situation, bounded by the assumptions in a given context and the individuals involved. An action is not indicative of a sense of self; it does not stem from one's "internationalization of external relations."[43] Rather, meaning is something that is produced and imputed by those social others in a situation and that is affirmed retroactively by the subject as an effect of institutionalized norms. The result of accepting behavior as epiphenomenal is that subjectivity is not something that is primarily internally produced but something that is produced for us. We are produced through the imputation of meaning ascribed by others—meaning that may be neither intentional nor meaningful to us but that is intended for those we interact with. This stresses the epiphenomenal nature of subjectivity, pointing to how subjectivity always depends on external forces and is not solely reducible to the material processes of the brain.

Behaviors are always interpreted after the event. When intent is ascribed to behavior, it is often inferred, both by the person who conducted the action as well as those observers who seek to make sense of it.[44] In their moment, interactions exist as a relation between two or more actors, which can be more or less intentional. But after the interactions, observers and participants are engaged in the project of making sense of them.[45] Gage's rude remarks or failure to make appropriate plans for himself are not something that he necessarily premeditated—and, if Damasio is correct, they are not things that he even could have anticipated, given his neurological disorder. But after the actions have occurred, those around Gage, as well as Gage himself, are left to wonder at the meaning and intent of his actions. The people around Gage make sense of him by comparing him to the Gage whom they had known previously. The historical Gage comes to motivate and contextualize the present Gage. In this way, Gage is authored by those in his social world—and, much later, by Damasio and others who would seek to use Gage as a case. Gage is ghostwritten as a particular kind of person and subject through the intentions of those who make him into a case. Damasio ghostwrites Gage to exemplify a neurological condition and set of behavioral difficulties; in making Gage's condition into a case of neurological disorder, Damasio seeks to interpret Gage's behaviors not as Gage would understand them, or even as Gage's contemporaries would understand them, but in line with Damasio's own ends, seeking to explain the relationship between localized functions of the brain and behavior, which can be interpreted to support a causal relation between matter and manners.

Neurological disorders are disabilities because they disrupt the ideology of independence produced by liberal capitalism and intensified by American neoliberalism. Neurological disorders show how interdependent individuals are and how society's orderly operation depends on the conceit of intentional, self-directed behavior as based in the subject. In the context of neurological subjectivity, Damasio uses

Gage to make clear that an abnormal brain can lead to social difficulties, at least because Gage's social relations become more difficult, but also because he appears to have difficulty holding down a job. Gage chafes against the capitalist ordering of society, or at least the conjectured version of his case by neuroscientists who would ghostwrite this difficulty into the historical record. Gage is a compelling early case for the neurosciences and the emerging understanding of neurological disorders in the twentieth century because his injury upsets his easy integration into polite middle-class society—or so those who ghostwrite his case would argue we interpret him as experiencing. For Damasio, Gage cannot be helped; his injury limits his capacities for polite social interactions and forethought. Even at the time Damasio begins to use Gage as a case in the 1980s, biomedicine would be unable to treat his condition as a result of the material damage to his brain. The best Damasio can offer to alleviate the experience of Gage and people like him is to argue for more humanistic engagement with the experiences of others. In this way, Damasio argues that abnormal brains require social sensitivity and accommodations. Given the organization of industrial capitalist society in late nineteenth-century United States, Gage could only be a burden, based on Damasio's view of his impairments. Accepting this social dimension of his disability depends on moving outside of the brain to conceptualize impairments as socially constituted disabilities; it also depends on recognizing that the order of liberal, and eventually neoliberal, capitalist institutions creates understandings of disorder that serve its ends. These institutional orders make individuals into burdens rather than possibilities for facilitation and connection. In the context of neurological subjectivity, neurological disorders are disorders because they trouble our conceptions of the individual, society, and order itself, and because they situate this conception of disorder in an irrevocable nature based in the material conditions of the brain.

TWO

Symbolic Subjectivity

How Psychoanalysis and the Communication of Meaning Disable Individuals

*I*n North Atlantic philosophical and scientific traditions, the use of language has long been considered a capacity unique to humans.[1] Communication through language, which might occur through gesture or speech, depends not only on direct conveyance of meaning but also on access to a symbolic register of shared interpretations of communicative acts.[2] In models of neurological order and disorder that understand access to communication as a fundamental human capacity, individuals are perceived to be disabled when they lack access to shared, normative ways to communicate. This lays the basis for symbolic subjectivity, which posits that access to a shared language is the basis for the elaboration of the self and the basis of personhood and subjectivity. In the context of symbolic subjectivity, communication alone is insufficient; rather, language as access to a shared, normalized interpretive repertoire is a necessary basis for personhood and subjectivity. In frameworks that assume that the unproblematic, clear communication of intention and interior worlds is a natural outcome of human development, neurological disorders are evident through an individual's inability to communicate in normative ways.

By focusing on two cases of individuals with nonnormative modes of communication, in this chapter I show how symbolic subjectivity relies on mimicry as a human capacity that exists prior to language.

For those who conceptualize subjectivity as primarily symbolic, to be human, to be treated as a person and subject, one must demonstrate a capacity for mimicry. The failure to do so leads to the imputation of neurological disorder. But seeing mimicry as a language unto itself moves it away from being an imitative behavior enacted by an individual and toward an interaction between bodies. This removes the burden of enacting subjectivity from the individual and places it squarely in the realm of social interactions. Noah Greenfeld's life as a child diagnosed with autism in the 1960s follows the early development of behavior-focused training in the psychological and neurological sciences. These practices focus on making children imitate the actions that are socially meaningful for their parents, physicians, and teachers, regardless of whether they are meaningful for the children. As Josh Greenfeld recounts in his family memoirs, what he sees as Noah's lack of access to the symbolic and shared interpretive frameworks makes him little more than an animal, first to the caregivers who work with Noah, then over time to the Greenfelds themselves. This erosion of Noah's personhood deeply troubles Josh and his family, and they struggle with how to care for Noah, a child whom they see as lacking access to the capacity to mimic performed behaviors based on his disinterest in imitative practices. The Greenfelds stand in contrast to the experiences of the Kisors, who, when Henry contracts meningitis at an early age, seek a personal tutor for him in order to help him to communicate with those around him in a way that passes for normal. This requires teaching Henry lipreading instead of sign language, a decision his parents make to mainstream him through oralism. In so doing, they actively choose to teach Henry to mimic those around him in ways that build an interactional capacity, unlike any of his hearing or deaf peers. Henry's mode of interaction depends on Henry and those around him embracing a more epiphenomenal understanding of communication, as they cannot rely on an institutionalized symbolic system to determine meaning in their interpretation of each other. Instead, they depend on a modular approach to interaction that works in what Félix Guattari refers to as a transversal way. Rather than an institutionalized and circumscribed basis for the interpretation of communicative acts, a transversal approach seeks to destabilize the interpretation of language and place emphasis on its epiphenomenal enactments.[3] All mimicry might be seen in the same way, having the power to disrupt institutionalized forms of meaning making and supplanting them with immediate, interactional means of communication. The therapeutic goal is not to instill a capacity for mimicry but to recognize that all language is necessarily mimicry, and that interpretation is a fundamentally situational act.

In the sections that follow, I first discuss the Greenfelds and the Kisors, then turn to a genealogy of the roles of meaning, language, and communication in psychology and neuroscience. The role of the symbolic as the basis for subjectivity, as catalyzed in psychoanalysis' emphasis on language in the early twentieth century, places too much emphasis on the historical situation of the individual and not enough on the epiphenomenal demands of communication that are governed by an individual's sociotechnical environment and its facilitations. As much as contemporary neuroscientists and psychiatrists might disavow the influences of Sigmund Freud and his followers, the reliance on access to symbolic language that motivates behavioralist understandings of personhood and subjectivity depends on conceptions of the individual and the individual's access to communicative forms that were central to Freud's early psychology and neuroscience. In concluding this chapter, I turn to two of Freud's followers, Jean Oury and Félix Guattari, and their experimental clinic, La Borde. Drawing on Guattari's writing about La Borde and a documentary film that depicts everyday life at the clinic, I argue that modularity is central to accepting epiphenomenal conceptions of subjectivity. Modularity here is based on Guattari and Oury's organization of La Borde as a nondisciplinary institutional space, which embraces nonnormative forms of social interaction that produce situations in which transversal disruptions of institutionalized power can occur. The openness of La Borde, contrary to its psychoanalytic origins, provides a way to conceptualize how communication might be facilitated through novel institutional forms rather than a reliance on historically determined forms of interpretation.

The Boy Who Can't Be Trained

RAISING A CHILD IN THE MEDICAL MODEL OF DISABILITY

Noah Greenfeld may be one of the most famous people diagnosed with autism in the world. The subject of three books written by his father, Josh Greenfeld,[4] Noah has also served as the basis of a book by his older brother, Karl, and segments on CBS's *60 Minutes*. I'm too young to have seen the original story featuring the Greenfelds on *60 Minutes*, which aired in 1978, but *60 Minutes* has followed the Greenfelds over time, and in 2000 the program checked in on their family. By then, as Josh recounts in his third memoir, Noah had been institutionalized for decades, having moved out of the family home when he was thirteen. One of the appeals of Josh as a memoirist is his unadorned writing, which is brutally honest about his experiences raising Noah. The memoir also recounts what life was like during a period in which living with the medical model of disability held sway over how people conceived of autism and related neurological disorders. Josh's feelings, based on his internalization of the medical model as well as the social challenges that his family faces, lead him to positions that are challenging by modern standards. In the 1978 *60 Minutes* story, Josh admits, "I've often thought about killing him. One of the reasons I wrote the second book was to say these things so that once I've said them, I can't do it. There's no way for me to beg a plea. I can't take Noah out and have an accident with him now."[5] In a field of earnest memoirists desperately seeking the child locked in the disabled body, Josh is frank about his experiences as a parent: Noah is challenging, and raising him in the 1960s, a period with less expert knowledge about autism, made Noah's care, and the family's stability, much more precarious. Each of Josh's books about Noah and their family takes the form of diary entries, often written daily, following their family as they care for Noah, seek medical help, and adapt to the demands of Noah's care that his facilitation requires. Josh's family memoirs thus call attention to how the presence of Noah disrupts the Greenfelds' expectations for an orderly, organized life through the medical imputation of a disorderly brain. In his 2000 *60 Minutes* interview, Josh draws explicit attention to this: "If you have a child, really appreciate normalcy."

By Josh's account, Noah started life as a relatively "normal" child, learning to walk, talk, eat, use the toilet, and participate in family life, even if his development was not as fast as they expected it would be based on their experience raising his older brother. But around age two, Noah began to regress. He lost his capacities for verbal communication, his attention to his need to urinate and defecate, and his ability to appropriately interact with the members of his family, friends, and strangers. For the Greenfelds, Noah went from being a "normal" toddler to an unruly one. The first of Josh's books, *A Child Called Noah*, follows Noah from his first year through his fifth. It largely focuses on the family's search for a diagnosis and treatment for Noah, and the effects that Noah's behaviors have on their family life. Having taken Noah to his pediatrician for his nine-month booster shots, Josh recounts their first brush with diagnosis:

> Noah now almost nine months, still does not sit up or turn over by himself. We expected the doctor to tell us that we had nothing to worry about, that we were being overanxious parents. But instead he asked us about Noah's speech—which is negligible. And whether Noah could pass objects from hand to hand—which he can't. He then voiced concern about Noah's motor development, suggesting that if Noah did not start to develop significantly with the next three months, we ought to have a specialist look at him. Afterward, in his office he tried to reassure us, saying that it was "strictly a gut reaction" but he didn't think we had anything to really worry about because everything else about Noah was so healthy.[6]

In this moment, the Greenfeld's expectations of Noah's development contrast for the first time with the clinical diagnosis of Noah, and from there they enter a period of intense scrutiny of Noah's behaviors as framed by the classificatory frameworks provided by American psychiatry and medicine in the 1960s. The Greenfelds come to interpret Noah's behavior as being without meaning; he seems more animal than human as he fails to meet social expectations. In this context, they begin to see the importance of instilling in Noah a capacity for imitation, for copying the actions of the adults around him in predictable fashion, even if the behavior he is copying is meaningless to him. Recognizing instead Noah's already existing patterns and how they might be modified through mimesis might have enabled other modes of communication and facilitation.

By the time Noah was three, he had been referred to a neurologist for evaluation. The neurologist writes, "Physical examination revealed a youngster who showed no true purposeful activity, and his motor function was often without direction. The child would jump up and down or on other occasions stare inappropriately at his right hand. On occasion the child babbled, but this babble was without inflection. At no time was there any evidence of true expressive language patterns."[7] The observations made of Noah are both physiological and behavioral. Given that he has no obvious physiological abnormalities, the conclusion is drawn that there is something abnormal about his brain, which can be inferred through Noah's behaviors and lack of language. Noah, like many children of his generation, lives under a variety of diagnoses, in no small part due to the lack of coherence in the category of autism at the time. Atonic diplegia, childhood schizophrenia, organic mental retardation, and eventually autism are all applied to Noah, but none of the categories that are used to make diagnostic sense of Noah helps alleviate the tensions in the Greenfeld home or bring an end to any of Noah's behaviors. Providing a child like Noah with a diagnosis of autism in the 1960s and 1970s—and today—is no solution; it offers no cure or even any causal explanation. But a diagnosis potentially offers a route for treatment, with the goal being the reduction or elimination of behaviors associated with the diagnosis. In the 1960s and 1970s, the remedies that are available are medications that treat symptoms and behavioral modification.

According to Josh, those around Noah see his behaviors as socially meaningless. His speech is incoherent to them, his gestures are perceived as largely self-stimulating rather than interactive, he plays alone rather than with others. As Josh writes early in Noah's life, "The fact remains that one can never quite reach him, and most of his babbling has almost no relevancy. One cannot get him to give a simple reply, to come when he is called, or to return the slightest modicum of affection. He accepts hugging and kissing but offers up no token of his own love. There is an opaque barrier, a filter or a jell, that he places between himself and the world."[8] Josh sees Noah as existing behind an "opaque barrier" that allows his caregivers to interact with him but that makes the interpretation and production of symbolic communication impossible for Noah. Whatever work is done with him to improve his language capacities through imitation, it seems to have little effect. He may or may not understand what people say to him, but in either case, his behavior is interpreted as entirely self-directed. Noah appears to his parents as totally disconnected from those around him, to the extent that Josh feels that Noah has no real connection with the family at all. Reflecting on a trip to the zoo, Josh writes, "[Noah] didn't seem to notice us at all. If we let him out of sight for a moment, he would attach himself to any adult thigh and wander away with it until I retrieved him. It was as if he did need *somebody*, but *anybody* would do. Not a very heart-warming feeling for a parent."[9] Josh's conceptualization of Noah in this event is precisely about the lack of meaning in Noah's social interactions, behaviors, and communicative acts: Noah does not care about meaning at all, yet he is still Josh's son, still a person, and the obligation for his care is deeply felt by the Greenfelds. But the challenge that Josh faces daily is that the bond he has with Noah is unreciprocated: he cares for Noah, but by the imitative standards of normative modes of communication, Noah seems to be entirely indifferent to Josh as a person.

The Greenfelds look for a school for Noah for years, visiting residential and day care facilities throughout the Northeast. By dint of history, the options are limited in the first place, and, upon interviewing Noah, administrators and teachers further limit the options that the Greenfelds have—some schools, they are told, are not good fits for Noah. Eventually, having ruled out or been ruled out of the options available to them around New York, the Greenfelds take a prolonged trip to Los Angeles to seek help from Ivar Lovaas, then early in his career at the University of California, Los Angeles. Lovaas developed a training regimen for children diagnosed with autism, used consistently since the 1960s, that is a subset of applied behavior analysis (ABA), a system of observation and intervention for producing socially recognizable behaviors in clients through imitation and rewards. The

Greenfelds are taught to parcel their desires for Noah's development into small, achievable goals: not whole words or sentences but single, imitated syllables; not sophisticated social interactions but simply being able to make eye contact with a parent or caregiver. Having parceled Noah's development in this way, Josh and Fumiko Kometani (Foumi) take turns rewarding Noah for his achievements, providing him with a sliver of potato chip each time he imitates the sound Josh is asking him to reproduce. In this painstakingly slow fashion, they seek to enable Noah to communicate, to interact meaningfully with his family and the world around him, and thereby to become a symbolic subject. Josh describes the plan this way:

> Make Noah pay attention, establish eye contact, by saying "look at me." And to reward such "appropriate" behavior with a cookie or a potato chip. So whenever Noah starts jumping on the couch as he prepares to take off into his own world, or starts to prance-dance about a room, I shout: "Look at me." If he persists in his self-stimulation, in his inappropriate behavior, I admonish him with a sharp "No," a "Stop it," and even an occasional smack.[10]

Josh likens the education they are to provide Noah with training that one might do with a dog—and in his desperation for Noah to achieve some level of normalcy, Josh resigns himself to treating Noah like more of an animal than a human. In considering Lovaas's prescribed operant conditioning, Josh reflects, "If nothing seems to work there, then we'll have to think hard about institutionalizing him. Otherwise our lives will be one long servitude. And that's something we cannot afford."[11] This is the decision that Josh and the Greenfelds wrestle with for years to come: to institutionalize Noah and release themselves from this servitude, or to continue to directly care for Noah and in doing so forego their own aspirations.

What stops the Greenfelds from institutionalizing Noah early in his life is Josh's view of the destructive potential of the residential hospitals that Noah would inhabit. Josh sees residential facilities as not so interested in making a subject of Noah as perpetuating him in his disorderly state. In weighing the decision, Josh writes, "Our lives must come first. Yet institutions mean cold, slow death to me, a surrender of a life to an organism that does not really care. Hospitals just as surely as they can heal and enhance life can wound and ultimately destroy it."[12] At the heart of the Greenfelds' experience with Noah is the question of his care, whether it is to be provided by the family or in a hospital. Both are institutions, but with radically different obligations toward Noah's personhood and subject formation. Moreover, the relationship between imitation and subjectivity, exposed in the Lovaas treatment's structured rewards for Noah—which are echoed in the performances of his parents and teachers—motivate the Greenfelds to keep Noah at home, imagining that the family is the best site for achieving Lovaas's goals. But this reliance on social reproduction through imitation fails to account for the patterns that underlie Noah's behaviors and communicative capacities; engaging with Noah's seemingly nonimitative patterns could provide the basis for communication through mimesis—and potentially accepting a nonnormative form of subjectivity for Noah.

Taken together, these concerns and motivations paint a portrait of American personhood in miniature. Families, the Greenfelds suggest, ideally provide the foundation for the development of an individual, who, over time, is able to express him- or herself through language that is recognized as meaningful in his or her social world, thereby developing a normative form of subjectivity. This process is purely imitative, reproducing personhood through strict social reproduction. But this ideological understanding of the making of the person into a subject elides the relational aspect of mimicry that makes an individual knowable to herself or himself as a subject predicated on processes of differentiation and repetition. It is not the nuclear family alone that accomplishes the goal of making a subject but rather a diverse network of facilitation enabled by society more generally that depends on more than mere imitation. Personhood depends on institutional recognition, but subjectivity depends on reciprocity, interdependence, and a robust sense of interpersonal connectivity that produces the individual as a subject through the facilitation of interactive capacities that mimic socially meaningful behaviors through practices of repetition and differentiation.

THE INSTITUTIONAL BASIS OF
PERSONHOOD AND SUBJECTIVITY

Personhood and subjectivity are facilitated through institutions. The family and the hospital produce particular forms of interaction, personhood, and subjectivity that are recognized as appropriate ways of being in the world and interacting with others. Embedded in the operation of institutions are normative expectations of how a person should develop, what an appropriate set of behaviors and forms of personhood are, and how this is internalized as subjectivity. In encountering an individual like Noah, someone on whom the disciplinary efforts of an institution do not stick, these normative assumptions about personhood and subjectivity are brought into relief, as are the processes through which personhood and subjectivity are normatively produced. Noah is not resistant to these disciplinary efforts in a purposeful, directed way—what some would conceptualize as willful. Rather, the problem is that institutions of the time fail to facilitate Noah's developing the capacity of mimicry as a necessary precondition to subjectivity. Instead, as in the case of Lovaas's treatment regime, they are focused on Noah's being merely imitative. In the 1960s, this lack of an imitative capacity is taken as indication of some kind of neurological disorder, which the experts that the Greenfelds consult increasingly see as organic and based in the brain rather than something that has resulted from bad or inadequate parenting or some unspoken trauma. In the context of developing neuroscience, Noah does not have a psychiatric problem; he has a neurological one. Noah's unintentional resistance to the efforts of his parents to make of him the child they would like him to be—speaking, communicative, interactive, behaving in an appropriate manner—exposes how tenuous the project of making a subject out of a child can be and how dependent it is on normative assumptions about human capacities as facilitated by the nuclear family as an institution. At the heart of Lovaas's and the Greenfelds' emerging sense of what a subject needs is the capacities for imitation. They see that the ability to duplicate the actions of others in a recognizable way is foundational to the ability to communicate; spoken language, communicative gesture, written words—all depend on the ability to reproduce the communicative acts of others. That Noah cannot do any of these things indicates, through his observable behaviors, that his imitative capacity is abnormal in some way. More important is his capacity for mimicry, the ability to reproduce with difference, based on difference. Josh and Foumi expose how parents take for granted the ability of imitation to work in crafting a person; they assume that a child will, through sheer natural processes of imitation, become a symbolic subject. That Noah is unable to undergo this process, that he does not naturally come to personhood through the facilitation provided by his family, begins the process of his diagnosis; his failure eventually leads to intervention on the part of Lovaas and his students, and the replacement of an implicit system of education in the family with an explicit attempt to instill an imitative capacity in the form of Lovaas's ABA treatments. What this project misses is that imitation is not enough to produce what the Greenfelds and Lovaas seek: mimicry, based on difference and rendering differentiation, is the basis for subjectivity and differentiation in the context of American individualism.

Lovaas's method consists of breaking down complex behaviors—speech, action, gesture—into their component pieces, and rewarding Noah for his ability to imitate his teacher. Functionally, Lovaas's method is seeking to create the imitative capacity in Noah; rather than rewarding Noah for meaningful speech or self-derived intentional gesture, Lovaas attempts to create a system in which imitation itself is the aim. The creation of this capacity in Noah, and other children who undergo Lovaas's therapy and similar efforts, is meant to be the first step in the eventual acquisition of full, socially meaningful communication, and by extension the ability to recognize what socially meaningful communication is and its importance in developing symbolic subjectivity. Implicitly, ABA treatments recognize that imitation is fundamental to what is accepted as human behavior. What Josh and his family seek is Noah's ability to interact, to speak and gesture in a meaningful way. What they invest themselves in is the belief that before Noah can reach these ends, he must first acquire the means—that is, the development of a imitative capacity. What this interest misses is that imitation is only reproduction, whereas mimicry's predication on difference is what will provide Noah with the subjectivity that those around him seek to produce. As the Greenfelds experience in their rearing of Noah, some individuals can only acquire limited communicative skills, even after years of training in the Lovaas method. Noah eventually speaks, but in a limited fashion. Even in adulthood, his speech requires extensive interpretive skills on the part of the people in his social world because it is not imitative enough.[13]

At their most basic, language and gesture are systems of imitation; they depend on the interpretive capacities of those around us to infer their meaning, and by extension their intent.[14] My ability to communicate through language is dependent on that language's being meaningful to those in my social world. We may not agree on the specific meaning of a word or phrase or on the intent of a set of gestures, but a collective understanding that words and gestures mean something and are intentional actions lays the basis for collective efforts at communication and interpretation. In this way, symbolic systems are institutions themselves. They produce particular kinds of subjects who can engage in the system and be recognized as intentional, self-directed communicators, thereby developing a subjectivity based on symbolic content and communication.[15] From this perspective, it is not only that Noah lacks an imitative capacity but also that he lacks a mimetic capacity that would indicate his ability to interpret the communications of others. It is not enough to make a sound; one must also be able to interpret the sounds of others. But the interpretive schemas of communication are embedded in the institutions of language that we are socialized into, and acquiring interpretive capacities depends on the existence of a mimetic capacity. In this model of symbolic subjectivity, meaningful interpretation depends on mimesis. Institutions depend on the ability of individuals to imitate the signals they receive to produce the basis for communication, and also to interpret the signals of others along the interpretive lines authorized by institutions. This latter capacity for interpretation depends on differentiation between speaker and audience, between signal and noise, between language and—as Josh puts it—"babbling [that] has almost no relevancy."

In considering Noah's communication, Noah is doubly disabled in this model. First, he is unable to imitate the signals that others take to be meaningful communication; second, he is unable to interpret the signals of others in meaningful, institutionally authorized ways. Caught in the institutions that comprise the contemporary United States—the family, schools, hospitals—Noah is institutionally recognized as a person, but he cannot return that recognition to others. In this model of symbolic subjectivity, there can be facilitation of and connectivity with Noah, but no reciprocity. Yet this reciprocity is critical both to the conceptualization of an individual as a person and for the process of subjectivation through mimesis. In this context, personhood can exist without subjectivity, because personhood is ascribed, but subjectivity cannot exist without facilitation through mimesis.

The institutions that the Greenfelds interact with are historically specific but are produced by capitalist demands; moreover, they were all designed to produce productive, individualized persons and liberal subjects. Yet as much as the Greenfelds have normative expectations of what kind of subject they seek to produce across these institutions, institutional actors have varied expectations of what the interactions with an individual will comprise and what constitutes orderly behavior—and by extension pathological behavior. In the American family, the independent individual as subject has long been the embedded norm, with the expectation being that an infant will grow into a child into an adolescent into a young adult, and during that process, this individual will mature in self-understanding and social relations, all of which will be able to be communicated to others in normative ways. In adulthood, an individuated subject should find a career, marry, and reproduce through parenthood. Variance from this norm has often been thought of in disparaging or pathological terms, from discourses around lifetime bachelors, old maids, mama's boys, and forty-year-old virgins to pathological psychological categories like narcissistic personality disorder and affect disorders that complicate meaningful romantic and social attachment. Similarly, popular discourses about slackers, deadbeats, hippies, and welfare recipients point to the moral value of being a productive member of society from a strictly labor-oriented perspective.[16] Abnormal behavior in each of these cases is taken as an indication of the failings of an individual to comply with or meet normative expectations of the person as a person, which, if the family does its job, should be produced through the naturalized emplotment of development. American hospitals seek to produce healthy individuals with a high quality of life—a process that relies on compliance to ensure that an individual is following the therapeutic protocols of attending physicians.[17] Individuals are meant to follow the norms embedded in social institutions and made explicit through categories of pathologization; if you are a bad subject, there are deliberate ways to make you into a good one, usually starting with changing behaviors. But Noah, and children like Noah, resist these normalizing efforts, not because of some internal drive against normalization but because of a lack of being facilitated in the development of capacities that undergird the ability to accede to, consent to, or resist these processes. Noah is an individual and he may be a person, but in the context of symbolic subjectivity, he cannot become a full subject. Subjection requires an acceptance and internalization of the interpretive schemas of dominant social institutions and the ability to reproduce and differentiate them. Through imitation, subjects become part and extensions of an institution, ensuring that the institution is enacted in everyday life, that it is productive, and that it is generative of the kinds of subjects the institution depends on. But mimesis is required to make the subject a subject through meaningful differentiation; social reproduction is not enough.

THE POLITICS OF DISORDER

At the heart of Josh's struggles with his combined roles as a parent, caregiver, and educator is his awareness of the function of capitalism in creating the difficult decisions he has to make in relation to Noah's potential institutionalization. As Josh writes, "The more money I have, the less of a problem Noah becomes—I can hire out the problem to others. Have a crazy kid and get to understand the gut meaning of a society."[18] Josh sees that to be free of Noah is only possible with economic support—and a willingness to be disconnected from the emotional burden of his care. The flip side is that with economic and institutional support, the Greenfelds might be able to develop a different connection with Noah, supplementing the need to facilitate him in the nuclear family with the support of an institution with the same goals. Finding the right institution would mitigate their need for ev-eryday care but is dependent on the economic means to do so. As Josh later writes, "If one has a child like Noah, one needs money. In order to get enough money, one must have the time and the energy to work. But a child like Noah drains away one's energy, takes away one's time. There is simply no way out. I must confess something: sometimes I hope Noah gets sick and dies painlessly."[19] Parenting Noah, for Josh, means residing in a trap created by society: yes, Noah is his child, a child who was born to Josh and Foumi, but the situation they find themselves in has been produced by the structure of the care of the dis-abled in the United States in the middle twentieth century. There are institutions available to them, but they are undesirable to Josh because he sees them as eroding Noah's personhood and continued well-being. In-home care is available, but this requires money and the right care-givers. Then there is the route the Greenfelds largely follow: devot-ing themselves to Noah's constant care and limiting their other goals accordingly. As this reality sets in for Josh during Noah's childhood years, he grows closer and closer to acceding to institutionalization, recognizing that it is his one route to freedom. Despairing at the mon-umental task of parenting Noah, he asks:

> Is it worth all the effort? The books I will not write, the paint-ings Foumi will not paint, the parental attention Karl will never get? And the answer is obvious. Of course, it is easy to senti-mentalize: how having a Noah gives meaning and definition to one's life. How people without Noahs are constantly searching for humanistic dedications. How a Noah teaches one the values of all the old verities. Bullshit! Without Noah we'd be freer to explore the boundaries of our own lives instead of constantly trying to pierce his perimeters.[20]

Josh is unlike other family memoirists in his answer to this question, which may be due to the influence of the dominance of the medical model of disability in the 1960s. Other parents, as Josh dismissively parrots, find some meaning in the rearing of their children, a discourse that is often intensified in the case of the care of the disabled. But Josh finds a quite different answer. "Bullshit!" he writes, puncturing the humanist desire to see the value in all human life, however difficult it may be. He is also puncturing the lie that it is a choice at all. Capitalist forces constrain the Greenfelds' decision making on each side, leading Josh to consider how systemic his situation is.

In the ethos of the post-1960s, Josh considers how disability and the care for the disorderly fundamentally thwarts the possibility of a radical reorganization of society. The choice the Greenfelds have to make, he realizes, is one that is provided for him and his family, not derived from an open field of possibilities. They must, thanks to history and social organization, choose a way forward, which will entail social, emotional, and economic trade-offs. Josh sees that this is an effect of the extension of American personhood, that by considering Noah a person at all, the options for Noah's continued care are necessarily circumscribed:

> If the pram in the hallway is the enemy of art, then the special child in the playroom is the enemy of revolutionary change. What happens to kids like Noah during a revolution? Even if the system is responsible for children like Noah in certain ways (because of restrictive abortion laws, because of a failure to enact birth-control legislation), ironically, as long as there are children like Noah, it cannot be stopped completely. To bring the system to a halt would require violence. And the first victims of any violence, the first to fall in any sort of a critical standstill, are the old, the sick, the handicapped, and the children. And a Noah fits three of those four categories.[21]

The system as Josh sees it—the matrix of institutions that make up everyday life and the ideologies that undergird them and are mobilized through them—annuls any attempt to change it, let alone overthrow it, at least for those who care about the old, sick, handicapped, and children. Despite themselves, Josh and parents like him come to embody the expectations and demands of the system, they seek to reproduce the social commitments and desires embedded in normative institutions because these institutions, however onerous they might be, recognize Noah and children like him as persons, and they slowly spread this recognition throughout society. Even if Noah cannot reciprocate with others through being an individuated subject, he nonetheless provides the foundation for these institutions to exist. Yet that does not predetermine what these institutions should look like or how they operate.

The Man Who Sees Voices

TEACHING A DEAF CHILD TO PASS IN A HEARING WORLD

In 1944, at the age of three, Henry Kisor experienced the "one–two punch" of meningitis and encephalitis, resulting in his hearing loss.[22] For years, Kisor had believed his hearing loss to be a result of just meningitis, but as an adult, his family doctor speculated that it was this one–two punch that left him deaf, but alive. Kisor was left profoundly deaf, but having been hearing for the first three years of his life, he held on to a rudimentary understanding of spoken language, which provided a foundation for him to develop lipreading skills. Unlike many children who are born deaf, Kisor grew up with a basic understanding of his own speech as well, and was able to communicate in spoken form in response to his lipreading. This was all fortuitous, as Kisor grew up in a period of U.S. history when deafness was largely treated as an insurmountable communication disability, a period in which American Sign Language had yet to acquire its institutional place as the lingua franca of deaf communities in the United States, although vernacular sign languages had been important throughout the United States for deaf communities up to that point.[23] The desire among many educators and families was to make their deaf child appear as "normal" as possible, which required the child to be able to communicate normally with hearing people—despite lacking the capacity to aurally understand what was being said to them. Kisor, like other deaf individuals, was impaired in a straightforwardly mechanical way: he could not hear in a society where communication is generally aurally signaled. Kisor, like other deaf individuals, was disorderly in that his inability to communicate in normative ways upset the ability for him to communicate with those around him, and for him to be communicated with. Over the course of his life, Kisor adapted to these communicative difficulties, first in acquiring lipreading skills and eventually in adopting new technologies made available over the course of the late twentieth century.

But throughout his life, Kisor needed to constantly work on his speech, on being able to be understood by other people—a recurring challenge for a man who served as a journalist and editor for his professional career at the Chicago *Daily News*.

Regarding his parents, Kisor writes, "For many parents, the verdict of deafness is like a death sentence for their child. How, they ask distraughtly, will their youngster be able to grow up to be a functioning member of society instead of being 'deaf and dumb,' a representative of a less-than-human species to be pitied and scorned if not simply ignored?"[24] Early in Kisor's deafness, his family falls into a relationship with an idiosyncratic, experimental educator. Doris Irene Mirrielees had spent years serving as a live-in tutor for deaf children while developing a theory of education for deaf children that sought to provide them with the "gift of language—the *whole* gift," as Kisor writes. He explains: "Miss Mirrielees believed that the educational establishment had failed the deaf. Inefficient, uncaring teaching methods had produced large numbers of semiliterate adults fit only for menial tasks. The underlying cause . . . was that most educators, especially those in the ubiquitous residential schools for the deaf, equated deafness with retardation. Of their charges they expected little and received less. Residential schools, therefore, seemed . . . nothing more than holding tanks for the hopeless." Kisor goes on to explain that "very young deaf children . . . needed the security and love of a life at home. Only in such a 'normal' environment . . . could a deaf child's intellect blossom."[25] Mirrielees's method involved exposing children to an item, action, or interaction, and repeating the term for it repeatedly in an attempt to convey to the child the mouth shapes and movements associated with the terms for the item, action, or interaction. Because so many terms are situational, Mirrielees insisted on regular field trips to expose students to new contexts and terms. Mirrielees would self-publish a memoir and eventually a textbook outlining her methods,[26] but her work never achieved widespread popularity. Mirrielees was an early advocate of mainstreaming,[27] introducing disabled children into mainstream classroom settings to ensure that they received the same education as other children in the community. Much later, this practice would entail special helpers for disabled learners, but during Kisor's childhood, it meant supplying him with the necessary skills to pass as hearing. By being able to lip-read, young Henry was able to attend school with his neighbors and friends, thereby maintaining social relationships. In contrast, children who were sent to residential facilities during this time were cut off from daily contact with family and friends; they relied on their local contacts with similarly deaf clients and their caregivers. Mirrielees centered the family as the basis for the elaboration of a child's intellect and provided the Kisor family with a set of routines, including regular field trips, to ensure that Henry was being introduced to new situations and things in the world, as well as strengthening the connections between family members—which would be vital to Henry's later movement in the hearing world, as his family would be called on to facilitate relationships for him. The goal for Mirrielees was to keep her students engaged with the world, confronting new contexts and people, and learning to develop an interpretive repertoire through which to discern the facial movements of family, friends, and strangers. In doing so, Mirrielees enabled her students to pass for hearing, as long as they were able to correctly interpret the oral gestures of those they interacted with. Yet because of the secondary effects of deafness, particularly the inability to hear one's own voice as others do, the ability to fully pass as hearing proved elusive to Henry.

Writing of his experience as a teenager, Kisor draws on his understanding of what kinds of speakers residential deaf-education facilities produced to explain,

> My speech was not unintelligible. If one listened, it was as understandable as good English delivered with a heavy Eastern European accent. There really was nothing to be ashamed of—but how can that obvious truth be conveyed to a youngster who has convinced himself otherwise? . . . Because I had not grown up around other deaf children, I had managed to avoid acquiring most of the obvious "deafisms"—telltale physical characteristics of the handicap. These include exaggerated facial and bodily expressions, which deaf children brought up together,

even in an oral environment, quickly learn in order to help them communicate with others. These often can seem grotesque to hearing people.[28]

Mirrielees's educational efforts helped minimize Kisor's outward appearance of deafness, but in any interaction that relied on spoken communication, Kisor was obvious in his difference from others: his speech is affected in ways that the speech of hearing individuals is not. Kisor's speech is a constant challenge for him, as he lacks the feedback loop that hearing people have in being able to hear himself speak and make adjustments to his vocal speech. As a result, in his youth he was teased, and in his adulthood he continued to work with a speech therapist on a weekly basis, ensuring that his control of his musculature produced the sounds that others expected to hear. Kisor's efforts to maintain his spoken communication was part of his daily routine, as he explains:

> At the bus stop on the way to work each morning, I peer around to see whether anyone's in earshot, then run through my drills, warming up for the day. To sharpen my "e"s, the vowel with which I have the most trouble—it often comes out too lax, almost like an "uh"—I'll concoct sentences full of "e"s. "Evil babies eat eels from the sea" is one of my favorites. Waiting for the bus one day, I reeled off a dozen shapely and orotund "evil babies" sentences, exaggerating that "e" so that the proper sound would stay with me all day even when I wasn't thinking about it. Then I looked around and saw that another commuter had joined me. She stared warily and kept her distance.[29]

However comical that anecdote is, it points to the ongoing maintenance that communication required for Kisor. The abilities to hear oneself speak and to control one's speech sounds that most hearing and speaking individuals take for granted in everyday speech were a matter of constant concern for Kisor. This leads him to make particular work decisions throughout his life, leading him away from reporting and toward an editorship at the *Daily News*—and also leads him to make specific kinds of decisions about how he moves about in the world, drawing him to a few, close interpersonal connections rather than to develop a more expansive social network. He attributes this decision to his challenges in normative modes of communicating. He writes, "Though it is intelligible in a quiet room, my low, nasal, breathy deaf speech easily gets lost in a forest of competing voices. My most troublesome sounds . . . are often too diffuse to be discerned against a noisy background. And when I raise the volume of my voice, the sounds tend to grow even more distorted."[30] The subtle effects of Kisor's voice—and his reflexive attention to it—inspire him to quiet, interpersonal interactions and a professional career that allows him to focus on connections with a small, tight-knit group of writers rather than an ongoing parade of new stories to report on. Mirrielees instilled in Kisor the capacities to discern communicative acts and to generally pass in the hearing world, but his inability to communicate in a fully normative way still encouraged his selecting some paths in life over others. Mirrielees's techniques facilitate Kisor's participation in an expansive community of people he becomes connected to—his natal family, friends throughout his education, his spouse, their children, and his coworkers. Yet like the maintenance of his speech, this requires an extensive amount of ongoing work on his part. Facilitation makes connectivity possible, but connection itself is laborious.

TECHNOLOGIES OF SYMBOLIC SUBJECTIVITY

Given the capacities for lipreading that he is taught, consider Kisor's recounting of his practices in school, paying attention to his teacher during class and his need to attend to the lips of those he is attempting to communicate with:

> Hearing students can relax and listen passively, eyes focused in the distance, soaking up auditory information as it washes over them. Lipreaders, however, must concentrate on a small visual point—the teacher's lips—actively hunting for clues to what is being said. "Listening" of this kind is extremely hard work. We cannot look out the window to briefly rest our eyes or to digest a piece of information; if we do so, we might miss something important and even lose the thread of discussion.[31]

He goes on to explain how the everyday functioning of a classroom— students asking questions and his teachers' responses—gives him "whiplash," as he looks back and forth from student to teacher in an effort to keep up with the conversation, only to find that he often misses the student's question, and misses the beginning of the teacher's answer as well. The result is that Kisor focused on his teachers, hoping to infer the question from the answer. In miniature, this shows the nature of Kisor's communicative capacities, caught as he is in a form of communication that depends on the intimate understanding of an individual's set of gestures. Whereas most hearing people can receive vocal signals from a room full of speakers and communicate themselves to that room through unimpaired speech, Kisor has no such ease of interaction. Listening for Kisor, unlike for many hearing individuals, is a full form of participation, requiring him to constantly monitor the mouths of the people he interacts with. Listening through lipreading requires Kisor to translate physical gesture into lexical meaning, a process that makes explicit the discrete interpretive work that hearing individuals do passively throughout their social interactions.

Lipreading, like Kisor does, depends on a complex chain of mimicry. Kisor infers from a person's gestures what sound she or he is making, and interprets those gestures alongside other similar gestures made by others in the past and the sounds he knows those people to have made. Moreover, he matches his interpretations of these gestures and sounds to the syntactic patterns he is observing. But rather than being able to rely on dominant, institutionally recognized schemes of interpretation, Kisor's ability to interpret the communicative acts of the people he interacts with is doubly idiosyncratic. First, Kisor needs to be able to translate a mouth movement into a syllable, but mouth movements are highly specific to individuals. A nervous tic, facial hair, a nonexpressive face—each can deeply frustrate Kisor's ability to discern what is being spoken to him, and each depends on his ability to understand the general appearance of a syllable's pronunciation as well as his ability to particularize his interpretation for each individual. Second, from that syllable and others, Kisor needs to derive the intended word or phrase spoken by his interlocutor. In the first case, each individual has her or his own set of communicative gestures that Kisor needs to decode, with the help of a visual lexicon of typical syllable movements. The second relies, by extension, on an interpretive scheme provided to Kisor by society—but only through his ability to relate the gestural cues to widely accepted words that are meaningful across society. Communication for Kisor is not easy, and it relies, like all communication, on a complex process of mimicry and interpretation, made possible by the institutionalization of symbolic meaning. In their institutionalization, mimicry and interpretation become technologies, ways of operating that facilitate interactions between people in unremarked-on ways. These technologies have embedded within them institutionalized assumptions, ways of mimicking and interpreting that are given to the individual rather than created by the individual. In that way, Kisor's form of communication brings into relief the unremarkable aspects of human communication that operate across all language, as well as the necessarily social aspects of mimicry and interpretation that make the institutional basis of communication possible. Kisor's mimicry is different than the desired imitative capacity for Noah, as Kisor has been purposefully trained to use mimicry in specific ways to interact with others through the differential recognition of patterns in communication.

Kisor always relied on the aid of others in his efforts to communicate on the telephone. In his teenage years, he depended first on his parents and friends to make phone calls for him, and eventually his younger sister played this role. In this way, his family sought to facilitate his connection with others, thereby enabling his symbolic subjectivity. As he writes,

> For a long time, when I was in high school, I had to ask my friends or Mother or Dad . . . to call my girlfriends to set up dates. This is no way to conduct a love life, having your *mother* ask if so-and-so would like to go to the movies, or maybe to Wimpy's for a shake, or whatever. . . . I am sure [Mother] was relieved when Debbie grew large enough to hold a telephone handset. . . . During the two years I lived at home while attending Medill, Debbie served as a very efficient social secretary, not only calling dates but reminding me when it was time to go out on them.[32]

Young Debbie served as Kisor's voice, allowing him to interact with people on the telephone, doubly mediated through Debbie and the telephone. Kisor relayed his message to Debbie, who then communicated it to whomever Kisor wanted to speak with on the telephone. Debbie then mediated for the person on the other end of the phone, communicating to Kisor what his friend sought to convey—this time, helpfully, with a set of speaking gestures that Kisor is deeply familiar with. Debbie served as a relay, embodying the processes embedded in a technology like the telephone, which similarly translates from speaker to listener in ways that for most people are not transparent. Telephony is a technology unremarkable in its modern ubiquity; but to have Debbie embody communication in a similar way exposes how she serves as a technology as well, one that communicates according to her own embedded logics, ghostwriting Kisor for others and vice versa. Kisor sees Debbie as serving as a precursor of much more complex forms of relaying information that deaf communities would come to use in the late twentieth century. As he explains,

> Deaf communities in many cities have organized "relay stations" of hearing volunteers, many of them physically handicapped and housebound. These volunteers take TDD [telecommunications device for the deaf] calls from the deaf and relay them by voice to their destinations, then call the TDD users back with the responses. . . . [In Illinois] the relay operators "translate" simultaneously between the two parties, and the better operators are so skilled that their service as go-betweens are virtually unobtrusive.[33]

As a technology, these modes of communication rely on the interaction of human bodies and technical systems, creating facilitating networks that enroll communities of individuals in making symbolic subjectivity possible for individuals whose social interactions would be more geographically circumscribed as a result of their communicative capacities and lack of social facilitation.

Throughout the twentieth century, deaf individuals used a variety of emergent technologies that enabled changing interactions with society and their environment. Cochlear implants, which serve as prosthetics for deaf individuals, functionally allowing them to hear a wider range of sound, albeit with a wide range of user experiences, gained widespread use in the 1990s and were further refined throughout the early twenty-first century.[34] In thinking about this history, Kisor writes,

> No deaf parents of a newborn, for instance, would be without a "baby crier," a microphone affixed to a crib that flashes a lamp when the infant wails. Or other such electronic visual attention getters as burglar alarms, wake-up alarms, fire and smoke alarms, pagers, phone and doorbell signalers, and more. . . . These devices were a long time coming—many of them had to wait for the invention of the transistor—but when they finally began to appear, they made the lives of deaf people immeasurably easier. Including mine.[35]

Kisor sees these relatively simple technologies as enabling new ways for deaf individuals to take care of their children, to know when they are in danger, or to learn when people are attempting to communicate with them. These basic functions of social obligation and connection make deaf individuals more fully symbolic subjects within the context of normative ideologies of communication and language; these technologies facilitate connection, moving away from the putative asocial effects of residential facilities and toward the normative ideal of full social integration through indexical signaling as the basis of communicative interactions.

Kisor suggests that technologies developed over the twentieth century radically remade the world of deafness, offering remedies that mediated the relationship between individuals and their environments in new ways. In recounting the history of technologies associated with facilitating communication for the deaf, from the teletype telephone system to more complex forms of relay,[36] Kisor sees the adoption of these technologies as enabling freedom on the part of once disenfranchised individuals, eventually resulting in the naturalization of these technologies as conveniences that are a part of everyday life in the United States, as ubiquitous and necessary as refrigerators and laundry machines:

> Modern conveniences are instruments of freedom. A life without something to cool perishables and freshen clothing would

be a very different one. We would need to devote a great deal of time and energy to basic survival tasks such as obtaining fresh food and clean clothes. Life without fridges and washers would be tolerable, but our spheres of activity would be severely limited. We would have less freedom to do things that matter—such as communicating with the rest of the world.[37]

In casting these facilitating technologies as enabling freedom and becoming mundane, Kisor implicitly argues for the technological drive in history creating new kinds of persons.[38] New remedies create new capacities for impaired individuals, and in so doing, they allow once-impaired individuals to integrate themselves in more robust ways with dominant social forms. In Kisor's view, where once a deaf individual was trapped at home, unable to communicate with the outside world, communication is now possible—at least with those who are able to use the same technologies. As Kisor recounts, the web of individuals, communities, and institutions that adopt these technologies—in no small part due to government requirements and support—allow deaf individuals to connect with broader and broader swaths of American society, and by extension to be recognized by that society as full persons and symbolic subjects. In this way, technology and personhood become permanently entangled in the production of subjectivity, enabling connectivity between more and more kinds of persons. In so doing, these technologies become necessary to maintain emergent social forms in order to ensure that who counts as a person continues to count as a person.

CONNECTIVITY AS THE BASIS OF SUBJECTIVITY

At the heart of Kisor's philosophy of life is the need for connection, an impulse that he draws via E. M. Forster. Kisor writes in closing his memoir, "*Only connect!* . . . In [E. M. Forster's] novels he showed how just a modest effort to communicate—to connect—could bridge vast chasms of indifference, bringing together people with little in common on a middle ground of mutual and sympathetic insight and understanding."[39] It is clear throughout his memoir that what he seeks in all of his communicative facilitations is a connection with other people—connections he sees as exceeding the expectations that Americans had of deaf people of his generation. His view of connection has largely been determined by the ableist, humanist, obligatory heterosexual and white norms of mid-twentieth-century American society, but connection should not be limited to human-to-human connections. Instead, focusing on the more-than-human connections bodies engage in and are facilitated through shows how animation creates the networks that connect persons. By American standards in the twentieth century, Kisor sees himself as an accomplished professional, having worked at a major newspaper throughout his career, maintained a marriage throughout his professional life, and raised two children. In retirement, he moved to northern Michigan, where he has a successful career as a novelist. Compared to many deaf people of his generation, many of whom were discouraged from acquiring sign language, Kisor sees himself as thoroughly accomplished; he has achieved what most Americans would regard as a "normal" life. Mirrielees's education, which stressed his upbringing in a "normal" family situation, may have been the primary motor for this achievement, but one might see Kisor's desire to connect as motivating his education, as well as his everyday life from childhood onward. As he writes of his young adulthood,

> Those who hear cannot imagine how grindingly lonely deafness often can be. A comfortable home can feel like a maximum-security prison if there is no easy means of communication with the outside. . . . Yes, I was living in the world of the hearing, and so long as I was in the presence of family, friends, and fellow workers, I connected. But I needed to enlarge the envelope of my life. As I grew older, like every other young man I needed to create and maintain my own physical and temporal space and from it communicate with the outside.[40]

The education that Mirrielees provided Kisor with, through her facilitation of his capacities to read lips and interpret the signals that others were conveying to him, made this connectivity possible. Kisor frames his desire for connection as largely human-to-human. Without the facilitating technologies that he interacted with throughout his life, these human-to-human connections would have been difficult, if not impossible. Kisor's desire for connection, and his ability to make those connections robust, allowed for his facilitated being in the world, which connected him to technologies, both explicit and implicit, to communities, the environment, and society generally. These technologies laid the basis for Kisor's personhood by American standards, but his desires for connectivity and reciprocation provided him with the means to become a subject.

Kisor sees his success as replicable but unlikely, given the contemporary institutional possibilities of education for deaf children, and the possibilities for education for American children more generally. He argues that the institutionalization of particular forms of education have limited the possibilities for connection for American children, resulting in a lack of capacity on the part of children to make the connections Kisor sees as so vital to life. As he writes,

> I am not wholly convinced that the failure, on the average,
> of the mainstreamed deaf community to keep up with their
> hearing peers is not part of a general failure of American
> education to serve broad segments of its clientele. It's the rare
> inner-city *hearing* high school graduate who can read even at
> fourth-grade level, and his peers who are bused to schools in
> middle-class neighborhoods don't do much better. Is a new
> segregation the solution? Or does the answer lie elsewhere, per-
> haps in the housecleaning of special education as well as general
> education?[41]

Kisor has a revolutionary spirit, in no small part due to his idiosyncratic experience as a student of Mirrielees. Rather than being disciplined by a specific institution at a young age, he was allowed to develop his capacities to communicate in his own way. Kisor was able to make do; he was capable of working with the training he received and mainstreaming into U.S. society. He sees this as possible for others as well—but not within the current configuration of education in the United States, which fails broad segments of its constituency, including disabled children and children born into underserved communities.

If Kisor despairs at the possibility of housecleaning the institution of American education in its entirety, then what he sees as more immediately beneficial is the creation of policies that shape the organization of U.S. institutions generally. He sees the need for a new interpretive framework that facilitates the personhood and subjectivity of those who would putatively be labeled as disabled, as embodied in the then-recent Americans with Disabilities Act (ADA). But lurking in that legislation and its expectations is a disabling premise that impinges on his claims to full personhood:

> I must confess to ambivalent emotions about the [Americans with Disabilities Act] provisions against discrimination in employment, as well as its sweeping application to all handicaps. It's obviously desirable that employers be prohibited from denying jobs to the handicapped on the basis of disability alone. But the law also obligates employers to provide "reasonable accommodation" to disabled workers, and that makes me uneasy. My deep-seated need for independence leads me to loathe the notion that my employer must spend money on me that would be unnecessary for a hearing employee. To me, that's charity forced by law, and an assault on my dignity.[42]

How does one square the distaste Kisor has for forced charity and the need for connection? Why would workplace facilitation be the sticking point for Kisor? The answer lies in the naturalization of the liberal subject as having a need for independence as embedded in the ADA. To be a student or to be a member of a society, Kisor sees that institutional transformations are necessary to recognize a wider swath of human variation as persons deserving of recognition and care. But to be a worker and to participate directly in the capitalist market, Kisor argues that facilitation should not be forced by the government. He suggests that the recognition of personhood is enough; enabling full liberal subjectivity through government subventions is unnecessary. Such a claim mirrors Kisor's experience of subjectivity and disability. What Kisor misses is that in order to fully participate in this way, individuals need to become symbolic subjects; they need to be able to find ways to interpret the communicative acts of the people around them in shared, meaningful ways. In this symbolic way of conceptualizing the subject, without the ADA's legal allowance for different modes of interaction that facilitate nonnormative modes of communication, disabled individuals continue to be ruled out by the lack of access to the symbolic. Their participation in society depends on acceding to the dominant mode of communication, meaning making, and intention. But what about children like Noah, for whom the symbolic will always be elusive and normative forms of subjectivity always impossible? Addressing this bias depends on expanding the nervous system to include the technologies, laws, and other institutions that enable diverse modes of being in the world. Moreover, it requires developing supple institutions that allow for modular interactions and socialities to emerge in contradistinction to the disciplined and controlled modes of subject formation that have marked earlier periods.

Sigmund Freud and the Tyranny of the Symbolic Subject
THE ROMANCE OF THE SYMBOLIC

Dr. Samson, a pseudonym for a senior psychiatrist at one of the neurology clinics where I conducted fieldwork, narrated his educational history to me after a grand rounds meeting in the neurology clinic where he worked:

> I was in medical school when people still kind of took psychoanalysis seriously. This was in the early 70s, and psychiatry was really exciting. On the one hand we had these big questions—how did the Holocaust happen?, why are people racist?, what will sexual liberation do for people?—and we had new scientific ways to answer these questions. It was like we were finally going to get answers to some really big questions. But then the science took over, and the big questions got replaced. Instead of being interested in human drives, people just wanted answers to physiological problems. It's like Freud just got thrown out the window. Look around. I'm the last of my generation here, and when I retire there will be a bunch of well-trained neurologists, but nobody to ask these bigger questions.

I thought about Samson's lament for a lost psychoanalysis while sitting through a weekly Lacanian training seminar.[43] Like Samson, I had read Freud during my graduate training, but by then, he was treated more as a social theorist than a scientific precursor to late-twentieth-century neuroscience and psychiatry. Like Samson, I developed a soft spot for Freud, especially the "big question" Freud. But where Samson's reading in graduate school had ended with Melanie Klein, John Bowlby, and Bruno Bettleheim in the 1970s, my own training had taken me into the work of Jacques Lacan and his students. Whatever pesky determinism undergirded Freud's conception of the human, Lacan's symbolic turn was too overdetermining for my taste. At the end of our conversation, Samson jokingly asked me, "Whatever happened to psychoanalysis?" I did not have an answer at the time, but now I do.

The symbolic is a prison. The interpretive schemes that we are provided with as a part of our acquisition of language provide the basis for the semiotic processes that we undergo in all of our communicative acts, laying the basis for the development of subjectivity within a world of shared, meaningful symbols. The meanings that we append to a given word may change over time, they may be played with through poetics or humor, or they may be made troubling through experience, but these changes depend on an understanding of the referentiality of a word. To be raised in a shared language is to adopt, through mimicry, the interpretive schemes we are provided with; we accept the sound and we accept the meaning. To be recognized in American society as a person means accepting this value of language, its codes, and its interpretive frames. For those who are partially or completely foreclosed from acquiring normative forms of language—as Henry Kisor and Noah Greenfeld are, respectively—the outcome is partial or complete foreclosure of normative personhood and subjectivity. For Kisor, this means finding mechanisms to bridge his capacities with the norms expected by society; he will come to know himself through his communicative difference as a form of mimesis, based on his ability to adopt spoken language and the other facilitating technologies that make verbal communication possible. For Noah, this means permanent foreclosure from normative models of symbolic subjectivity, as he never fully develops the ability to communicate in normative ways. At least, this is the model of symbolic subjectivity that has been developed over the course of the twentieth century, heavily informed by psychoanalytic approaches to consciousness, cognition, and personhood.

The symbolic subject—which is not so different from the neurological subject—is one who is constrained by history, albeit a largely social history, rather than a primarily biological one. In a challenge to neurologically reductive forms of subjectivity, this moves the space of subjectivity outside of the lone individual and places it squarely into the matrix of social connections and relations an individual is born into and maintained through, particularly in the context of communication. But Kisor and Greenfeld show that how personhood and subjectivity are defined affects the kinds of facilitation available for the elaboration of symbolic subjectivity.

Sigmund Freud had two founding myths that he deployed to conceptualize the relationship of the individual to society, both deeply symbolic. The first and most famous was that of the Oedipal conflict, in which a boy child's primary affection and desire is directed at the mother but comes to be thwarted by the presence of the father.[44] In frustrating that affectionate connection, the child turns his desire outward to find another source of passionate interaction. The child–mother dyad opens into the child–society relationship, which facilitates the child becoming a full person and subject. But this transition can go awry, perhaps leading to a host of neurotic disorders—which is why Freud relies on the Greek myth of Oedipus to tell this story. Oedipus accidentally marries his mother, Jocasta, after freeing the city of Thebes from the threat of the Sphinx. Much later in life, when he realizes that his primary romantic interest is his mother, Oedipus blinds himself and spends the rest of his life as a shattered version of his former self. For Freud, it is not the literal reenactment of this drama that each child goes through, but rather a symbolic recreation of this founding relationship and its transition to a focus on social relations more generally—and the creation of subjectivity as based in the individuated person mediated through symbolic relationships.

The other founding myth of Freud's that is less well known is the story of the primal horde.[45] In that tale, Freud imagines an early epoch of human prehistory in which a patriarch has made a harem for himself of the available women in a community, depriving his sons of mothers for their children. The sons band together and murder their father, dividing the women among themselves, and thereby create a more egalitarian society (for the men). In doing so, they also install the prohibition of incest, ensuring that women will be distributed among the community rather than hoarded by any one man. Like with Oedipus, whether or not there was ever a primal horde is beside the point; the important thing is that the symbol of the father stands in for the organizing principle of society itself. The symbolic makes sense of the organization of social relations, both in the implicit mimicry individuals engage in through their subject formation and through their interpretation of social norms as rooted in a historical situation, even if that situation is itself fanciful.

A third story more important to Freud's adherents in the late twentieth and early twenty-first centuries relates to an unpublished book that Freud began in 1895, his "Project for a Scientific Psychology."[46] The earliest part of Freud's career was spent working in a physiology lab focused on the brain. Freud came close to being able to offer the first accurate description of the neuron as a biological object, as well as how neurons work through the conduction of electric signals. Freud was an early neuroscientist, even if he is rarely remembered as such. Like many contemporary neuroscientists, Freud was working on finding a material basis for neurotic experiences, attempting to show how the actual physiological functioning of the human brain might be impeded or created by social experiences. "Project for a Scientific Psychology," which was only published posthumously, is significantly unlike other books written by Freud in that it attempts to posit an entirely materialist basis for mental distress, and Freud goes to great lengths to describe these mechanisms using scientific language and causal logic. Ultimately, Freud would abandon the "Project" in favor of his more social and symbolic conception of how neurological disorders operated, seeing in symbolic explanations the possibility of cures that were impossible in a strictly biological system. Advocates of neuropsychoanalysis use this early Freud,[47] both to identify his unnoticed contributions to neuroscience as it would develop throughout the twentieth and early twenty-first centuries, and to point to the possibilities for integrating Freud's symbolic understanding of neurological disorders with materialist conceptions of biological determinations of impairment. But the symbolic underlies all neuroscience that relies on the communicative capacities of individuals to make themselves known through language and that accept the lack of communicative capacities as a symptom associated with particular disorders.

Although Freud would at times traffic in biological determinism,[48] a primary concern for him was the symbolic basis of communication, both between individuals and between the unconscious and the conscious mind. Freud's conception of dreams relied on our unconscious mind's ability to construct a narrative, sometimes seemingly nonsensical and often in code, in order to relay messages to our conscious selves.[49] Freud allowed for the symbolic to be shared and to be intensely personal. Without the symbolic and its interpretation, for Freud we would live in a world of brute representation, where a pipe is always simply a pipe. For Freud and those who follow in his wake, for humans, the symbolic produces a necessary distinction between us and other animals. Other animals might be able to communicate in some rudimentary fashion, but they lack access to the symbolic. Existing as we do in the symbolic, interpretation is the basis of all communication; it suffuses every communicative act. The necessity of interpretation allows for the complexity of our dreaming lives, but also for the sociable wordplay of joking, innuendo, and everyday communication.[50] In this view, interpretation and the symbolic make humans human through everyday forms of mimesis. This communicative mimesis marks our fundamental difference from other animals and serves to differentiate among humans, as some individuals have more nuanced symbolic and interpretive faculties than others—hence the difference between the psychoanalyst and the neurotic, the latter disabled by an inability to see the world as it truly is, whereas the former can pierce the symbolic veil and thereby facilitate healing. The symbolic, following Freud, both differentiates humans from other animals in their cognitive capacities and makes possible the complex processes that compose civilization,[51] which helps to maintain normative social forms, thereby suppressing baser animal instincts but also creating a social world wherein access to the symbolic is necessary as part of normative forms of subjectivity. With these assumptions as the basis of subjectivity, nonverbal individuals like Noah are immediately foreclosed from normative subjectivity, and nonnormatively verbal individuals like Kisor must find remedies to supplement their partial access to shared institutions of interpretation, symbolism, and meaning making.

However disabling lack of access to the symbolic is for Freud, in the hands of Jacques Lacan, the symbolic order becomes the very web of human life, tying humans throughout history to a dominant institutional organization of meaning making and interpretation.[52] For Lacan, the symbolic order also makes social life possible, simultaneously barring individuals from accessing particular expressions of nonnormative desire and channeling the pursuit of desire into generative, normative behaviors. In Lacan's work, the symbolic becomes both the basis of neurosis and neurosis' potential remedy; the symbolic divorces humans from the real and also protects humans from it, but humans are driven, through the pursuit of desire, to attempt to come into contact with the real, to pierce the edifice of the symbolic. For Lacan, it is not simply that all social interaction is symbolic and depends on the interplay of mimicry and interpretation but that all human history is shaped by structural relationships embedded in the symbolic order and that this symbolic order comes to structure the subjectivity of individuals, imprinting on them the normative order of society and making them metonymic extensions of that order. To lack access to language exempts individuals from the symbolic order, suggesting that subjectivity is externally derived—at least to the extent that they know themselves through the symbolic. For Lacan, any access to communication necessarily partakes of the symbolic order, as the structural basis of the symbolic order entails that the fundamental structure of language and subjectivity finds its logic in the relationship between the real and the symbolic.[53] The structure of the symbolic order is necessary to make subjects of individuals and to reproduce society: individuals need to be moved away from their brute animal understandings of the world and toward the symbolic referentiality of words, ideas, and communication. For Lacan, those who cannot make this move from mere imitation to complex forms of mimesis are hopelessly impaired, unable to communicate with others and unable to create a subjective understanding of the self.

In psychoanalytic understandings of the individual, language, and society, history is paramount, which has been inherited in neuroscience through trauma studies and theories of epigenetics. This historical contextualization of the symbolic in individual lives moves neurological disorder outside of the individual and into society. Individuals are disabled not solely due to their inability to communicate but because the nature of communication is intrinsically symbolic—that is, it is necessarily institutional and predicated on the practice of interpretation. The symbolic subject is not the neurological one; the symbolic subject is not based on an individual's reflexive awareness of the material action of the body, as Antonio Damasio argues. Instead, the symbolic subject is one that is willfully created by others who participate in the symbolic ordering of society and its continuance. Such a conception of subjectivity is just as species specific as the neurological subject; other species lack access to the symbolic, and only humans become persons through the symbolic. In these formulations, nonhuman animals may be able to communicate, but their forms of communication can only ever be instinctual, such as responses to a predator.

In making the anthropocentric claim that only humans have access to symbolic language, the symbolic subject and the neurological subject are equally moored on the distinction between the animal and the human, making the neurologically or symbolically impaired more animal than human. It is here that Freud's founding myths of Oedipal conflict and the primal horde come into play. In both of these myths, the father plays an important role, first in helping to redirect desire away from the mother and toward society more generally, and in the case of the primal horde, by constituting the foundation of society itself. Society and subjectivity exist because of the intervention of the father, who, symbolically speaking, becomes aligned with the superego, civilization, and culture—the forces of repression that compel the productive investment in the future of the individual and the species. In both myths, this production of social investment and sociality is based on a foundational history. In this psychoanalytic and symbolic view, humans do not live in history so much as recreate it.

BEYOND THE PRISON HOUSE OF THE SYMBOLIC

Neuroscience might offer a way out of symbolic subjectivity toward a conception of the self that is intrinsically material, if not for three problems. As Antonio Damasio argues, any knowledge of the self depends on language. Indeed, Sigmund Freud and Jacques Lacan argue that language is always situated within history, and, most important, that the brain is not simply a material processor but rather a heavily regimented symbol in its own right. That the brain is taken, popularly and scientifically, as an object has to do with its symbolic reification; it is an organ that can be referred to as a whole or by its component parts as an actor with intentions. That "neurological disorder" is meaningful as a term relies on the shared conception that the brain is central in a particular set of biological phenomena, and that the brain itself is unitary in its spatialization and universal in its capacities—at least as they are idealized. The symbol of the brain is indebted to the history of medical semiotics, which, in allopathy and biomedicine, conceptualizes the body through strict localization.[54] This is in contrast to other medical traditions, including practices from South Asia, East Asia, and Africa, that conceptualize the body not as a series of discrete organs but as a set of systems or humors that individual organs are a part of, and which are not reducible to a specific organ or an organ that North Atlantic biomedicine would identify as such. This is not to deny that lesions are spatial but to point to the belief that a lesion in one location may be the result of a systemic condition and produce specific, recognizable effects. Biomedicine is reaching similar conclusions, as the growing awareness of the microbial colonies of one's body affecting organ processes is pointing to the possibility that organs are not easily reducible to a particular body space but are rather subsystems within a larger system.[55] Failing a paradigm shift in how biomedicine conceptualizes organs, the brain exists as a sign that refers to a set of processes and functions that regiment how symptoms are interpreted and acted on. As a symbol, the brain limits interpretation and action to a definable set of categories conceptualized as neurological disorders. It also motivates specific kinds of interventions, although these interventions have changed over time: psychoanalytic talking cures, invasive surgeries like lobotomy, treatments like electroconvulsive therapies, and most recently pharmaceutical interventions. The symbolic associations of the brain have changed over time in tandem with the therapeutic technologies used to act on the brain and its disorders, but the brain as a material object continues to hold symbolic heft. When neuroscientists like Damasio refer to subjectivity as based in an individual's reflexive understanding of the brain and its functioning, such claims rely on this symbolic construction of the organ as a stable, unitary object that can be referred to in a meaningful way.

As much as the neurological subject exists outside of history and is a function of an awareness of biological processes, attention has been increasingly drawn to neuroplasticity, the possibility for the material structure of the brain to change over time.[56] Discussions of plasticity have been focused on the positive aspects of these changes, which encourage individuals to train or exercise their cognitive functions in ways that enhance the brain. Such a view accepts that biology is not destiny and that the brain can be changed in subtle ways; neuroplasticity also accepts that the brain can be changed by the environment and social interactions in ways that shape its capacities. At its most benign, this leads to ideas like the Mozart effect, which posits that exposing an infant to certain kinds of classical music will foster genius-level cognitive capacities, although there is no evidence to support this. Neuroplasticity's more serious implications suggest that periods of severe deprivation and trauma might adversely affect brain growth and cognitive development.[57] At first glance, this would seem to replace a transhistorical structure of the human brain with a more individualized history; it would also seem to allow for the self-help possibilities of cognitive training, leading individuals to be able to overcome any disadvantageous situation they are raised in through dedicated practice. Neuroplasticity accepts that to be born into poverty or an abusive family shapes the brain in material ways, but it offers the promise that these material impoverishments can be overcome—if only individuals are dedicated enough to the project of reshaping their neural pathways and connections. This is a typical neoliberal fantasy, displacing onto individuals the burdens placed on them by society. In the context of neuroplasticity, this displacement makes the burden of personal development exquisitely material, structured into the very stuff of the brain. Can trauma that has shaped the brain actually be overcome? Neuroplasticity would appear to offer an affirmative answer, even if sociological conceptions of social stratification would suggest otherwise. It is not brains alone that allow individuals to overcome structural inequalities, and any recourse to neuroplasticity as a panacea for social inequities ignores the entrenchment of inequities in the United States.

The invocation of these two regimes of history—symbolic, structural history and individual, material history—lays the foundation for the moralization of the neoliberal subject through behavior. The symbolic subject is one that is produced, first through the structural relations embedded in human sociality and second by the enactment of symbolic relations in any given family. Being normal means enacting these family dramas unerringly, reproducing society generation after generation. An abnormal individual points to a failure in this system of reproduction—not the structural relations of society, but in the family unit.[58] In this psychoanalytic model, an abnormal individual is the fault of a family, most likely the mother and father, who have somehow mangled the symbolic reproduction of the subject. A psychological disorder is not the individual's alone but something shared by parents—and potentially ancestors stretching back generations.[59] Disorder in the individual speaks to disorder in the family, and although individuals can overcome this generational disorder through therapy, they are indebted to this family history, which displaces the need for moral evaluation away from the individual and toward the family. Bad families produce bad individuals, but virtuous individuals might overcome this history through good acts, including therapeutic commitments to betterment.

However retrograde such a conception of disorder and subjectivity appears to be, scientific understandings of hereditary illness and epigenetics are not wildly different in their causal explanations for the source of disorders. Where they do diverge is in their moralization of the individual: psychoanalytic understandings of disorder implicate families and sometimes the whole social order, whereas biological understandings of disorder place it squarely in the body of the individual. In either context, the burden of seeking normalcy falls on individuals, which, in biomedical frameworks, means seeking some remedy to mediate the relationship between individuals and their environment. Individuals who do not use a prescribed remedy, whether pharmaceutical, surgical, or prosthetic, can be construed as noncompliant, its own form of bad behavior; individuals who cannot use a remedy are marked as impaired and in need of care, whether in the form of a family or kin network or institutionalization. This need for remediation can throw onto the family responsibilities and obligations, which, when unmet, cast the family in a moral light. The failure of an individual to meet normative standards, as in Noah Greenfeld's case of failed language acquisition, has the consequence of casting his lack of achievement as a failure on the part of his parents to meet the standards set forth by Ivar Lovaas and his colleagues or to take seriously the family's need to shape Noah's behaviors in normative ways. As much as the neurological subject and other biological ways of conceptualizing human subjectivity attempt to vacate the family from consideration in the production of subjectivity, it is important to note that in both neurologic and symbolic models, the individual is never alone. The actions of others are reflected in the individual's failures to realize full human potentials.

EXTERNALIZING SUBJECTIVITY THROUGH EPIPHENOMENAL INTERPRETATION

Regardless of psychoanalysis's or neuroscience's attempts to sidestep these moralizations of the individual and the family, one solution is to adopt a view of subjectivity that is epiphenomenal—that judges an individual not through the lens of a personal or family history but in the context of the individual's present. Such a view depends on adopting understandings of communication and the symbolic that are less historical and more contextual. In Noah Greenfeld's case, his communication is immediate, responding directly to his environment and needs. Yet as Josh Greenfeld reports, Noah rarely communicates even in this most directly referential way. Noah seems unbothered by a full diaper, unmotivated by hunger. Noah wants what he wants. He seems unperturbed by the need to communicate to others what his intents or desires are. He may exist outside of language, outside of subjection, but he remains an object of attention—from his parents, his physicians and educators, and eventually the care workers who facilitate his life at the residential hospital where his parents house him. Noah is not a full subject in either the neuroscientific or symbolic model because he lacks language and interacts with institutions that rely on the metric of linguistic self-expression as the basis for judging subjectivity. Noah is foreclosed from subjectivity by these institutions, either because he lacks the capacity to develop a subjective sense of self, or because the social world he is a part of has failed to facilitate him in some irrevocable way. No expansion of symbolic conceptions of the subject will find room to include Noah as a full subject. But he is treated as an individuated person because of dominant American ideas about the individual and personhood.

Henry Kisor, on the other hand, has a contextual, epiphenomenal understanding of the symbolic based in his learned mimetic capacity. His lipreading depends on his ability to interpret a gesture in its context and infer situational meaning. The mode of interpretation that underlies Kisor's social interactions is transversal, cutting across the horizontal and vertical institutionalizations of interpretation and meaning, providing him with a modular basis for social interactions based on situational experience. Kisor's social participation in this way—limited in specific contexts by environmental forces and modes of interpersonal interactions—entails his treatment by others as an individual and as a subject in his own right. Deaf people like Kisor, potentially with less capacity for lipreading, have been progressively recognized as full persons and subjects despite their treatment in the early part of the twentieth century and for generations before that. Kisor argues that this change in status depended on the growing set of technological remedies for the communicational difficulties associated with deafness, as well as the ADA and institutional support for deaf people, all of which simultaneously make personhood possible and facilitate it through an expanding nervous system that includes legal statutes and practices, novel technologies, and social affordances. In a strict model of symbolic subjectivity, Kisor and individuals who rely on the facilitating technologies that provide access to normative forms of communication share in dominant symbolic understandings of the world only partially; they conceptualize their world through the mediating powers of the technologies and institutions they interact with. In the symbolic model of subjectivity, they are symbolic subjects of a different order than those who do not rely on these mediating technologies, despite the attempts of these technologies to work their way into the fabric of everyday life and disappear therein. This elides how all communication and interpretation is not strictly imitative and that every symbolic subject exists in some variance from institutionalized norms as an outcome of mimesis. Every symbolic subject is discretely disabled through the slippery processes of mimesis and interpretation.[60]

In this symbolic view of subjectivity, Henry Kisor's epiphenomenal semiotics allow him an idiosyncratic access to the dominant symbolic world he lives in. All symbolic systems depend on interpretation, but for most speakers, interpretation is constrained by the historical context of symbols. However, for Kisor, symbols need to be interpreted on the basis of the immediate situation he finds himself in, which can lead to confusion on his part and that of the people he interacts with. The title of Kisor's memoir, *What's That Pig Outdoors?*, derives from one of these confusions: Kisor's five-year-old son rushes into the room where he is sleeping to ask, "What's the big loud noise?" Kisor mistakenly interprets this as, "What's that pig outdoors?" The mouth gestures look the same, and with an abstract referent—and in this case one that Kisor cannot hear—Kisor's interpretive options are expansive. That the appearance of a pig is more likely than a loud noise makes Kisor's misinterpretation comedic, but such misinterpretations are rife in his interactions with other people. This is not to minimize Kisor's linguistic and social achievements but to point to the ways that all individuals depend on epiphenomenal semiotics in their interactions with other people and that Kisor's experiences offer an intensified version of everyday practices of mimesis and interpretation.[61] How we interpret others, and by extension ourselves, is dependent on the facilitation of others; how we interpret is based on the historicity of language but also the constraints of the social interaction we find ourselves a part of. This is true at the level of everyday social interactions as well as an individual's moment in history, and Kisor's narrative of technological advancements in the facilitation of deaf individuals points to how he sees the personhood of deaf individuals changing over the course of the twentieth and early twenty-first centuries as a result of finer and finer access to the dominant symbolic order through a technologically expansive nervous system. Kisor is not foreclosed from symbolic subjectivity, but his experience—and that of others with sensory disorders that are seen as interfering with normative forms of communication—is idiosyncratic and depends on the explicit facilitation of technologies, human and nonhuman. Kisor's experience is an intensification of the nature of symbolic subjectivity: language is a facilitating technology, and all speakers depend on the historicity of shared meaning as the basis for communication. Kisor's is an exemplar of an experience that all symbolic subjects share. But what of those like Noah Greenfeld, who are foreclosed from access to the symbolic as it is usually conceived?

Based on the assumptions of normative communication in symbolic forms of subjectivity, Noah is a nonsymbolic subject. Unable to communicate his intentions and desires in normative ways, his father is led to wonder whether he has intentions and desires at all. At one point in Noah's early training with Ivar Lovaas and his students, the suggestion is made that Josh and Foumi withhold food in order to inspire Noah to meet their demands. Rather than grow hungry and capitulate to the requests that are being made of him, Noah simply does not eat; he seems to have no desire to eat, but he will respond to food when it is placed before him. Rather than grow hungry and in his hunger become aware of his needs, he simply grows hungrier. This may be a state of Lacanian jouissance, a state of pure pleasure, beyond the prohibitions of his family and society more generally, but it is one that is dangerously close to death. Josh and Foumi see in Noah a capacity to forego eating to the point of starvation. In recognizing that drive in Noah, they abandon the experiment of withholding food. Noah cannot be coerced through any typically behaviorist method. For Josh, Noah not only lives beyond language but also lives without desire. Similarly, for Josh, Noah not only does not mimic in a communicative way but also fails to imitate in ways that make him a recognizable person by normative standards, troubling the ability of others to see him as a person. There is seemingly no internalization for Noah, no symbolic register to engage with and to use to mediate his relationships with his environment or other people. Theories of subjectivity that depend on the symbolic, on language and self-referentiality, miss Noah and people like him. Symbolic theories of the subject render those without normative forms of communication as mere objects—animals at best, obstacles at worst. This is the very heart of the problem for Josh as he wrestles with his competing desires: at once, he wants to care for Noah, to nurture him into a speaking, symbolic subject, a recognizable person for society, yet all indications are that Noah will never achieve this symbolic capacity, that he will never be a full symbolic subject, even if he is treated as a full person. The Greenfelds' decision to institutionalize Noah is based on this assumption. In the symbolic regime, Noah will never be a full subject, and pretending that he will be only seems to lead to the reshaping of Josh's ambitions, as well as continued distress within the family. As Josh writes, they see it as better to accept Noah's limitations and adopt an institutionalized solution that will at least care for Noah, if not labor under the expectation that he can ever become a fully symbolic subject.

The problem here is implicit: if access to the symbolic is something only humans have, how can individuals with neurological disorders be subjects in any normative way? At worst, foreclosure from symbolic subjectivity is tantamount to treating individuals as mere objects rather than as persons—things to be talked about but not communicated with. Once removed is the position that nonverbal individuals are more animal than human, able to understand simple commands, even if they cannot communicate with anything other than following directions or immediate indexes of intent, captured in Ivar Lovaas's reliance on imitation. Then there is the possibility that individuals understand most of what is communicated to them, but they are unable to communicate in a dominant language, making them interpreters without being fully mimetic. This is the position that Henry Kisor's teacher seeks to overcome by ensuring that he can both be communicated with and communicate himself to others in ways that help him pass as "normal" through oralism. To be a fully symbolic subject means being able to acquire dominant forms of interpretation and mimicry to the extent that any communicative act can be not only understood but also responded to appropriately. It is in that matrix of interpretation and mimicry that an individual can elaborate a normative symbolic subjectivity, and any variance from full capacity in either of these qualities—mimicry or interpretation—invariably results in less than full, normative subjectivity. The question remains open as to what those with nondominant forms of mimicry and interpretation make of themselves. What forms of subjectivity are made possible by not trafficking in dominant modes of communication? One answer might lie in forms of indexical communication,[62] in which the relationship between sign and referent is immediate rather than representational. As scholars who argue that there is a difference between human and nonhuman communication suggest, when a dog whimpers in pain or a dolphin whistles to indicate an interest in playing, there is no interpretation other than the immediately indexed referent. So far as we know, a dog or dolphin cannot deceive itself or others, cannot trade on an inferred meaning to humorous ends; communication is immediately referential and purely indexical. Subjectivity might be read as existing in the same temporal frame, always constrained in the present without any future or historical frame to situate itself within.

Interpretation in a dominant symbolic framework is a static understanding of a sign and its referent. Subjectivity likewise is largely static, in that the categories and relations that lay the basis of individuals' subjective understanding of themselves are static in their referentiality. These static views of language and subjectivity are the groundwork for theories of social interaction that depend on recognition,[63] as recognition relies on individuals' fitting neatly into dominantly understood categories of identity and relational forms. Nonnormative forms of subjectivity risk being unrecognized by individuals and institutions, which is why diagnostic categories become so vital in the attempt to address the needs of nonnormative individuals. In order to achieve recognition, accepting these categories and relations becomes a disliberal necessity. But the acceptance of these categories depends on individuals or family members who understand the dominant category they are laboring to utilize as the basis of recognition. In this respect, consider the elaboration of the politically satirical category "neurotypical." The category was initially developed by activists in an attempt to point to the ways that neurodivergent individuals were treated as fundamentally different from the majority of the population; "divergent" here substitutes for abnormal.[64] A category like "neurotypical" works as a means to unravel assumptions about neurological disorders, but it is the tool of those who can create a meaningful play on language. It is not the tool of those foreclosed from symbolic subjectivity— individuals like

Noah Greenfeld—although it may speak for him. Similarly, the term "neurodiverse" is an attempt to destabilize the categories of neurological disorder that would restrict the lives of individuals with a neurological disorder that might necessitate institutional interventions. If neurodiverse people can be seen as inhabiting a form of subjectivity that is nonnormative and can be recognized as a basis for personhood, then dominant society can expand to embrace a greater breadth of nonnormative experiences of the world, eventually making these other modes of subjectivity recognizable variations.

However, there is another possibility, and that is embracing the kind of modular epiphenomenal semiotics of Henry Kisor, a semiotics of the present that depends on the immediate situation rather than history and the institutional regimentation of signs. Making the symbolic modular in this way renders it supple in its interpretation and manipulation; it renders it transversal and more open for interpretation. To reach this end, moving beyond imitation and recognition is vital. Instead, seeing facilitation as the basis of social interaction, personhood, and communication opens up possibilities for nonnormative subjectivities that defy becoming vertically and horizontally institutionalized. Symbolic subjectivity—and neurological subjectivity to the extent that it participates in the economy of medical, scientific, and popular symbols—depends on the construction of a continuity of the subject. This view holds that individuals are situated within history, theirs and society's more generally, and that any behavior in the present is informed by the historicity of subjects and their interpretations of the symbolic interactions they are having. A modular, epiphenomenal semiotics unmoors the individual from these institutional histories of interpretation; it bases mimicry not in historical interactions but in the immediate context of communication. Such a conceit levels the communicative field, rendering the communicative acts of all participants to be equivalent in their meaning, or lack thereof. In this framework, meaning is immediate; it indexes not history but the desires of the present, and potentially the future. Epiphenomenal semiotics focuses attention on collaboration, on the interactive relations that make communication possible, which recognizes the need for shared projects that can be communicated about, even if they are constantly changing in their constituencies, roles, and goals. One such experiment in communication is the psychoanalytically inspired La Borde, a residential hospital in France, which captures, in an everyday way, the revolutionary spirit Josh Greenfeld is warned away from and that Henry Kisor sees as fundamental, which is an attempt to facilitate wider ranges of human variation as persons and subjects.

How to Make a Modular World

EXPERIMENTAL INSTITUTIONS FOR
EPIPHENOMENAL SUBJECTS

The first thing that might strike a visitor about La Borde is its emplacement in nature. The yard is expansive and free, birds chirp and sing, bugs trill and squeak. Everyone ambulates each to his or her own gait. Uneven strides, dragging feet, shuffling, open zippers. A lone, idiosyncratic walker might not strike anyone as exceptional, but a parade of idiosyncrasies points to the nature of the community at La Borde. La Borde is an experiment in psychiatric care designed by Jean Oury in the 1950s to work against the debilitating institutions that composed the contemporary landscape: residential hospitals more interested in interring patients for their lifetimes than in facilitating their participation in society. As an institution, La Borde was conceived as a society unto itself, a collection of diverse individuals—clients, their families, manual workers, clinical staff—brought together by the institution and motivated by shared projects. Rather than the cellular structure of a hospital or prison, where each client or pair of clients is confined to a room with small, shared spaces, La Borde was conceived as a shared home. Clients were housed in barracks-style bedrooms, with several sharing one space; common spaces, like dining and living areas, were designed to be open, allowing people to participate as they desired to, but also able to be molded to specific ends as needed by a collaboration—an art project, group cooking, therapy. Likewise, the grounds of the institution were intended to be open, allowing for people to walk, play, and congregate as they saw fit, as well as being open for meetings and performances. That the grounds of La Borde are filled with wandering clients who would otherwise be treated as disorderly is part of the plan, just as the collaborative project of staging Witold Gombrowicz's *Operetta* is part of the therapeutic design of La Borde,[65] which provides the narrative basis of Nicolas Philibert's documentary *Every Little Thing (La Moindre des Choses)*.[66]

From its inception, La Borde was thought of as an experiment, moving away from the kinds of institutions that permanently housed individuals with neurological disorders. Psychoanalytic philosopher Félix Guattari, who played a central role in La Borde's organization and day-to-day operation, sees these earlier hospitals as "quasi-zoological," reducing the institution's clients to the status of animals by stripping them of their human capacities, particularly those relating to communication: "Psychotics, objects of a system of quasi-zoological guardianship, necessarily take on an almost bestial allure, turning in circles all day long, knocking their heads against walls, shouting, fighting, crouching in filth and excrement. These patients, whose understanding and relations with others are disturbed, slowly lose their human characteristics, becoming deaf and blind to all social communication."[67] By Guattari's account, La Borde regularly housed approximately a hundred clients and employed about seventy workers, including clinical staff and manual workers—chefs, groundskeepers, janitors, and other staff that helped the clinic run on a day-to-day basis. As Guattari argues, in a typical mental hospital of the time, the divisions between the staff, workers, and clients were rigidly maintained, and clients would only see clinical staff during group or individual therapy and consultations. Workers were tasked with maintaining the order of the hospital, but not necessarily interacting with clinical staff or potentially the clients. La Borde sought to disrupt these tendencies by ensuring that the manual workers found themselves in work situations that were not part of their usual tasks, and that clinical staff would help with manual labor. Putting clinical staff into these everyday situations—sweeping, cooking, tending the garden—forced them to step out from behind the curtain of medical expertise and objective remove; they could not stand apart from the community, but had to be integral members of it. For clients and their families, workers, and other clinical staff, the goal was to demystify medical experts and put them on the same hierarchical level as everyone else by disrupting the typical social structure of the clinic.

The clients at La Borde represent a wide set of diagnostic categories, including schizophrenia and autism, but Guattari refers to them all as psychotics.[68] Many of them communicate in nonnormative ways. Some have full verbal capacity; some are nonverbal. All of them—and this is what Guattari is indexing in his use of the term "psychotic"—are disorderly by the standards of contemporary French society. If not housed at La Borde, they would be institutionalized elsewhere or taken care of in their family home by family and caregivers. As an institution, La Borde was designed to facilitate personhood and subjectivity, albeit personhood and subjectivity that are nonnormative. This facilitation was predicated on the expectation that shared projects provide individuals mechanisms to understand themselves and each other with, and that these projects become the basis for collective forms of collaboration. They become ways to upset the seriality of everyday life and replace it with a trajectory that motivates individual and community action.[69] Besides Guattari's and Oury's firsthand reports of life at La Borde, *Every Little Thing* is the one document of the institution in its day-to-day operations. Released in 1997, a few years after Guattari's death and while Oury was still the head of La Borde, *Every Little Thing* follows the community as they set about rehearsing and eventually staging *Operetta*. Philibert makes no distinction between the staff at La Borde and the clients. He labels none of the speakers; nor does he go to any length to situate the scenes of everyday life he provides the viewer. Instead, it is as if the viewer were simply dropping in on the actions at La Borde over the course of several weeks. Scenes, much like life at the institution, are languid and unrushed; the inhabitants of La Borde are simply living their bucolic lives outside of the confines of mainstream French society.

Philibert captures the contradiction of La Borde: the European formality of the place—a mansion from an earlier age, ornately built yet filled with a hodgepodge of cheap furniture, accumulated less by design than by utility, peopled by the inhabitants of La Borde who might be dressed strangely, either abiding by their own sense of style or costumed for a play they are rehearsing. La Borde is at once deeply formal in its appeal to European classical aesthetic standards yet shot through with the informality of a society that rules itself. The building that houses La Borde is foreboding in its whiteness, an enormous home set among an expansive green yard, lined on each side by trees. Arrayed in front are the vehicles used by the staff: white vans with three or four rows of seating, ready to transport members of the community to town for a shopping trip, to the mountains for skiing, or to visit an exhibition or museum. As much as the clients might be wandering the grounds or lounging in the mansion, they might also be hard at work, building a set for *Operetta*, helping cook a meal for the community, cleaning, gardening, or helping with some other institutional chore. The clients and staff might also be hard at work rehearsing lines or practicing music to accompany a performance. Throughout these daily activities, they might also make apparent the conditions that have brought them to La Borde: nervous tics, lack of affect, speaking loudly and out of turn, banging on furniture or walls, guttural noises in place of language, public self-stimulation. The list of symptoms is long and not particularly of interest to anyone there. There are no strict divisions between the clients and the staff, to the point where a quirky clinician might be mistaken for a client, or a well-composed client might be confused for a member of the clinical staff. Maybe most glaring in the converted mansion are the incongruities between the secondary consequences of the clients' neurological disorders—lost teeth, bruises and other wounds, messy, greasy hair, generally disheveled states of being—and the ornate architecture. As with the rehearsing players assembled to warm up, chanting "the stools of Lord Blotton," it is clear even to a casual observer that La Borde is not a French mansion fallen into disrepair and taken over by squatters but an institution organized with a shared purpose, however uncommon its assemblage of characters might be.

CHANGING THE SUBJECT THROUGH REORGANIZATION

If you call La Borde, you are likely to talk to a client assigned to the switchboard, who is tasked to redirect your call. Likewise, the person mopping the floor of a shared dormitory might be a staff member or a client. An individual might be instructing another in a musical performance, or learning to use stilts. Everyone takes turns cooking. There is a fluidity to the community, with staff and clients working side by side throughout the day to meet their collective needs, and this shared purpose suffuses communal life, as everyone takes turns rotating through shared chores. Staff work on the daily need to provide clients with all their necessary medications, sitting in the pharmacy, breaking up blister packs of pharmaceuticals and putting them into bowls and bottles destined to be redistributed. Group analysis is organized throughout the week, and clients have one-on-one meetings with clinical staff, sometimes in private offices or unconventional settings, like the garden. Everyone seems to smoke—or at least everyone seems to carry cigarettes. Everyone drinks coffee. There are seemingly no divisions within the community, with everyone participating to the extent that he or she can, facilitated in their efforts by the staff and other clients. As Guattari writes about La Borde and its organization, "It is through this activity alone that individual and collective assumptions of responsibility can be instituted, the only remedy to bureaucratic routine and passivity generated by traditional hierarchy systems."[70] The radical nature of La Borde is that it takes facilitating nonnormative persons and subjects seriously, and the community recognizes that facilitating persons and subjects depends on shared projects and responsibilities that work transversally. The clear statement of intent and conveyance of meaningful information is secondary to the collaborative process of the institution's ongoing molecular revolution, constantly refashioning itself and the individuals who call it home to meet the collective interests and goals of the community.

As an institution, La Borde is organized by a facilitating technology referred to as the grid, a means of scheduling events, roles, and duties to distribute them across participants, regardless of their institutional role. This destabilizes social roles, with physicians and nurses put onto the same level as cooks and gardeners, as well as the clients. In this way, La Borde embraces a concept that Guattari referred to as transversality, the active disruption of vertical and horizontal arrangement of power and social roles. In the hospital, Guattari saw that the vertical arrangement of power and decision making—from nurses to physicians to administrators—resulted in each hierarchical level being more remote from the level below it, and most important, from the needs of the clients and their families. On each level of this hierarchical structure, Guattari saw individuals being organized horizontally in relation to others who share the same status and role. At worst, this leads to the segmentation of relations, so that, as Guattari writes, senile clients are stuck on the same ward as only other senile clients, and in their aggregation as a group of people, they come to be treated uniformly by those above them in the power structure. Individuals at every level are organized through these horizontal relations, leading to conservativism in the arrangement of the institution and the means of interpretation they have before them. All interpretation becomes concretized by the horizontal and vertical arrangements that depend on categorization. Guattari sees this as a form of blindness, like the blinders of a horse, limiting vision and leading to decisions and actions that stem from this skewed conception of the institution and the needs of its clients. To disrupt this, transversality seeks to unravel both the vertical and horizontal structure of institutions, placing individuals in roles they might otherwise eschew and putting them into contact with other individuals in the institution that they might otherwise only interact with in specific roles, like the patient–clinician dyad. The goal for Guattari is to produce new subjectivities, new understandings of the self and each other, and this relies in no small part on the dismantling of semiotic regimes of interpretation that keep individuals locked into specific understandings of themselves—as expert doctors, dutiful workers, and pitiful patients—and each other. Loosening the regimes of interpretation allows behaviors to enter into new interpretive schemes and moments of modular collaboration.

From its inception, La Borde relied on a 1901 law that allowed individuals to put together social clubs, a law that was utilized for the clients of La Borde to organize in collectives of shared interests. These clubs were legally recognized and allowed alliances to be formed between clients, workers, and medical staff at La Borde, which served as bridges to communities outside of the clinic. They also provided individuals with a project, a trajectory for their activities and relationships with one another and the world. In one case, this led to the formation of a club entitled La Borde–Ivoire, initially intended to help a cook from La Borde resettle in the Ivory Coast but eventually leading to ongoing relationships between the community at La Borde and the chef's village in Africa. As Guattari narrates it, this project led to a profound change in the institution as well as the individuals involved:

> In a period of time in which everyone was very unhappy, an event sprang forth which, without being able to know precisely why, changed the atmosphere. An unexpected process led to the secretion of different universes of reference; one sees things otherwise. Not only does the subjectivity change, but equally the fields of possibility change, the life projects. For example, a cook, originally from the Ivory Coast, decided to return there. However, he had no means to establish himself again in his village. He worked at La Borde for a number of years and was much loved. A group formed to help him. . . . They collected twenty thousand francs to assist him in his move. Later a doctor and nurse went to visit him. Then, in turn, a kind of village came to visit La Borde for three months. Now there is a group of six patients who are going there for three weeks of vacation. Here we have a *process of institutional singularization.* . . . In each case, the local subjectivity was profoundly modified, especially its latent racism.[71]

Guattari sees in these shared, ongoing projects the production of new desires—and in these emergent desires, the opportunities for individuals to become invested in relationships that did not previously exist become available. In so doing, these projects create institutional singularizations, new possibilities for subjectivity for the clients, workers, clinical staff, and those they come into contact with. His invocation of "latent racism" here is meant in precisely this way: bringing people into contact with those whom they would not normally interact with, particularly in the context of postcolonial Africa and France, can change beliefs about the self, and new beliefs and practices can be articulated as the basis for subjectivity and claims to personhood. Although this project is an expansive one, crossing continents and enrolling a variety of individuals in France and the Ivory Coast, smaller projects lay the basis for everyday life in La Borde, including the production of *Operetta.* Guattari sees in these projects profound effects in the expressive capacities of the clients at La Borde, particularly nonverbal communication as made evident through art, including drawing, painting, and sculpture. La Borde will not make anyone "normal," but through transversal modularity, it creates alternative means of association and relation that open up new possibilities for subjectivity and communication. La Borde takes as its therapeutic project the goal of making clients as well as manual and clinical workers all part of the same community, of making them feel at home and becoming, as Guattari puts it, "one of us." The projects that individuals participate in are intended to do just that, positioning individuals as part of a shared interest rather than standing apart from a community they would like to be a part of—a situation that Guattari sees as being endemic to the horizontal and vertical organization of capitalist society. By creating transversal relationships between individuals, "home" becomes located in the shared projects that communities build themselves around, which, as Guattari argues, lays the basis for behavioral change in the individual. He suggests that

> it is a fact that if a boy is to learn to read or to stop wetting
> his trousers, he must be recognized as being "at home," being
> "one of us." If he crosses that threshold and becomes re-
> territorialized, his problems are no longer posed in terms of
> phantasy; he becomes himself again in the group, and manages
> to rid himself of the question that had haunted him: "When
> shall I get to be *there*, to be part of *that*, to be 'one of them'?"
> As long as he fails in that, his compulsive pursuit of that goal
> prevents his doing anything else at all.[72]

Implicit in Guattari's conception of these associations is the need for facilitation; not every individual will be able to participate as fully as other individuals, but those who are participating seek to allow everyone to participate to the extent that participation is possible. A play like *Operetta* allows a wide variety of people to participate, as anyone interested in playing a role can always be costumed as an extra to fill a scene, and any set of behaviors that do not fundamentally disrupt the action of the play can be contained in the diegetic world of the performance. It might be hard to see how an individual like Noah Greenfeld could participate in any of these projects, or even simpler ones like peeling vegetables for dinner or helping with gardening chores, but Guattari's response would likely be that outside of the social expectations of La Borde and the treatment of Noah as full member of the community, he has never been allowed to develop the capacities necessary for these kinds of participation; he has remained an object of his parents, educators, and medical support staff rather than becoming a subject himself, which is only possible outside of the symbolic overdetermination of normative subjectivity.

As an institution, La Borde is designed to thwart institutionalized forms of interpretation, which Guattari sees as producing the desire for clients, families, and staff to maintain the quasi-zoological character of the residential hospital. Patients are not meant to get better or behave differently. In vertically arranged institutions, patients are meant to be maintained until their eventual death. For disciplinary hospitals, new possibilities are not as important as maintaining the status quo. To ensure that nothing changes in the treatment of patients or the expectations of the staff of the hospital, modes of interpretation are held static as well: patients fit diagnostic categories and are treated appropriately—as patients. However, in La Borde, the goal is to create a space of interpretive possibility, and in so doing create a space of emergent subjectivities. As Guattari writes, this depends on the deliberate construction of La Borde as an institution that facilitates the epiphenomenal interpretation of signs. He explains, "The whole of La Borde must function as a concrete machine in order that, at a given moment, some peculiarity, a way of taking a cigarette or of handing someone a dish, can relate to the level of conjunctions effected by psychotics' modes of semiotization. Conversely, however, those same psychotics must be able to function as concrete machines to make La Borde the kind of *agencement* [arrangement] that it is."[73]

The figure of concrete machines is one that Guattari deploys elsewhere to describe the ways that an action becomes either subject to interpretation, upholding already existing organizations of relations, or instead disrupting the institution in such a way that a new interpretive event becomes necessary.[74] Creating this space requires not only a change in disposition on the part of the employees of La Borde and the families of the clients who live there, but also a change in the disposition of the institution itself, which, in its arrangement, helps to foster expectations on the part of all the members of the community that they are "one of us." Guattari explains that it is through the inclusive nature of the institution that changes in subjectivity can occur, although this requires not only social inclusiveness but also the deliberate construction of facilitating spaces. He explains, "The most heterogeneous dimensions contribute to the positive development of a patient: relations to architectural space, economic relations, co-management by the patient and care giver of the different vectors of treatment, the seizing of all opportunities of exposure to the outside, and the processual development of factual 'singularities'—finally, everything that can contribute to the creation of an authentic relation to the other."[75] For Guattari, communication is not so important as collaboration, and it is through shared projects that the community of La Borde creates itself as a collective. The singularities that Guattari sees La Borde producing are new subjects in relation to these shared projects—subjects that would have been impossible in another social arrangement.

Guattari's portrayal of La Borde is its ideal form: its negative qualities or unsatisfying outcomes are downplayed in favor of the positive outcomes of the experiment. Similarly, in *Every Little Thing*, the frictions of everyday life together are unapparent, with emphasis placed instead on the steady collaboration of the community in staging *Operetta*. Most troubling about La Borde, both for its contemporary critics but also historically, is the continued use of electroshock therapy, a treatment that many critics in the antipsychiatry movement found abhorrent and which Jean Oury staunchly defended, largely on the grounds that the critique of its use was baseless.[76] In condemnation of his critics, Oury writes, "What is traumatic in electroshock? For me, it's the word 'shock.' And above all the phase of awakening. But what is traumatic there, can be by contrast of an extraordinary interest on the level of reconstruction of contact . . . thus, the problem of contact, it matters."[77] Oury's dismissal of electroshock therapy's critics exists in contradistinction to Guattari's nuanced attempts to construct a social and environmental space for the articulation of nonnormative subjectivities—but it might also be read as participating in the same project. Electroshock may not be integral to La Borde, but, as Oury's language of "reconstruction of contact" indicates, electroshock therapy similarly disrupts the interpretive schemes of individuals, albeit in a violent way. Ideally, La Borde facilitated transformations in individuals and communities through gentle institutional arrangements. But La Borde still participated in the mid-twentieth-century therapeutic conceptions of the brain as a material organ that can be acted on in specific ways to disrupt its pathological operation. As much as La Borde attempted to create a new space for the articulation of subjectivities that defied institutionalized forms of interpretation, it could not be entirely removed from the social and scientific currents of France at the time and the neurosciences in the North Atlantic more generally. Oury could not extract himself from the materialist conception of the brain and its therapies in much the same way that Guattari could not entirely divorce himself from his psychoanalytic training.

As Guattari writes in his appraisal of La Borde and what it has taught him over the years, "The ideal situation would be one in which no two institutions were alike and no individual institution ever cease[d] evolving in the course of time."[78] La Borde is an experiment, and to a degree it has been successful in making new modes of interaction and subject formation possible. But if it is not an institution that can be recreated in a universal way, its lessons about interaction can. To borrow Guattari's language, communication tends to rely on vertical and horizontal interpretive frameworks; the mimicry that individuals rely on is transmitted and interpreted in vertical and horizontal relations of power, parent to child, and child to child. Embracing epiphenomenal, interactional semiotics like Henry Kisor's is tantamount to instituting Guattari's transversal basis of relations. Rather than accepting the meaning of a term in its historical frame, a transversal, modular approach to language allows a sign to attach to new referents. Communication becomes unlocked from its histories and instead becomes understood through the shared collaborative projects that individuals are engaged in together. This modular semiotics is a means of facilitating communication, relying on the active participation of communicators in making meaning in an immediate and future-oriented way through interactional projects.

La Borde, as an institution, is a technology to make this facilitation of communication operable, but other technologies are available that act in more discrete ways, making communication possible outside of the confines of facilitating institutions. In the next chapter, I address this question of facilitating technologies by turning toward the explicit engagement with media—particularly social forms enabled by communication technologies—that throw into relief how facilitating technologies animate persons through social relations.

THREE

Materialist Subjectivity

How Technology and Material Environments Make Personhood Possible

*M*aterialist subjectivity builds on the assumption that subjectivity is fundamentally rooted in the material that composes an individual's world. More expansive in its conception of the material world than neurological subjectivity, materialist approaches move beyond the brain to the environment and its influences on an individual. They include the spaces that an individual inhabits, the food eaten, the social interactions engaged in—everything is material. Like symbolic subjectivity, however, materialist forms of subjectivity are deeply deterministic, and individuals struggle to transcend the material situations they find themselves in. Materialist understandings of neurological disorder rely on technological remedies that change an individual's capacities for interactions with the environment. Without material interventions, some individuals are impaired in their capacities for communication. By focusing on how technologies mediate interactions and shape subjectivity, materialist views of subjectivity are helpful in exposing the role of ghostwriting that occurs in the ascription of personhood and the development of subjectivity. Ghostwriting is generally taken to be a transparent form of translation, as ghostwriters put individual and family experiences into readable prose. But ghostwriting might also be understood as the basis for all material interactions in the world, as the material stuff we interact with has been authored by individuals other than ourselves and shapes personhood and subjectivity in intended and unintended ways. It is not that ghostwriting is positive or negative, but a recognition that all being in the world, all interactions, are necessarily mediated. Ghostwriting is not limited to writing but rather addresses this necessary mediation as the basis of language, communication, and interaction.

I turn first to Peyton Goddard, who as a young woman is diagnosed with autism and a variety of other neurological disorders. Unable to speak with her voice, Peyton comes to use facilitated communication (FC) through the assistance of her mother and caregivers. Peyton's use of a keyboard to provide her with a voice depends on a diverse network of technologies, from the keyboard to the individuals in her life who manually assist her in her communicative acts, as well as the institutions that support her and her family and the medical care she receives. Peyton's experiences point to the nature of facilitated personhood and subjectivity, or how personhood and subjectivity are achieved through the network of care that constitutes the nervous system that an individual is a part of. This personhood is not given but rather made in a continual process of interactions that support particular kinds of being in the world—which, in the cases I discuss, depend crucially on producing some form of communication between an individual with a neurological disorder and the social world she or he inhabits. From this facilitated personhood, subjectivity can follow, but both are indebted to the material world that an individual exists within.

I follow Peyton's case with that of Cecelia "CeCe" Bell, a noted children's book author who lost most of her hearing when she was a small child—an experience that is at the center of much of her writing. Bell used a variety of hearing aids throughout her youth, which she depicts in her memoir. These hearing aids enabled her to hear and develop social connections with her parents, siblings, teachers, neighbors, and peers. Like Peyton's experience with FC, itself mediated by technology, Bell's use of hearing aids connects her to a social world that both facilitates particular forms of personhood but disables others. That she is able to make the connections she does exists in tension with expectations about her as a deaf child and about what she can and cannot do, both with and without her hearing aids.

From Peyton and Bell, I turn to a minor figure in the history of neuroscience, José Delgado, who used a novel technology in order to alter materialist subjectivity. Delgado's technology, largely ignored in his time, has been reinvented recently, which I use as a way to conceptualize the role of technology—and its social functions—in the facilitation of personhood and materialist subjectivity. Far from a benign technology, Delgado's controversial "stimoceivers" bring into relief how social expectations of normative personhood and subjectivity are embedded in the technologies that produce them. Throughout this chapter, I suggest that facilitating personhood is a kind of ghostwriting, a practice central to memoirs about disability. Ghostwriting, like facilitation and epiphenomenal conceptions of communication and subjectivity, puts the crafting of personhood outside of the individual and is enabled by social technologies that make normative forms of personhood and subjectivity legible. In memoirs of disability, like with other technologies, personhood is something that is made, rendering individuals into recognizable persons through facilitation that produces specific capacities, and is dependent on disliberal claims to recognition. I use this discussion of ghostwriting and facilitation to discuss the nervous system as a replacement for materially reductionistic views of the brain as the source of disorder. In so doing, I seek to externalize the forces that make individuals into persons and subjects, and to consider what the stakes are in displacing agency from the internal brain to an external world of facilitating technologies, relations, and institutions. Materialist subjectivity sees the material infrastructures individuals are a part of as laying the basis for—if not wholly determining—the development of an understanding of the inside self and the outside world, thereby helping erode the distinction between individuals and their world and demonstrating their integral relation to each other. Where materialist approaches fall short is in addressing the human and nonhuman behaviors and desires that are the unexpected or unintentional outcomes of material legacies. This is most evident, as the cases I focus on show, in situations where technologies are used not as they were intended by their creators but in creative and surprising ways that unravel social expectations and possibilities for subject formation.

The Woman Who Speaks without a Voice

UNLOCKING THE SUBJECT THROUGH FACILITATION

Peyton Goddard was thirty-seven when her memoirs were published in 2012. They were entitled *I Am Intelligent*, a title translated from her first experience of facilitated communication (FC), in which she wrote "i am intlgent" with the help of a caregiver. Peyton grew up at a time in Southern California when, for most of her childhood, adolescence, and young adult life, she was categorized as mentally retarded and was cared for with the help of state institutions that relied on that categorical designation—care supplemented by her parents, with whom she lived. She started in mainstream schools, only to experience a loss of communicative capacities and bodily control that eventually led her to state-run, special education facilities until she was in her early twenties. As an adult, she was diagnosed with autism, but even that category seems like it fit her poorly: autism tends to include communication impairments, motor fixations (like hand flapping), sensory sensitivities (including aversion to touch), and asocial behavior. Peyton is nonverbal, has some motor control issues, fixates on complex behaviors (like picking up all the lint and dust bunnies in a room), does not seem particularly perturbed by most sensory experiences, likes touching others and being touched, and is intensely social. She experiences frequent, long-term insomnia, manic and depressive periods, obsessive-compulsive disorder, attention deficits, and epilepsy. To aggregate Peyton's behavior and symptoms under any one rubric is difficult, so a diagnosis of autism at least provided the basis for continued medical care and institutional support for her and her family. Although she acquired some speech in her earliest years, she lost that capacity as she aged, until, at age four, she was entirely nonverbal. At twenty-two, however, she began to use FC, which allowed her to find her voice.

FC is controversial to those who ascribe to the ideological view that communication is an unmediated expression of the self through language. The facilitator uses a hand as a brace for the communicator's arm or hand, loosely gripping the elbow or wrist, and helping to maneuver the communicator's hand to a keyboard button or tablet application that uses simple iconographic content indicating the desire to eat, go to the bathroom, play, or other common activities. But FC is more encompassing than that, and can include any direct mediation of an impaired communicator's language, which may involve interpreting eye or limb movements, tapping, or other means of interaction. In Peyton's case, she uses a Lightwriter, a small keyboard and speaker that vocalizes for her, and her mother or one of her other caregivers helps her control her body so as to communicate with the device. The controversy around FC is based on the skeptical view that the communicator is not authoring the communication but rather the facilitator. Debunkers have established this to be the case in a number of situations, as desperate caregivers seek to find the voice of their disabled friend or family member, and instead provide their own voice, masked by technology and FC. But consider Peyton's psychiatrist's attempt to outdo the debunkers:

> I had Peyton's parents leave the room, while I told Peyton
> a specific phrase for her to type when her parents returned.
> Each time I did this, over several weeks, there was 100 percent
> accuracy in Peyton typing the correct answer to my question.
> There was no possible way for Dianne [Peyton's mother and
> primary facilitator] to know what I had asked Peyton, and it was
> clear then Peyton was communicating her own thoughts and
> feelings.[1]

Peyton, like many other impaired communicators, relies on direct facilitation of her communication. This does not invalidate her communicative acts but should instead be seen as analogous to all communication, ghostwritten as it is. This more expansive view of all communication as facilitated by others moves away from ableist conceptions of communication and language as necessarily only following normative models predicated on the liberal subject. Recognizing instead that all communication is facilitated provides grounds for accepting nonnormative forms of communication as equally valid and in need of social support.

As a memoir, *I Am Intelligent* is a collaborative effort between Peyton, her mother, Dianne, and, for lack of a better term, a ghostwriter named Carol Cujec. I call Cujec a ghostwriter here because it is unclear how much of the book she wrote, and how much rewriting of Dianne's and Peyton's writing she did; although she's named on the cover, her actions are diffuse and potentially profound. If one compares Peyton's unedited writing—which can be found on her blog—to the writing in the memoir, there is significant polish, both in terms of spelling and syntax, but also in phrasing. Peyton writes in a kind of free-form, verseless poetry that Cujec has a talent for turning into more direct statements. On her blog, Peyton writes of trying to relearn how to speak: "After 25 silent years, I'm trying ready I initiater again my freed very great voice. I was muted by heartbreak of hubbub trauma as it tipped red emotions epoch in I. My red awe I answered by truth teethed together I told by typing my book. Now I'm returned to me. My quest I'm on is freeing red as I'm lip tried join in. Heartbreak tread is healing."[2] When Cujec edits Peyton, minor typos that lead to syntactic misunderstandings get ironed out, and phrasing is parsed so as to produce more straightforwardly meaningful sentences, even if they are filled with Peyton's poetic wordplay.

I Am Intelligent is constructed around the interplay of Dianne's and Peyton's voices, with the majority of each chapter focusing on the events in their family's ongoing struggles with Peyton's undiagnosed condition, told from Dianne's retrospectively omniscient perspective, which is interrupted from time to time by Peyton's reflections on the events discussed by her mother. Cujec ghostwrites for both mother and daughter, editing the interplay of Dianne and Peyton to produce a narrative that flows from one event to the next, following Peyton through public school, her eventual adoption of FC, her enrolling in local community college, and eventually her graduating and participating in the dissemination of FC as a reliable method of communication for the nonverbal. There are moments of drama and crisis throughout the book, largely told in Dianne's voice, but based on Peyton's experience. Temporally, they occur before Peyton begins to use FC, but they are told from Dianne's omniscient perspective. These include, most importantly, what is happening to Peyton in school or at home when her parents are away, including a series of abuses by older cousins and school staff members. There might be other ways to convey this information instead of making Dianne omniscient, but the conceit of the text as a family memoir depends on the story being told in a familial voice—which is actually a time-traveling, ghostwritten Peyton as voiced by her mother and written by Cujec. This practice of ghostwriting is analogous to other technologies that facilitate the construction of personhood and subjectivity through communication. What Cujec is doing in ghostwriting is not unlike the claims made against FC as a legitimate form of communication. Yet in some contexts ghostwriting is accepted, if not wholly expected; when it is obvious in the case of an individual with a neurological disorder, as in the use of FC, however, it can become controversial.

Like so many memoirs of disability, *I Am Intelligent* follows a generic trajectory: there is a problem with a child, parents seek a diagnosis and cure, physicians and psychiatrists are befuddled, the child is in distress—usually institutionally and interpersonally—and so is the family, and eventually there is a breakthrough. In Peyton's case, it is learning how to use FC with the help of her mother. Although Peyton's family's life proceeds in fits and starts, for Peyton, while she is without communicative capacities, no such progression is felt. At one particularly low point, without access to verbal communication, Peyton recognizes her impulses as suicidal, as do her mother and psychiatrist. What Peyton lacks is a way to break the repetition of her everyday life. She cannot break the seriality of being trapped in the same role. She has become an object of other people's actions rather than an actor in her own right. Consider her mother's description of speaking with Peyton before her total loss of language, and the way that mimetic uses of repetition and difference become critical in their conversational interactions:

> If I repeat a word that Peyton has said spontaneously, then she can avoid getting "stuck" on it and move on to say a second word, even though she may be unable to put the two words together on her own. Every day after school, I sit with Peyton on the sofa to work on reading phrases or verbalizing from pictures. When Peyton says, "Read," I repeat, *Reeead* with a rising inflection and this unlocks Peyton's voice to say a full phrase: "Read the book," much to my glee.[3]

Dianne's use of language unlocks Peyton's everyday interactions in a way that is analogous to how FC unlocks Peyton as a communicating subject. Once Peyton is verbal again, once she is able to communicate in a facilitated way, she is able to build relationships, define her intentions, and interact with her environments in ways that had previously been obscured by her inability to speak. There are problems in communication as well, but communication serves to free Peyton—and her family—from the seriality of their everyday lives of disorder.

SOCIAL INCLUSION THROUGH FACILITATION

In her earliest days, Peyton seemed to be a typically developing child, moving, walking, and speaking as emplotted in scientific understandings of child development. But Peyton slowly begins to lose her sense of coordination, and her speech begins to regress. Where once she could put together a modest sentence, she begins to get stuck on individual words; rather than being able to communicate in a transparent way, she has increasing difficulty making her intentions known to others. This leads to behavioral issues, including tantrums and toileting accidents, which only seem to exacerbate the tensions between her and her family. Eventually, the Goddards seek medical help for Peyton, but no one can provide any definitive answer for what is wrong with her other than describing the symptoms, which importantly include aphasia. After a series of tests, the Goddards accept that Peyton is developmentally delayed at best and mentally retarded at worst, and they acquiesce to her enrollment in a special education preschool. As Dianne writes, "I have bought into the conventional wisdom that segregating Peyton into special-education classes will allow her to gain the skills necessary to someday rejoin her peers in general education. Realistically speaking, segregation is the only option offered. . . . Segregation is the only known road, and we never ask for proof that it will lead back to rejoining the community."[4]

This becomes the central motif in Dianne's concern for Peyton: that she will one day overcome the ostracization that she experiences as a result of her impairments and rejoin the social fold. But being ostracized at school is only part of Peyton's social rejection. She is similarly cast aside from church outreach programs, a situation Dianne feels is hypocritical and damaging. Told by their pastor that "it will be impossible for me to have Peyton come when fellowship starts in September. I have only two or three Sundays to engage the regular kids and encourage their joining,"[5] Dianne's response is to think, "You see others as valuable and Peyton as not."[6] Through negotiations, Peyton is allowed to attend the teen fellowship meetings with Pat, her father, monitoring from the sidelines. Over the course of a few meetings, he sees that the other attendees casually ignore Peyton, making her attendance merely symbolic. Seeing this failure to integrate Peyton into the community as emblematic of the church's failure to accept Peyton as a full person, the Goddards split from the church, but not before Pat can deride the head pastor: "Having Peyton as part of the church was an opportunity—for the church. And the church blew it!"[7] Dianne's invocation of "value" and Pat's use of "opportunity" indicate what they find so troubling about segregation: it is not only Peyton who gains something from social inclusion, but society itself. For the Goddards, it is evident that embracing people like Peyton as persons, as members of the community, makes the community more humane and makes individuals like Peyton full persons.

Peyton disrupts the orderly flow of social life, both for her parents and for those she comes into contact with. As social as she is, she is also intensely disorderly in her social engagements. In order to facilitate Peyton's inclusion in activities throughout her childhood, Dianne volunteers to teach the children's Sunday school class, and eventually agrees to lead the neighborhood Brownies group. Pat is always also in attendance in case Peyton needs to be cared for—or, more likely, distracted from behaviors seen as inappropriate by others. As Dianne writes, "In all situations, we are there to swoop Peyton up or sweep her aside whenever her constant attempts at connecting with others are viewed as scary or inappropriate—like placing Brownie beanies on any uncovered heads, or buttoning all undone buttons on others' Brownie shirts and sweaters."[8] Peyton disrupts the easy ordering of a Brownie meeting or Sunday school, and for Dianne and Pat, there is some value in this disruption; it forces the community to address Peyton as a member of the community, and in so doing adjust expectations of what personhood and connectivity are and can be. Other children can fend off her attempts to button their Brownie shirt, or they can facilitate her participation in the community by allowing her to button their buttons. Such an engagement makes allowances for Peyton's behaviors while asking members of the community to be modular in their responses to Peyton. Peyton may be noncompliant, as some of her teachers and physicians label her, or she may simply be abiding by an order all her own.

When Peyton is eight, enrolled in special education at a local school, Dianne is asked to help with Peyton's classroom behavior by a particularly strict teacher, Ms. Waters. Dianne explains,

> I am forced to watch Peyton's daily activities—not participate in or support them. I sit, stiff and wooden. Peyton knows I am there, but she must be stiff and wooden, too, never allowed to go back to talk to me or ask for help. Ms. Waters is stiff and wooden in her approach to teaching as well; Peyton must be the one to conform—without support—to Ms. Waters' mold. When she does not, I am asked to escort her home.[9]

Ms. Waters and her classroom are a caricature of institutional inflexibility. Ms. Waters is rigid in the behaviors that she expects of her students and the way that behaviors are interpreted. Any variance from the institutional expectations that Ms. Waters has established leads to Peyton's being regarded as noncompliant, as not meeting the demands of the classroom—and, by extension, her own needs as a student. This institutional inflexibility is founded in an ideology of equality not based in individual capacities but in institutional expectations, which Dianne explains: "Peyton has to adhere to the rules, and in the name of equality, the rules must be the same for everyone. But as Peyton will proclaim years later, *equal* doesn't mean that everyone should get the same treatment; it means that everyone should get what they *need*."[10] Dianne is here making two arguments simultaneously, one for institutional modularity and the other for facilitation. An institution that seeks to foster capacities in its clients might organize itself differently, minimally allowing Dianne or another caregiver to aid Peyton in her classroom tasks; an institution that seeks to facilitate an individual's participation would seek to supplement an individual with the necessary technologies—human, institutional, and mechanical—to meet the expectations of the institution. After years of struggle with the teachers and administrators at Peyton's school, Dianne summarizes her understanding of the institution's logic this way: "We will break you in order to control you. We measure only what is important here. We measure deficits. We chart each time you are asked to sit down and you do not. But we do not measure your sitting down when we facilitate your wandering body to come to a desk that holds things of interest to you because, bottom line, we do not believe you can learn."[11] Against the inflexibility of the institution, Dianne posits the need to facilitate Peyton and her fellow students. There is no making the students at the school "normal," but there are ways that the students can be facilitated to participate in the institution and the broader community.

Pat and Dianne see the central need for facilitation as being the fostering of Peyton's ability to talk, which would also make Peyton a recognized speaker, a full person and subject. In a meeting with a school administrator, Pat argues, "Peyton needs a strong, credentialed professional who will focus on communication—not just getting her to listen and obey, but to *talk*."[12] Pat and Dianne seek Peyton's release from the school that she had been attending, given the school's failures in facilitating Peyton's efforts at communication. They instead place her in a nearby public elementary school where she is assigned a full-time aide in the hopes of mainstreaming her. What follows are a few good years of Peyton making steady progress in developing her physical skills, that, at their best, include learning to ride a bike, which she happily does with her father. At their worst, Peyton starts bolting from her parents, sometimes running out into busy streets. But while her physical abilities are maturing, Peyton's ability to communicate is still hampered. Three years after Pat and Dianne's confrontation with the school administrator about Peyton's learning to talk, Dianne and Peyton come across a PBS *Frontline* episode on FC, which Dianne eagerly anticipates will provide a solution for Peyton's inability to speak. But within minutes, the *Frontline* reporter is deriding the claims made by the proponents of FC, showing footage of clearly staged efforts at communication. Dianne is disappointed and abandons her hope that FC might provide a way forward. Peyton, looking back at the event, voices her despair: "Your dismal dismissal of touch I pouted. / I am a person who needs touch to move. / If the physical resistance to my

hand, wrist, forearm, or elbow, / which is a necessary accommodation for the success of my / purposeful movement, is not being sup-
plied, / then the hulk of my life is insanity."[13] Some four years later,
in 1997, Peyton would finally adopt FC with the support of her family.
Despite this early discouragement, as a result of an intervention
by Jackie Leigh and Darlene Hanson—a psychologist and speech pa-
thologist, respectively—Peyton is eventually initiated into the process
of FC. As Hanson explains, "I am going to offer your arm support . . .
to see if this might help you to communicate with us by typing. I'll
adjust my support and pull back a little until I feel you pointing to the
letter you want."[14] Leigh then asks Peyton what her favorite food is,
and slowly, with Hanson's support, Peyton ekes out "pppizza" on the
keyboard. Peyton then responds to a handful of questions, ending with
Leigh asking if Peyton has "anything else you want to say?" Peyton
responds by writing "i am intlgent," followed by "i type to tell people"
and "i think mom think i smrt."[15] That Peyton can type and spell with
modest mistakes is chalked up to her early and constant exposure to
the written word. As Peyton later explains, it is not that she could
not understand people communicating with her but that without facilitation she lacked the ability to communicate back.[16] In her earliest
efforts at communication, spelling and syntactic errors abound, but
Peyton is undeterred and sets about acquiring finesse in her communication so as to better express herself. Within weeks, she is being invited
to address audiences interested in her life as a communicating person.
In response to a question about what it feels like to be autistic, Peyton
responds, "i am not able to control my body. i cannot talk. i need help
to do most things. but i can open my heart to most people. can you do
that?"[17] With the introduction of a viable means of verbal communication, Peyton transcends her years of lack of communicative capacities,
able to speak for herself, and arguing, in her way, for facilitated ways of
being part of a community.

UNLOCKING THE SYMBOLIC SUBJECT

With her newfound abilities to communicate, Peyton eventually grad-
uates from high school and enters a local community college. The pro-
fessors and administrators all support Peyton's educational pursuits,

and they allow her to bring facilitators to class and tests, and to develop learning and testing aids. Starting part-time taking a developmental psychology class, Dianne and Peyton, along with her other caregivers, snap into action, escorting her to class, making flashcards to help her study, helping her with her reading and other assignments. After a discouraging start, earning a 64 percent on her first test, Peyton resolves to commit herself fully to her education, thereafter earning an A in the course overall. In reflecting on the dramatic change to Peyton's life, Dianne ruminates, "What a switch for Peyton from having only dead time to having no time to waste."[18] Dianne brings together the seriality of Peyton's previous everyday life, trapped as she was in a noncommunicative, disorderly experience of the world, with an experience of "dead time," of ordered nothingness. College provides Peyton, her family, and her caregivers with a project, and one that Peyton throws herself into with aplomb. At the time of her graduation, Peyton is asked to serve as class valedictorian and to give a mediated speech.[19] Rather than have her type the speech in real time and thereby attempt to simulate a live speech, one of Peyton's friends, Hollyn, is asked to read the speech for Peyton, while Peyton stands at the podium on stage with her. Peyton's speech is full of poetic allusion to the geopolitics of 2002, encouraging peace and neighborliness over xenophobia and revenge for the September 11, 2001, attacks. After decades of struggle against institutional expectations, Peyton is recognized as finally having met them—but only in the context of an institution that is willing to accommodate her, and only with the facilitation of her writing technologies and her various caregivers.

During her time at college, Peyton begins to use facilitators who are not her mother, which include a young woman named Tricia. In Dianne's retelling of Peyton and Tricia's partnership,[20] Tricia is immediately interested in helping Peyton, and over time she and Peyton begin to talk about the possibility of rooming together, the first time Peyton would live separately from her parents. But Dianne and Pat "notice that when Tricia facilitates, Peyton's comments are more humorous and even include bold requests about wanting to be independent of us."[21] Things come to a head when Peyton has a guest, Gabriel, who similarly relies on facilitators for his communication. Tricia sits between Peyton and Gabriel at dinner, and facilitates for both of them simultaneously. After dinner, they adjourn to a nearby sitting room where they can close the door for privacy, ostensibly to have a private conversation without parents eavesdropping. After the conversation, both Peyton and Gabriel are visibly disturbed, with Gabriel behaving in an agitated way and Peyton "quiet, almost frozen."[22] After Gabriel is taken to his mother and Tricia to her dorm, Peyton tells her parents that Tricia had used her hand to type "lewd comments" to Gabriel and that she now fears Tricia. Peyton writes to her parents, "She is insane. Various times I tell Tricia not to. Saw joy in Tricia in not listen to I."

A cynical reader might suggest that Tricia's inclusion in the text is meant to serve as an inoculation against criticisms about FC: Tricia's behavior is clearly unethical and manipulative in making Peyton into her mouthpiece, whereas Dianne's use of FC is truly enabling of Peyton, similar to the experimental psychiatrist Peyton sees. Tricia stands in for all of the impure-of-intent facilitators who corrupt FC in the public eye. But this would be to ignore the potential social worlds that are being enabled by this facilitator, however onerous they might be to Peyton, her family, and friends: Tricia is attempting to create a world despite the interests of those who will be forced to inhabit it. Tricia is the ghostwriter revealed, her intentions impure, her manipulations transparent. If Dianne is the benign conduit through which Peyton's personhood is facilitated, Tricia is the controlling technology that produces only a normative subject, aligning with expectations of romantic intent and young bawdiness. Peyton could choose to inhabit these roles, but given her ability to communicate with her mother's help, chooses not to. She had become able to craft her own subjectivity, moving away from the disabled subject Tricia would treat her as and toward full personhood through the use of FC, thereby able to articulate a sense of self with the help of her mother and caregivers.

Tricia is not the only person who would abuse Peyton; nor is she the most grievous in her actions. What FC enables Peyton to communicate are two historical incidents of sexual abuse, one at the hands of employees at one of her special education schools, the other at the hands of her second cousin, Duane. Duane's rape of Peyton is the most dramatic passage in the book, taking the form of a series of cut scenes between her experience at home, ostensibly being babysat by Duane and his sister, and Dianne and Pat attending the centennial ball at the San Diego Yacht Club.[23] Duane's abuse is enabled by his sister, Connie, and when Peyton shits on her bed during the rape, Duane and Connie call their mother for help. They bathe Peyton forcibly, launder her pajamas and bedsheets, and greet Pat and Dianne when they return home as if nothing had happened. Despite being ten and toilet trained with only the occasional accident, Peyton begins to urinate and shit in her bed, the site of the attack causing her no end of distress. Eventually this leads to Dianne and Pat disposing of the bed and replacing it with "two barren twin beds,"[24] which stand in symbolic opposition to the "frilly pillows" and "fluffy comforter" of the old bed—symbols that were intended to signify Peyton's admittance into adolescence. Instead, after the rape, she regresses.

Nearly a decade later, Duane, "full of alcohol, self-destructs, his car spinning out of control and crashing head-on into a palm tree."[25] Peyton's family drives to Arizona for the service, about which Peyton writes, "God is present here now,"[26] a cryptic acknowledgment of the delayed justice that Duane's death provides. But it is only a year later that Peyton is finally able to tell her parents what had happened to her,[27] a confession that they bravely face, realizing that for Peyton, facilitated use of language has become a wellspring for her articulation of her subjectivity and the recounting of events that shaped her experience. But rather than dwell on the event or Duane, she encourages her parents to "not go to revenge"[28] and proceeds to tell her grandmother about the event. "I tell truths will set I free," she writes,[29] accepting that her confession will not kill her grandmother, as her abusers had warned her would happen, and that her newfound status of full personhood and symbolic subjectivity through facilitation depends on others understanding why she had been behaving in the ways that she had been without the benefit of language to convey her traumas.

Peyton is successful in becoming a symbolic subject and person, albeit on her own terms and through FC. Despite the efforts of those like Duane and Tricia to shape her to their desires, Peyton flourishes thanks to her use of FC and the facilitation that she is provided by her caregivers. In spite of Tricia's "lewd" and "bawdy" attempts to bond

Gabriel and Peyton, she and Gabriel are able to develop a close, romantic friendship. Peyton also seeks out alternatives to medical treatments. She consults with a "shaman," who explains that she is the perfect realization of what he calls "expanded consciousness," an awareness of her intimate connection with the world.[30] This leads her to "meditation, prayer, hypnosis, relaxation, and reading ancient texts."[31] As much as these practices help Peyton to manage some of her symptoms, as Dianne explains, "there is still something beyond her control that flares up in a rage, sometimes daily, sometimes weekly,"[32] and for that, she takes propranolol, which helps her to control her otherwise uncontrollable behaviors. Peyton's life makes clear the various kinds of facilitation she requires, all of which provide her with the foundation to be a recognizable person by the standards of her community and which lay the basis for subject formation. She relies on technology and the physical aid of others to communicate, she relies on medication to control her bodily outbursts, and she relies on modular institutions to facilitate her capacities as an individual. Without this wide array of facilitation through a diverse nervous system, she would have continued to live an existence of what Dianne referred to as "dead time," the blank seriality of disorderly everyday life—not as a recognized social subject but as an individual disrupting the order of everyday life for others. Peyton the person and subject is made possible by those people and technologies that facilitate her; she is ghostwritten through these facilitations, some benign and others abusive. Peyton makes all of this facilitation visible, but facilitation is universal in social worlds, as individuals, institutions, and technologies aid in the creation and maintenance of social others.

The Girl Who Could Hear through Walls

ORGANIC IMPAIRMENTS AND PROSTHETIC CAPACITIES

Cecelia Carolina "CeCe" Bell experienced hearing loss at the age of four as a result of a bout of meningitis. Hearing loss is often associated with bacterial meningitis, which can result in anything from mild hearing loss to profound deafness. In Bell's case, her hearing loss is almost total. But in 1974, she is offered hearing aids that augment her remaining capacity to hear. Over time, with lipreading, she is able to understand most face-to-face communication. Bell's memoir, *El Deafo*,[33] is a graphic novel, and she is able to use the language of graphic media to convey her experience of hearing loss—and its augmentation with hearing aids—with visual tools that are unavailable in a textual memoir. For example, Bell recounts her experience of losing her hearing, which occurred while she was hospitalized with the bacterial infection, by making voices appear to become fainter and fainter, until the television is silent, as are the people around her. Bell's experience of near-total hearing loss at a young age leaves her to guess what has happened to her; she's too young to read, too deaf to hear. The world is suddenly silent, and Bell is able to communicate this to the reader through the use of empty word bubbles and the inscrutable behavior of the adults around her—her parents, the hospital staff, and eventually the audiologist who fits her for hearing aids. The graphic novel form also allows Bell to depict herself and the people around her as anthropomorphic bunnies, their faces mostly human except for a pink, triangular nose, ears extending up from their heads in an exaggerated way. Filled with anthropomorphic bunnies, Bell's memoir is intended to appeal to young readers, and a world full of long-eared creatures points to the centrality of hearing as a sense, means of communication, and token of personhood.

Weeks after she has been discharged from the hospital and is at home with her family, Bell goes to see an audiologist, who runs a series of tests on her to identify her range of hearing and fits her for hearing aids. Because Bell had been hearing for the first four years of her life, she has a handle on spoken language that many of her deaf peers lack, both in modulating her voice and in making herself understood to hearing peers, as well as in understanding the speech of others with the help of hearing aids. This nascent communicative capacity lays the basis for her eventual lipreading, which supplements her hearing aids. Her first year of school is at a school for the hearing impaired, the J. B. Fisher Model School, and she works closely with a teacher and peers on improving her lipreading skills. Her teacher explains, "I see a bear. I see a pear. 'Bear' and 'pear' look the same coming out of a person's mouth, don't they? You can't just watch a person's lips. You have to be a detective and watch for other clues, too."[34] Such encouragement entices Bell's imagination, and she depicts herself embracing a detective's role, wearing a Sherlock Holmes deerstalker cap and carrying a magnifying glass and pipe, as she discovers the rules of lipreading: "(1) Must see person's face at all times! (2) exaggerated mouth movements are confusing! (3) shouting is *not* good (4) moustaches and beards are bad news! (sorry, dad.) (5) hands in front of mouth are also bad news! (6) when it gets dark, give up! (7) group discussions are impossible to understand."[35] This is Bell's first portrayal of her young self as prone to flights of fantasy, which, with the help of her Phonic Ear, she eventually elaborates into her superhero identity, El Deafo. Bell's experience shows that the material technology of her hearing aids, like the FM system of the Phonic Ear, and the microphone and amplifier behind-the-ear system she uses at home, supplement her capacities for communication in specific ways, shaping her subjectivity through the buried intents of the makers of the technologies, as well as the explicit intents of Bell and her peers. It is not that her subjectivity is inborn in her brain or wholly symbolic. Rather, it is that it is made through the material world she interacts with through the prosthetics she uses to facilitate her social inclusion and interactions.

Bell requires her teachers to wear a special closed-circuit FM microphone system called the Phonic Ear, which is linked to a receiver and headphones Bell wears. This enables Bell to hear the teacher wherever he or she might be in the room, and it helps her isolate her teacher's voice from the noise of the other students. When her teachers leave the room, they often continue to wear the microphone, enabling Bell to hear the teacher as she or he moves around the school, talking with other teachers, smoking in the teachers' lounge, making copies of assignments, going to the bathroom, heading back to the classroom. Writing of her first grade teacher, Bell explains, "The Phonic Ear makes Mrs. Lufton's voice louder, just for me. It even *clarifies* her voice—really sharpens it! Even when I don't see Mrs. Lufton's face, I understand *every word she says* without having to lip-read at all."[36] She goes on to consider the role that the Phonic Ear plays in her abilities, accepting the prosthetic as enabling her to be more than human: "I have *amazing abilities* unknown to *anyone!* Just like Bruce Wayne uses all that *crazy technology* to turn himself into Batman on TV."[37]

Bell keeps this newfound superpower to herself for fear of drawing more attention to her deafness and her reliance on the Phonic Ear. Most important in a classroom setting, however, is that the Phonic Ear transmits a speaker's voice with such clarity that Bell does not need to be able to lip-read in order to understand what is being spoken. By her account, this means that Bell can clearly hear lectures and class discussions, and she can also hear her teacher talking with other students in the classroom. Her behind-the-ear hearing aids, which she wears while at home, lack this kind of fidelity, and, later in elementary school, when the Phonic Ear is accidentally broken and she has to wear her behind-the-ear hearing aids, she finds herself adrift, unable to hear her teacher speaking clearly enough to succeed in school. Frustration sets in, in no small part because she has become dependent on what the Phonic Ear provides her. As a facilitating technology, the Phonic Ear becomes integral to how Bell communicates as well as how she thinks of herself. The Phonic Ear is the foundation of Bell's social connectivity and her materialist subjectivity.

El Deafo follows Bell through elementary school, ending with her year in fifth grade. Central to her experience of deafness in elementary school is her sense of social exclusion, which she accepts as largely the result of the obvious Phonic Ear she wears in the classroom. After Bell's kindergarten year, her family moves and enrolls her in a mainstream elementary school. Bell experiences her difference from the local children as they turn on a radio to sing along to music. One of the kids tries to help Bell by turning up the music, to which she replies "Uh . . . thanks." What she wishes she could say is, "Thanks, but I can hear the radio with my hearing aid just fine! I just can't understand it, because I can't see the faces of the people who are singing and talking!"[38] This is the first of Bell's experiences of social loneliness, which intensify in her earliest days of first grade. As she explains, "Superheroes might be awesome, but they are also different. And being different feels a lot like being alone. With the Phonic Ear, I have super hearing. Without it, I can't hear. Am I deaf? Maybe? First grade is lonely at first. Wherever I am . . . it feels like I'm always inside my bubble. Is everyone staring at the hearing aid? At me?"[39] Bell visually depicts her loneliness as a bubble that she exists within, carrying it with her wherever she goes: the schoolyard, the lunchroom, the gym. It is in this experience of loneliness that Bell becomes friends with a girl in her class, Laura, whom she later begins to think of as Super Bossypants. Laura takes advantage of Bell's loneliness, cajoling her into situations she might not otherwise desire and often criticizing her art projects, play styles, and imaginative flights of fancy. What seems like a fun proposal from Laura has the tendency of being revealed as a sadistic ploy, as when Laura convinces Bell to walk slowly around her family's dining room table. After being lulled into thinking it is just an insipid game, Laura sets her family dog on Bell, with the dog lunging at Bell and biting her leg. Similarly, Laura convinces Bell to wear identical outfits as her to school, saying how fun it will be to be twins, and eventually criticizing Bell for not picking the right clothes to wear. Rather than confront Laura about her feelings, their friendship is dissolved when Laura and Bell are assigned to different second-grade classrooms, where Bell meets a new friend named Ginny.

Ginny is drawn to Bell in no small part because Bell can be Ginny's "deaf friend." Ginny is intensely aware of Bell's deafness, and Bell draws Ginny communicating with Bell in an exaggerated fashion: Ginny's words are drawn larger than normal, and every word is broken down into its constituent syllables. Neither loud speaking nor slow enunciation helps Bell to make sense of what is being spoken to her, and although Ginny has redeeming qualities—she is quirky and more fun to be around than Laura—she offers a model of facilitation gone awry. Introducing Bell to her friend Kristen, Ginny says, "cee-cee, this is kreee-sten! cee-cee is my deaf friend. she is act-u-a-lly one of my best-est friends!"[40] Bell resolves to confront her friend about her loud, slow talking and her self-congratulatory tokenism of Bell as her deaf friend, but it is only when Ginny insists on listening to her brother's Monty Python record that Bell snaps. Like listening to the radio, listening to a record is an alienating experience for Bell: she can hear the voices speak, but without faces to attach the sounds to, the context of speech is missing. With comedic speech, this is exacerbated. As Ginny relays what the Python Players are singing, Bell finds herself driven deeper and deeper into a feeling of difference. Bell explodes: "This secondhand Monty Python stuff is driving me crazy! And what's more—

you don't have to talk to me so loud and slow! I can't stand it!"[41] This exchange leads to the temporary estrangement of Bell from Ginny, resulting in Bell developing a deeper relationship with her television and finding comfort in TV shows. However difficult TV shows are for her to understand, they offer an outlet for Bell's social imagination. It is ultimately through television that her self-conception as El Deafo congeals. During an after-school special about a deaf child, the main character is referred to as "Deafo" by bullies. At first stumped at what is funny or hurtful about the term, Bell decides to appropriate it for herself, christening her Phonic Ear–aided alter ego "El Deafo."[42] Once alienated from media technologies like the radio and record players, Bell's sense of self is able to crystallize around what the television offers her, from after-school specials to Batman shows. TV offers her a way to conceptualize her world, her difficulties with communication, and her relationships with other people.

MATERIAL CAPACITIES BEGET SOCIAL INTEGRATION

Bell thinks of her more-than-human self as a young superhero. She does not fight crime, but she does use her difference as the basis for conceptualizing herself as potentially more than her neighborhood and school peers. This plays into the recurrent trope in memoirs of disability of the recuperation of a perceived stigma or impairment into the basis for some claim to being more than human—what has been referred to as the supercrip.[43] Children—and sometimes adults—come to learn that what they first perceived as a limitation on their claims to full personhood and subjectivity enable capacities that mere "normal" people do not share. In memoirs of deafness, these tend to include the ability to lip-read and thereby eavesdrop on those who thought they were safe behind glass or on the other side of a room, and, as Bell discusses, the ability to use prosthetic hearing aids to enable more-than-human hearing. But unlike other supercrip narratives, Bell's superhero imaginary applies to all of her friends as well. Laura, the pushy, sadistic friend is renamed Super Bossypants. Her fifth-grade crush, Mike Miller, is thought of as Supercrush. And her friend Martha, who sees past Bell's deafness, is portrayed in a Robin costume, similar to Batman's sidekick, and thought of as True Friend. She also views her relationships with her mother and her gym teacher through the same highly dramatized lens, imagining the powers of her Phonic Ear as being able to subdue or mind-control her enemies.

Bell's relationship with Martha comprises the narrative spine of the second half of *El Deafo*: first their connection as friends beyond the tokenism of Ginny or abusive manipulation of Laura, and then its dissolution as the result of an unfortunate accident. While chasing one another, Bell is poked in the eye by a low-hanging branch, an injury that results in her having to wear an eye patch temporarily. Martha is deeply disturbed by the injury, seeing it as her fault—and thinking of it as profoundly damaging to Bell, as it endangers one of her otherwise "normal" senses. Martha cannot bring herself to be around Bell, despite Bell's attempts to placate Martha's sense of wrongdoing. Bell's one solid friendship becomes frayed, and it is around the same time that her eyesight begins to have difficulties as well. Bell ends up in prescription glasses, which only seems to deepen Martha's sense of guilt, leading her to avoid Bell whenever they see each other. And to make matters worse, one day in gym class, Bell's gym teacher accidentally drops the Phonic Ear, breaking it. Bell recounts thinking, "The next morning, for the first time ever, I actually miss putting on the Phonic Ear. I feel so . . . so naked!"[44] Bell resorts to wearing her hearing aids to class and begins to fall behind, as she is unable to understand most of what is spoken in class. However, she is undeterred from thinking of herself as her alter ego, declaring, "With or without superpowers, I am still El Deafo—and I am outraged!"[45] She sets about overcoming her gym teacher's disregard for her physical abilities during a Presidential Physical Fitness Test, but then finds herself relating to her friends and neighbors awkwardly—including Mike Miller—most likely as a result of the situation she finds herself in at school, having gone from being confident and self-possessed to anxious and underachieving. It is in this context that the final act of *El Deafo* begins to develop, leading Bell to use her Phonic Ear in ways that capitalize on her more-than-human hearing abilities to impress her friends and classmates.

Amid her late elementary school crush on Mike Miller, Bell explains to him the powers the Phonic Ear bestows on her, and he quickly sees ulterior uses for the technology. During their shared homeroom class, their fifth-grade teacher, Mrs. Sinklemann, often leaves the children in the classroom for twenty minutes unattended, during a period she refers to as "quiet math." As one might expect, students take liberties during this period, sometimes getting caught when Mrs. Sinklemann returns early and catches them out of their seats and playing. With quiet math seen as an opportunity to be exploited, Miller convinces Bell to conduct a small experiment: Miller takes the Phonic Ear's microphone for a walk to see what its range is. Once they have established how far its powers reach, Miller hatches a plan: "When Mrs. Sinklemann leaves today for quiet math, you can use your stuff to listen out for her. We can all have fun until you tell us she's coming back! You'll be a *hero!* What d'ya say?"[46] Bell reluctantly agrees to the plan, and finds herself the enabler of her peers' delinquent behavior—not necessarily behavior benefitting El Deafo. El Deafo might have problems with Bell's new role, facilitating the bad behavior of others, but Bell experiences social inclusion—predicated on her prosthetic technology—easing what moral frictions there might be, and leading to a rewarding reunion with her estranged best friend, Martha, who shares in the excitement of the experimentation with Bell's Phonic Ear technology. Miller's strategy for delinquency works, and *El Deafo* ends without Bell facing any repercussions for her facilitating of her classmates' unruly behavior. Instead, Bell seems to finally enjoy unfettered social inclusion, enabled in no small part by her acceptance of the Phonic Ear and the capacities that it provides her with.

The Phonic Ear facilitates communication and social interactions for Bell and allows her to connect with her environment. Although she can lip-read with some proficiency, especially in person, the Phonic Ear enables forms of sociality that would otherwise be difficult or impossible. The Phonic Ear expands Bell's sensory capacities—it makes her able to hear what she otherwise could not—and expands her sociotechnical environment. She becomes, if not the same as everyone else, at least as capable as her peers, and in some ways more so. As a technical object, the Phonic Ear bundles together sets of relations that enable it as a technical object, but it also enables new relations for its wearer. At first it is the intimate, one-way relationship that Bell has with her teachers, enabling her to eavesdrop on them as they go about their extraclassroom business. Eventually it bridges Bell's relationship with her sought-after neighbor, Mike, albeit not in the way that Bell had hoped would come to pass. When she finally uses the technology to enable her peers' less-than-studious behavior in the classroom, Bell garners their respect as well as inclusion into everyday schoolyard sociality. In these emergent social relations that Bell enjoys, the relations bundled into the Phonic Ear that make it an effective actor become invisible; they become ghosts, animating their host with new social possibilities that are built on sociotechnical histories focused on facilitating the individual as a locus of personhood, self-determination, and agency.

José Delgado and Technological Facilitation of Material Subjects

BYPASSING NEUROLOGICAL AND SYMBOLIC REDUCTIVISM

In 2008, Dr. Gibson—a young neuroscientist who worked in a large research facility that focused on rehabilitative sensory implants—and I sat down to lunch at Café Gratitude in the Mission District in San Francisco. We were sitting down to talk about recent experiments in his lab at a nearby university. The lab was well known for having done work on various prosthetics, especially cochlear implants, and had recently moved its attention from the senses—Gibson's appointment a few years before had been based on his work on vision and optical implants that transmitted images from cats to computers—to mental health, broadly conceived. The conversation began as so many of ours did: I asked, "What are you working on now?"

> "We're starting to work on implants that produce emotion. It's intended to be therapeutic—you don't want to smoke anymore? We can put a chip in your brain so that whenever you start to smoke, you feel sad. Soon you won't be smoking anymore."
> "How do you even do that?" I asked.
> "It has to do with interrupting neurotransmitters. Whenever we turn the implant on, it will stop certain messages from reaching the brain and replace them with other messages. So a

stimulus can be changed to produce a negative effect, and the person's behavior will change."

"Does the technology actually exist?"

"No, not yet, but we're working with engineers to produce a microchip that can be grafted to mice that will do this."

"Isn't that kind of a dangerous technology?"

"It has a lot of therapeutic implications. There's the whole world of addictions that it can be used for. It could also be used for people with rage problems, or depression. Why be depressed when you can just bypass the impulse? It might even mean that people with affect disorders like schizophrenia can be helped with it. Or autism or narcolepsy."

When I asked Dr. Gibson years ago what he thought were some of the most important publications in his field, he mentioned José Delgado's *Physical Control of the Mind: Toward a Psychocivilized Society,*[47] a cult classic among some neuroscientists. Long out of print, pristine copies routinely sell online for hundreds of dollars. Delgado, born in 1915, spent his early career at Yale and returned to his native Spain shortly after the publication of *Physical Control of the Mind,* ostensibly to help establish the Autonomous University of Madrid. His return to Spain may have also been due to the controversy around his book, which came out at a time when electroconvulsive therapy was being debated and the legacy of lobotomies was near at hand. Delgado had invented what he referred to as a stimoceiver, a radio-activated implant that produced electrical stimulation in the brain of those it was installed in, which included cats, monkeys, bulls, chimpanzees, and eventually humans.[48] The stimoceiver was effective, and according to Delgado, it could produce feelings of calm, elation, and sadness. For many readers, Delgado is compelling not simply because of the invention he engineered and the applications he thought to apply it to. He is compelling to many readers because he is deeply invested in what control of the mind could allow in humans, arguing throughout *Physical Control of the Mind* that the next stage of evolution for humans depends on our turning technology inward, on making new "minds" through the use of targeted material interventions. Even if his ethics are problematic to most modern readers, Delgado's understanding of the individual is contemporary. He sees the mind as a function of the relationship among environmental stimuli, personal histories, and the physical structure of the brain. Delgado also makes plain what might be implicit in other people's thinking, namely that humans are always subject to the control of others, and what Delgado is providing in his technology is a means to level the field, to ensure that our leaders are as subject to control as the rest of us. In making this argument, Delgado elaborates a view of materialist subjectivity that intimately depends on interpersonal connectivity and facilitation, of ghostwriting the other through technologies. Delgado's technology shows how neurological reductivism misses how the technologies that facilitate us alter our capacities in profound ways, making new forms of subjectivity possible. His technology also shows how the symbolic fails to capture the material influences that shape how the symbolic is interpreted. However troubling Delgado's scientific practice is, he helps to show the necessity of conceptualizing the material environment of subject formation, including mediating technologies.

This is an example of what Delgado would do. After sedation, electrodes, which are implanted directly into a bull's brain, are able to deploy a low-voltage electrical charge targeted at a specific area of the subject's brain. In this case, the areas of the brain associated with pacification are targeted, and the electrical stimulation can be achieved through the use of a remote control. During recovery, the bull is placed in a pen where it is allowed free movement. Eventually it is confronted with a human interlocutor—not a farmhand or a bullfighter, but Delgado himself, acting as scientist-showman. Delgado sets about provoking the bull, taunting it verbally and pelting it with small rocks. The bull turns to face Delgado, then lowers its head as if to charge. On that cue, Delgado presses a button on the remote control he has, which initiates electrical stimulation of the bull's brain. The bull is pacified, looking momentarily dazed, and the scientist is now safe—until, that is, Delgado begins to taunt the bull again, at which point the bull's nostrils flare and it lowers its head as if to charge. Again, the scientist stimulates the bull's brain, and again, the bull is momentarily pacified. This process is repeated for hours, then over days. Eventually the bull's impulse to attack its human interlocutor—even when verbally taunted and hit with rocks—is entirely suppressed or eradicated. By all accounts, the attempt to modify the bull's behavior is successful. Ever the showman, Delgado often demonstrated the profound powers of the stimoceiver to interested audiences, culminating in the publication of *Physical Control of the Mind*. What Delgado can do for a bull, he also suggests we can—and should—do for all of society, albeit through slightly different means.

Consider Delgado's description of another experiment, one specifically designed to test what stimoceivers could do to ensure that an egalitarian society could be maintained:

> A monkey named Ali, who was the powerful and ill-tempered chief of a colony, often expressed his hostility symbolically by biting his hand or by threatening other members of the group. Radio stimulation in Ali's caudate nucleus blocked his usual aggressiveness so effectively that the animal could be caught inside the cage without danger or difficulty.... A lever was attached to the cage wall, and if it was pressed, it automatically triggered a five seconds' radio stimulation of Ali. From time to time some of the submissive monkeys touched the lever, which was located close to the feeding tray, triggering the stimulation of Ali. A female monkey named Elsa soon discovered that Ali's aggressiveness could be inhibited by pressing the lever, and when Ali threatened her, it was repeatedly observed that Elsa responded by lever pressing. Her attitude of looking straight at the boss was highly significant because a submissive monkey would not dare to do so, for fear of immediate retaliation.[49]

At their worst, stimoceivers would seem to only offer a new mode of domination, with those already in power mandating their implantation in those they dominate, to ensure that the power of the few is never threatened by the masses. But Delgado offers the opposite possibility—or at least a series of variations. What if we instead implanted those in power, so that their most dangerous impulses could be curtailed? Or what if we implanted everyone, ensuring that all dangerous impulses could be stopped? Delgado sees in these possibilities the ability to progress civilization to a more utopian point, finally overcoming a history of war and violence with discrete technologies that facilitate our better natures rather than leave us to our animal instincts. Delgado had been publishing his research related to the use of stimoceivers since 1952. *Physical Control of the Mind* summarizes his work, and it considers the many physiological and social impacts that his research might lead to. There is an enormous social history to consider in relation to Delgado's research and the timing of his book's publication, including the rise of fascism in Europe, his view that physical control could overcome passionate manipulation of the masses emblematized in National Socialism, and the student activism and counterculture movements of the 1960s. Delgado saw in his research a liberatory possibility, freeing us from our Alis and the violence endemic to human social life. Delgado's broader research program focused on electrical stimulation of the brain (ESB). While he was contemporaries with lobotomists and those who performed electroconvulsive therapies, Delgado saw his work as qualitatively different. For him, lobotomy and electroconvulsive therapies were nonspecific attempts to modify the physical structure or composition of the brain, whereas what ESB offered was precise, careful, and well researched. Throughout his work, Delgado is interested in the constitution of a psychocivilized society through the use of psychogenesis, an understanding of the material shaping of human behavior. This psychogenesis could be enabled—as in the case of the bull and Ali—through the use of technologies that shape the brain and its impulses in direct and deliberate ways, thereby facilitating particular ways of being in the world.

What underlies Delgado's work—and the work of many of his contemporaries in the neurosciences in the middle twentieth century—was a form of strong materialism that stood in opposition to popular ideas about psychology and culture, emblematized in post-Freudian psychoanalysis and its interests in symbolic subjectivity. Rather than ideation and mind being created by some symbolic order that lies outside of the individual and the world into which he or she is born and shaped through, strong materialists like Delgado see the raw material of the brain—and to a lesser degree the rest of the nervous system—as determining the actions and affect of individuals, not unlike

Antonio Damasio's neurological subjectivity. Strong materialists argue for a form of materialist subjectivity, of the self being determined by the material experience of the world. This was the conceit of Walter Freeman in his work on lobotomy, which literally scrambled parts of the prefrontal cortex of those who underwent the surgery to produce therapeutic effects. Talk therapy was unnecessary when the brain's fleshy material could be rearranged so as to change the way an individual interprets the world and behaves within it. In this paradigm, the mind is reducible to electrical currents and impulses in the brain, and the modification of those material factors produces the kind of subjects the therapy is seeking. "Mind" is an epiphenomenal effect of the brain's material processes, and strong materialists seek to act on these material factors to produce the right kind of mind. Such a position does not entirely dismiss the symbolic as an important, even vital, part of social life and subjectivity. Materialist subjectivity instead argues that the content of symbolic interactions is not rooted in historical, institutional human experiences but is merely subject to individual histories and the interpretive frameworks provided by society. Delgado is not so different from contemporary neuroscientists in his conception of what the individual is. Where he differs is in his views of what this understanding of the individual allows for the management of society.

It would be easy to dismiss Delgado, along with contemporaries of his like Freeman, as hubristic scientists and ethically ignorant butchers, but Delgado and his research are more complicated than any simple reading of science and history might allow. As much as he is like proponents of lobotomy and electroconvulsive therapy in his materialist ontology, he is quite unlike them in his sociological imagination. Delgado anticipates many of the ethical critiques of his work in *Physical Control of the Mind*, and however he might be characterized, he cannot be seen as ethically ignorant. However, his ethics are driven by utopia. His ethical postulates are quite clear, drawn from historical and cultural materialism as articulated in the midcentury. Importantly, his experiments share assumptions about material technologies facilitating particular forms of personhood and subjectivity. Whereas many technologies of facilitation are presented as already invented black boxes of sociotechnical relations, the stimoceiver is a technology of facilitation that has its inner workings—and potential future effects—laid bare by its maker. In Delgado's case, the ghostwriter has written his own social exegesis. Focusing on Delgado and his technology makes obvious what is at stake in these technologies of facilitation and how, given their social situation, they succeed or fail in making the right kinds of persons and subjects.

EPIPHENOMENAL EXPERIENCE AND MATERIAL SUBJECTIVITY

For Delgado, as for any strong materialist neuroscientist, consciousness, the mind, personality—whatever it is called—is epiphenomenal. That is, first there are chemicals, neuronal structures, and their interactions, and secondarily there is consciousness, which is a by-product of these interactions. These neural and chemical interactions are produced as reactions to the social and natural environment. Delgado begins with this premise in an effort on his part to differentiate material being in the world and what is popularly accepted as the mind:

> The newborn brain is not capable of speech, symbolic under-standing, or of directing skillful motility. It has no ideas, words, or concepts, no tools for communication, no significant sensory experience, no culture. The new born baby never smiles. He is unable to comprehend the loving phrases of his mother or to be aware of the environment. We must conclude that there are no detectable signs of mental activity at birth and *that human beings are born without minds.*[50]

Delgado explains that his conception of the mind and its material basis depends on feedback as the fundamental motor for consciousness: "The mind is not a static, inborn entity owned by the individual and self-sufficient, but the dynamic organization of sensory perceptions of the external world, correlated and reshaped through the internal anatomical and functional structure of the brain."[51] What is accepted as consciousness—and particularly the realm of the symbolic—is a secondary production of these environmental stimuli. Delgado writes, "Our only way of being in touch with external reality is by transducing physical and chemical events of the surrounding into electrical and chemical sequences at the sensory receptor level. The brain is not in touch with the environmental reality but with its symbolic code transmitted by neuronal pathways."[52] This materialist assumption is necessary to motivate and explain how ESB can produce profound changes in personality and behavior, and how dominant ideas about meaning are secondary to the material basis of life itself.

Delgado's view of individual behavior is inseparable from his conception of materialist subjectivity. Individual actions are not meaningful outside of the understanding that they are a response to a stimulus. In this view, behavior is not something that is internally predetermined but rather is a reaction to the environment; this stretches from autonomic responses to creative output like art, literature, and science. Delgado reaches this claim in part through experimental design. Using animals in which he has implanted stimoceivers, he restrains their ability for movement; a cat provoked to jump has its leg held so as to frustrate its ability to act. Yet the behavioral impulse is experienced, and the cat finds a way to resolve the impulse by moving its body into another position so as to resolve the behavior.[53] This drives Delgado's conception of behavior as something that is mediated by the senses but that is a response to the environment: "Individual reactions are determined by environmental factors acting through sensory inputs on neurophysiological processes and are manifested through appropriate motor output as behavior."[54] Reactions to one's environment are not difficult to see in this frame, as one might shade one's eyes from a bright light or hold one's breath while walking through an odiferous space, but Delgado argues that more complex, symbolic behavior is equally a by-product of one's environmental and sensorial context. What makes complex behaviors—art, literature, science—legible as behaviors are the shared historical contexts of the maker and the consumer. They share an institutional history that shapes their interpretive understandings of behavior, and these institutions are deeply material in their presence in people's lives.

One report of Delgado's is worth reproducing by way of demonstrating how precisely he sees ESB operating on personality and what its futures might be:

One of the moving pictures taken in this study was very demonstrative, showing a patient with a sad expression and slightly depressed mood who smiled when a brief stimulation was applied to the rostral part of the brain, returning quickly to his usual depressed state, to smile again as soon as stimulation was reapplied. Then a ten-second stimulation completely changed his behavior and facial expression into a lasting pleasant and happy mood. Some mental patients have been provided with portable stimulators which they have used in self-treatment of depressive states with apparent clinical success.[55]

Delgado explains elsewhere that "automatic learning is possible by feeding signals directly into specific neuronal structures without conscious participation."[56] Taken together, it is clear that consciousness just seems to get in the way. For strong materialists like Delgado, humans are a collection of chemicals, structures, and impulses that comprise physiological functioning. Consciousness can be produced—and more important, altered—as needed, and the more direct the means of this production, the less likely there will be interference from the environment. For Delgado, happiness can exist outside of our social conditions as long as the brain is acted upon directly, which ESB allows.

This conception of consciousness is all due to what Delgado refers to as "functional monotony."[57] For Delgado, the active response to an environmental stimulus is not pregiven. For example, implanting a stimoceiver into a cat and stimulating the cat's brain so as to produce the set of reflexes normally associated with swatting at an enemy—which is the basis of an actual experiment—means only that the cat will enact those actions, not that it will spontaneously find an enemy in its environment and act against it. The same stimulation can occur a number of times, and each time, the result on the brain is the same, but how the stimulation is extrapolated to the world will vary. If a target is nearby, then the behavior may be directed at it, regardless of what the subject thinks of that target; cognition comes after the action in an effort on the part of the subject to make sense of the action in the context of what he or she thinks of him- or herself. What matters in each case is that the biological strata that are being acted upon are experiencing an actual, profound effect, and that over time, this effect might be able to be retained without direct stimulation—as in the case of the bull, Ali, patients, and the many other experimental subjects Delgado worked with. Consider Delgado's claim regarding the patient able to produce "a lasting pleasant and happy mood." It seems not to matter that the patient is in an asylum, removed from family and friends, work, and everyday life. These possible influences on the patient's mental state are removed from consideration. Instead, what actually matters for Delgado is the stimulation of the patient's brain and the effects this produces. Happiness begins in material being and is extrapolated from there to the world. This inverts dominant ways of thinking about emotions—that they begin in interactions and lead to effects on the brain—but is there anything necessarily wrong with this conception of the material basis of the self?

The implication of Delgado's thinking about the tripartite relationship among material brain, environment, and individual interpretations leads him to the claim that *"The individual mind is not self-sufficient."*[58] He makes this claim in direct refutation to the belief in "Occidental cultures" that "the individual personality is a self-contained and relatively independent entity with its own destiny, well differentiated from the surroundings, and able to function even when isolated from earth and traveling in an orbiting capsule."[59] Delgado makes the claim that individuals are deeply rooted in their environments, that any sense of an independent self is ideological illusion, and that removal of individuals from an environment leads to the deterioration of "normal mental functions." One of the implications of this view is that the subjectivity that individuals experience is the subjectivity produced by the deliberate or accidental production of an environment, a process that Delgado sees as a function of governance with a goal of producing "civilization."[60]

Delgado points to the practices of blood testing engaged couples to ensure they are free from disease and relation, ensuring that travelers are properly vaccinated ahead of travel, adding chlorine and fluoride to municipal drinking water, and regulating the inclusion of iodine in table salt.[61] His point is that Americans tolerate all of these interventions, largely without protest, and they shape the material experiences of bodies as well as relationships to society and the environment. These governmental interventions create, however unevenly, materialist subjects and the civilization into which they fit. He argues, "Human health has improved in a spectacular way precisely because official agencies have had the knowledge and the power to influence our personal biology, and it should be emphasized that health regulations are similar in dictatorial and in democratic societies."[62] This view ultimately leads him to the claim, "The mother certainly teaches the baby. The policeman imposes order on city traffic. To discuss whether human behavior can or should be controlled is naïve and misleading. We should discuss what kinds of control are ethical, considering the efficiency and mechanisms of existing procedures and the desirable degree of these and other controls in the future."[63] The question for Delgado is settled. Control of the individual for the betterment of society and the ultimate goal of an orderly civilization are already being done, but in ways that the individual has little or no control over. Stimoceivers, and ESB more generally, make control a reciprocal function of social life; they make explicit what is otherwise implicit—that subjectivity depends on control. What Delgado is arguing for is a deeply materialist subjectivity. Individuals become subjects through environmental interactions that depend on their normative physiological functioning. Moreover, their environment is something that is crafted to produce particular expressions of subjectivity. Knowing this, the ethical thing to do, Delgado suggests, is to take control of the ways that the environment shapes our brains. If we cannot change our environment, at least we can change the way that it materially affects us with the help of facilitating technologies.

Reading Delgado today, it is difficult not to see the historical controversies associated with midcentury materialist approaches to the brain and its treatment. Delgado exhibits a nuanced, if idealistic, view of ESB and its implications. As one might expect of a resolute materialist, Delgado sees ESB as existing on a continuum of all extant means of acting on the brain, including pharmaceuticals, electroshock therapy, and psychoanalysis. The realm of the symbolic, which psychoanalysis traffics in, is too slow to effect the kinds of changes needed in the lives of most people; moreover, its process is inexact. Similarly, electroshock therapy is too unpredictable in its effects to be useful for "normal" people.[64] Pharmaceuticals, although they hold promise, also entail unpredictable side effects. ESB, Delgado argues, produces exactly the effect desired. For Delgado, the ethical consideration is not why we should not use ESB technologies but how we can possibly refrain from doing so when all of the alternatives are less effective. Stimoceivers promise to make us all the individuals we hope to be—maybe with a remote control for ourselves, and a matching remote control for all those we interact with throughout the day, so that we can facilitate for others "a lasting pleasant and happy mood."

How to Ghostwrite a Person into Being

EXTERNALIZING THE NERVOUS SYSTEM

Neuroscience holds that the nervous system is interior to the body, that it extends from the brain, through the brain stem, to the spinal cord, to the nerves throughout our bodies. The nervous system, like our bodies, is bounded. A conception of the materiality of the brain and its interactions with the environment—like Delgado's—raises questions about the reality of this boundedness. Is it ideological, like the construction of the individual that Delgado points to, and if it is, what are the alternative possibilities for conceptualizing the nervous system? Delgado's materialist view of subjectivity is only partial; he seems to discount the symbolic as being mere ephemera, as immaterial. But what both Peyton Goddard and CeCe Bell help to show is that communication and the symbolic are predicated on material infrastructures. The facilitating technologies they use are obvious—the Lightwriter and the Phonic Ear—but all communication depends on material interactions, through gesture and sound, and to ignore the materiality of communication is an ideological sleight of hand that Delgado uses to marginalize some mechanisms of social change, like talk therapy or political movements, in favor of stimoceivers and ESB. Delgado's conceptualization of subjectivity as based on the material interactions of individuals and their environment is not materialist enough. According material power to the infrastructures that enable communication as well as communication itself renders Delgado's materialism more robust. It shows what is at stake in materialist conceptions of subjectivity. Delgado is not wrong in his understanding of built environments and infrastructures influencing individuals. He is also not wrong that these material factors have been authored by those in power, or neglected by those in power to produce particular results.[65] However, he does not extend his conception of matter far enough. Humans are connected to each other and their environments through material interactions, and these interactions provide the basis for the development of subjectivity and sociality. Peyton and Bell make this clear. They are shaped by the connections that their particular modes of communication make possible for them, just as they are negatively affected through connections that are impossible, difficult, or abusive.

In conceptualizing the consequences of a more materialist view of subjectivity, consider the figure of the ghostwriter, those often invisible authors who make communication possible for memoir writers. Ghostwriting depends on a set of relations that become obscured in the technological object of the memoir, and that construct a recognizable life for the subject of the memoir. In the case of Peyton Goddard, the ghostwriting accomplished by Carol Cujec is profound. Peyton's use of FC might be conceptualized as being based in the same logic. Peyton is able to write on her Lightwriter and thereby communicate, but only with the aid of a facilitator. Ghostwriting fundamentally makes Peyton's life legible for her readers, at the syntactic level as well as at the level of Peyton's everyday life. Critiques of FC are based, in no small part, in the visibility of ghostwriters, both in their physical assistance of facilitation and in the content of the written text. There is something unsettling about making the ghostwriter too apparent, too visible, because it makes clear that individuals communicate only with the facilitation of others—especially so for communicators like Peyton but equally true for all interactional communication. It is also true that technologies like the Lightwriter are authored; they are designed using assumptions about how communication works, both in terms of how people interact with a keyboard and what a graphical interface should look like. Technologies like the Lightwriter and Phonic Ear are designed with embedded assumptions about communication, which are fundamentally about the relationship between individuals and their environment. The term "ghostwriter" might also be used to name those often invisible individuals and groups who have authored built environments, infrastructures, technologies, and languages. Ghostwriters, in the immediate sense, are those who author for another, but the mimicry that individuals partake in to model socially meaningful interactions depends on ghostwriting too. Subjects are authored through others who reward successful mimicry and ignore sounds and gestures with "no relevancy," as Josh Greenfeld puts it. This authorship extends throughout interactions with environments, infrastructures, technologies, and languages, as the remote authors of those materials shape their capacities as facilitating technologies in ways that render particular forms of communication and subjectivity possible. Authorship in this way sees writing as any manifestation of intent, concretized in a technology. Writing, then, is the materialization of history, creating the institutionalized contexts for meaningful mimicry and interpretation.[66] When institutions make specific modes of communication illegible, or when particular modes of communication are derided—like FC is—individuals are foreclosed from even attempting to inhabit forms of subjectivity supported by dominant institutions.

The stimoceiver makes plain the role of the ghostwriter. Our social others hold in their hands the ability to change our experience of the world. They are able to facilitate for us in ways that are transparent. "Why be depressed when you can just bypass the impulse?" my neuroscientist friend, Dr. Gibson, rhetorically asks, and Delgado provides the answer: with the push of a button, replace your depression with a "a lasting pleasant and happy mood." This naked facilitation of other people's subjectivity—and the ability to explicitly control their experience of society—makes the stimoceiver and related technologies challenging for American ideas about the individual. Should we be able to self-determine our affective states, even when they are self-destructive or asocial? What if the intents of our remote control-wielding social others have our best interests at heart but chafe against our self-understanding or intent? This is clearly the problem many see in FC and that Peyton Goddard's experience with Tricia makes plain: facilitation is indebted to the intentions of our facilitators as well as the methods they have at their disposal for facilitation. When a facilitator is intention free—and this might be the case with Peyton's mother and psychiatrist, as exposed in her psychiatrist's experiment in communication—the technology is liberated from these suspicions of its impingements on the agentive powers of the individual. The appearance of transparency in communication creates the illusion of freedom and independence. But no technology of facilitation is intention-free. If, as Delgado implies, our material world is authored for us, then materialist subjectivity is never free of the intentions of others. Materialist conceptions of subjectivity imply that there is no outside of materiality. It follows that what is possible in the present is always determined by what has preceded it.[67]

FC offers the most robust example of the deeply embedded nature of communication in material networks. Peyton is able to communicate only because another person is able to facilitate her movements into conveying information, which, for Peyton, depends equally on her Lightwriter. If subjectivity is produced through the material conditions of everyday life, then the people who facilitate for Peyton are as dependent on those who facilitated them, on backward through the whole of human history. If one accepts this materialist hypothesis, human history is embedded in planetary history, stretching back to the earliest chemical and geological formations on Earth. Similarly, the technology that Peyton relies on is indebted to the whole of planetary history, and that Peyton and the technology exist at the same time is a matter of contingency. Another time, another place, and Peyton would have never "unlocked [her] voice." That Peyton's consultation with a shaman leads her community to think of her as experiencing universal consciousness is no mistake: her embeddedness in human and technological facilitation makes evident to her how precarious her ability to communicate is, how deeply material it is in its underpinnings and expressions. That Dianne is willing to experiment with FC is in large part due to the desperation that she and Peyton each privately face, a possibility that emerges in the wake of Peyton's suicidal urges and Dianne's despair. Dianne and Peyton do not break from history; they do not emerge into a new world. But their willingness to experiment with FC is predicated on their exhaustion of other means of communication. Peyton's unghostwritten prose makes evident how profoundly different her relationship to communication is, how two decades without a socially recognized means of expression has shaped her experience of herself and her world. The material shaping of Peyton's subjectivity is profound, and its effects are ongoing. That she can communicate, even with the explicit facilitation of other people and technology, does not make Peyton "normal," but it does mean that she can participate in her world as a subject and not merely a person.

CeCe Bell's experience with her Phonic Ear provides an example of a benign facilitating technology that allows her to experience the world of her friends and family. Although the technology itself seems to be exempt from questionable intentions, once the technology is introduced into Bell's social world what it facilitates in terms of her relations with others, might begin to raise questions about the social value of the technology and its uses. The makers of the Phonic Ear have a clear purpose for the technology in mind: the communication between one speaker and one listener. The context of the dyadic relationship can vary, but the relation remains the same: one listener, one speaker. The Phonic Ear works to facilitate this relationship, with a microphone for the speaker and an earpiece for the listener. The microphone can also pick up the sounds that the speaker hears, transmitting those to the listener without differentiating them from the speaker's voice. The Phonic Ear compresses the environment into one channel that the listener experiences. The assumptions here of a speaking communicator and a listening audience depend on a vocal speaker; deaf-to-deaf communication might not be facilitated by the Phonic Ear in the same way and would depend on a different means. The Phonic Ear also depends on radio and electrical technologies that power the device and that provide the medium for the components to communicate, meaning that the Phonic Ear works in modern environments that support these requirements and cannot work elsewhere. One of the Phonic Ear's material qualities that chafes against Bell's desires is its obviousness: its bulkiness, wires, and earpieces all make the technology apparent to her friends and classmates, something that she is extremely conscious of but that its designers disregard as either unimportant for the user's experience or as impossible to design away as a result of the technology's requirements. As Bell recounts, her social experiences throughout elementary school are shaped by her anxieties around the appearance of the technology itself. While it enables her to communicate with her teachers, it also makes her self-conscious of her appearance and her communication needs. As a result, she finds friendships not with those whom she would normally seek out but with those who either see her social vulnerability as a means to control her, as in the case of Laura, or, as Ginny does, to use Bell's deafness to reward themselves with the pride of having a deaf friend. This shaping of Bell's social world has consequences for how she thinks of herself and her relationships with other people; it is deeply indebted to the technology that facilitates her communication with her hearing friends and teachers. The effects of the technology are material in their consequences, shaping Bell's experiences of herself, her relationships, and her environments. Not all of these consequences can be anticipated, and many of them may be unique to Bell's experience with the technology, but all of them are shaped by the facilitating technology that she comes to rely on.

If the Phonic Ear and other hearing aids hide much of the assumptions of their authorship, they still remain obvious as technologies that are facilitating communication for their users. The stimoceiver, and ESB more generally, offer the possibility that facilitating technologies might be rendered almost entirely invisible. Indeed, Delgado's interest in the everyday ways that our material experiences are shaped by governments points to the ubiquity of attempts to render individuals unaware of the technologies that facilitate their experiences of themselves and their worlds. Consider his examples of fluoride in drinking water and iodine in table salt. Fluoride ensures modest protection against tooth decay, and iodine is important for thyroid health. Both create bodily conditions for individuals and communities that shape their experiences of themselves, their environments, and their communities, but, most likely, the fluoride and iodine and their powers are obscured for the communities that consume them. Pharmaceuticals offer another example of a similar process, although individuals are generally aware of the pills they are consuming, if not their chemical composition. Pharmaceuticals shape the experiences that individuals have of their bodies, and by extension the worlds individuals inhabit.[68] People with epilepsy who take anticonvulsants can experience fewer or no seizures, women who take birth control pills do not often get pregnant, and people with insomnia who take sleep aids might experience consolidated sleep. Each of these small chemical technologies has embedded in it ideas about what normal bodily comportment and experience is, and the pharmaceuticals seek to produce these normalcies in their consumers. What Delgado hopes for in the stimoceiver is even more discrete than these pharmaceutical or additive attempts to materially shape subjectivity: a fully actualized version of his world, with everyone enjoying a stimoceiver implanted in the skull, would ensure that individuals could act on one another—despots could be brought low, friends could be cheered—and that individuals could act on themselves. The technology, he suggests, would create freedom—freedom from tyrants, freedom from the seriality of everyday life, and freedom from the material determinants of our physiologies. But to make the stimoceivers work, especially at the level of a whole society, would depend on a massive infrastructure to support the devices and their facilitations. Like the Phonic Ear, stimoceivers are only possible in particular kinds of societies: those that would tolerate them as a pervasive technology for facilitating personhood and subjectivity. That no society has adopted such an explicit attempt to make specific kinds of subjects may be due in no small part to the naked mechanism of facilitation: discrete technologies help to maintain the liberal ideology of the individual, and a society built on stimoceivers would make plain the material indebtedness of persons to the technologies and environments that produce them as subjects.

It is not simply that facilitating technologies allow individuals to interact with their sociotechnical worlds but that worlds interact back, that facilitating technologies are able to fill the facilitated individual with the technology's intents and expectations. Bell gets caught up in the social possibilities and expectations that the Phonic Ear enables, however childish they might be, but this makes obvious how being part of a social world means being facilitated by others. The stimoceiver, FC, and Phonic Ear are all obvious technologies, but humans are equally facilitated by largely invisible technologies like language, institutions, and society itself, which have been brought into being and which control our experiences of self and world through often invisible yet highly determining forces. The individual is not to be conceptualized as independent versus dependent, but as always facilitated by a whole range of technologies—human interlocutors, the discrete stimoceiver, Lightwriters, caregivers, pharmaceuticals, and prosthetics, as well as the institutions of everyday life, and conventions of language and communication. All of these facilitating technologies in our nervous systems have been authored for us, even if the authors are no longer so apparent; they have become ghostwriters, making communication and subjectivity possible and then disappearing into the material technologies that their authorship has created. These facilitating technologies make us not what we will in some idealist sense, but into the kinds of persons that the technologies make possible. We are subjects—not solely of personal histories but also of the facilitating technologies that compose our worlds.

If, as materialist conceptions of subjectivity hold, subjects are indebted to their external nervous systems—that humans are fundamentally impossible to disconnect from their worlds—then personhood is trapped by historical conceptions of the individual. Peyton Goddard and CeCe Bell both provide ways to conceptualize how breaks from this materialist determination might occur. That the desperation of the Goddards and the play of Bell and her peers disrupt the possibilities that individuals see in their situations should be no surprise.[69] Both desperation and play are central to mimicry as a social form, leading to what Roger Caillois conceptualizes as forms of camouflage, of attempts to fit in with one's environment and play with this capacity for mimesis.[70] Mimicry as a social practice strives toward duplication and repetition, but when these drives prove fruitless, one possibility that remains is to mimic differently, to produce duplication with variations. Bell and Supercrush Mike Miller's innovations for the use of the Phonic Ear are not so much total breaks from Bell's historical situation as they are minor variations on the use of the technology to produce different effects. By using the Phonic Ear to report to her classmates what she hears, she subverts the intended use of the technology. What the designers of the Phonic Ear had anticipated—a receptive listener in a dyadic relationship with a speaking teacher—becomes perverted by the social designs of Bell's other authors, her classmates and Supercrush. One set of mimicry practices, of teacher and student, becomes supplanted by another, of eavesdropper and observed. Bell and her friends animate the use of the technology—and their social forms—differently than expected, producing predictable results. Even with their innovation, how Bell can conceptualize herself is constrained by the media that facilitates her. From Bell's perspective, she is the superhero, yet her teachers and parents might feel differently. Peyton is more complicated, and her ability to break from the situation she has found herself in—what her mother refers to as dead time—is entirely contingent on the availability of novel technologies, willing psychiatrists, and facilitating caregivers. That she can become a speaking subject, however she inhabits that role, is thanks to the willingness of her network of family and caregivers to disrupt her experience of dead time by animating her differently. By taking Peyton's arm in hand, Peyton becomes animated in a way she had not been before. Desperation bleeds into play as Peyton's family and caregivers allow her to experiment with FC and the Lightwriter. That play breaks Peyton from her situation, making new possibilities emerge. As I discuss in the next chapter, animation makes emergent social possibilities, as play with and through facilitating technologies disrupts normative situations, changing the situation of the nervous system that individuals inhabit, and their subjectivities too.

FOUR

Cybernetic Subjectivity

The Fusion of Body, Symbol, and Environment in the Facilitated Person

*I*n this chapter, I theorize how animation as a process makes individuals into persons and produces communicative subjects able to use language, but this language may defy normative conceptions of symbolic subjectivity. Instead, communicating subjects are interacting subjects, embedded in animating social connections through which they are facilitated and by which they facilitate others. The two case studies in this chapter focus on the Suskinds and Karasiks, both families with boys diagnosed with autism who grow into men with an intimate relationship with media technologies. In the case of the Suskinds, their son, Owen, develops an intense interest in Disney movies, and with the help of his family, he is able to create a novel form of communication that depends on textual references, memorized dialogue, and a theory of the sidekick. David Karasik comes to develop a relationship with television shows from his youth in the 1950s and 1960s, which do not allow him the same kind of technological manipulation that Owen has access to with recording technology like VCRs. Instead of being able to memorize whole films, David depends on highly repetitive, serialized television shows. In his youth, his family is unable or unwilling to fully integrate David's modes of interaction into the family despite caring deeply for him. This inability to forge a communicative channel with David until later in his life may contribute to his continued frustrations and disorderly behaviors, as well as the family's view of him as disruptive.

What these two cases help show is how animation depends on a reciprocal relationship between individuals and the technologies, environment, and other persons they interact with in order to produce reciprocally animating subjects. In furthering this argument, I turn to two very different sets of psychological research. First, I look at Harry Harlow's experiments with maternal affection—and eventually the affection of whole kin networks—to put forward a theory of the family as predicated on the animation of persons. In focusing on Harlow's work, which uses both animate and inanimate models as the basis for socializing young monkeys, I argue that despite the many things that Harlow gets wrong about development and social connections, what his work shows is that reciprocal animation through material connections is vital to producing relations between individuals, as well as the production of personhood and subjectivity. Drawing on Harlow's work about child–parent bonding, I turn to Gregory Bateson and his theory of the double bind as the basis for the production of affect disorders. Bateson's theory has been widely influential in a variety of fields associated with cybernetics despite having been discredited as the cause for schizophrenia and other affect disorders. I follow his influence through contemporary cyberneticists and family therapists who provide a set of tools for developing a theory of social relations that displaces the brain as a determinative object and moves toward a conceptualization of the nervous system as a living, animating organ that can produce and sustain a variety of nonnormative personhoods and subjectivities.

Animation and the nervous system help to develop cybernetic subjectivity beyond the deterministic view held by Bateson and his contemporaries as emblematized in their use of the double bind. Instead, following Mony Elkaïm, a cybernetics-influenced family therapist, I suggest that cybernetic subjectivity provides a means to pull together the neurological, symbolic, and material views of the subject into a robust framework that recognizes the diversity of influences in making persons and subjects. Such a view does not privilege any one of these forces as primary in the production of personhood or subjectivity. Rather, it recognizes that bodies and their capacities are the result of complex worldly interactions that exceed the brain, language, and the sociotechnical environment. Cybernetic subjectivity provides a way to conceptualize how connections among persons, their kin, environments, technology, and communicative infrastructures maintain individuals as persons and produce particular forms of subjectivity predicated on reciprocal animation. Moreover, cybernetic subjectivity moves away from the view of individuals having inborn capacities—a presumption in neurological, symbolic, and materialist views of subjectivity—and moves toward the foundational conception of capacities being facilitated through an individual's connections with the world.

The Animated Boy

CHANGING THE SUBJECT THROUGH PLAY

This is the Suskind family: Ron, the father, and Pulitzer award-winning journalist; Cornelia, the mother, a dedicated homemaker and educator; Walt, their older son; and Owen, their younger child. The Suskinds are firmly upper middle class, living in the Washington, D.C., area so that Ron can be close to the U.S. government, which is the basis of much of his reporting. They have available to them a wide array of professionals—educators, physicians, psychiatrists—who support them in their diagnosis of Owen, as well as in Owen's caregiving and education. Born in the 1990s, Owen benefits from decades of neurological and psychiatric research, and his symptoms—aphasia, erratic behavior, lack of eye contact, fixations—quickly add up to a diagnosis of autism. Owen has regressive autism. During his first couple of years, he seems to be developing along normative lines, but around the age of three, things change. As Ron reports, Owen's use of language erodes to the point where he can say very little, and what he does say seems to make little sense. He runs around, frantic, then stops, stands still, and cries. Then he starts running around again, repeating the same sequence. Where once he would make eye contact with his playmates and family members, his gaze no longer seems to fix on others. Instead, his eyes seemed preoccupied with something invisible. From a rather typical little kid, interested in others and in play, Ron sees Owen's personality recede to the point of disappearance. Yet from his earliest exposure to them, Owen loves Walt Disney movies of all kinds, from the earliest hand-drawn cartoons to the more recent computer-animated and live-action films. The Disney films offer Owen a safe space to inhabit, where every narrative tension is resolved and every character finds a role in the social fabric. The films also offer, over time, a way for Owen to interact with his family and others. The films animate Owen; they provide him with scripts for social interactions and with frameworks for interpreting himself, other people, and the world. The Suskinds show how subjectivity is facilitated through a modular and playful epiphenomenal interpretive framework based on a shared, animating, material environment—in this case, Disney films and their generic conventions.

Ron narrates their family's search for treatments for Owen's behaviors. He and Cornelia both throw themselves into caring for Owen, knowing that there is no cure but that there might be ways to shape his interactions with others and his environment in socially recognizable ways. By the 1990s, Ivar Lovaas had established himself as a leader in the field of applied behavioral analysis, which Ron describes as relying on "rewards and verbal 'aversives'—stern language and sometimes shouts—[that] forces changes in the child's behavior. It's pure behavior modification. . . . It looks to the untrained eye like animal training."[1] During the same period, Stanley Greenspan had introduced a competitor to Lovaas's behavioralism, referred to as Floortime.[2] Ron explains that Floortime is "basically following the kids—driven by their intense self-directed urges—wherever they go, and in whatever they utter, and try, with various methods, to draw them out."[3] Ron rightly notes that both Lovaas and Greenspan share a conception of the therapeutic intervention as relying on "a one-on-one model of intense engagement with a goal of bringing these kids into the world."[4] The Suskinds reject Lovaas's approach, referring to it as "monkey training."[5] They see something in Owen unlike other children, something "compensatory." Ron writes, "Like the way Down syndrome folks often have highly evolved sensory equipment. There's something about the way one area of challenge, a blockage, often creates compensatory skills somewhere else. No different than blind people with powerful hearing, but, in this instance, in subtler areas of emotion or expressed sensitivity."[6] If Lovaas's behavioralism is primarily designed to make the children into "normal"-seeming children, Ron's invocation of compensatory skills indicates the Suskinds' willingness to let Owen develop his capacities for social engagement in nonnormative ways. It may be this rejection of normative treatments for Owen that allows him to develop the relationships with the Disney films that prove so animating for him.

Owen's relationship with each of the Disney films is intimate: he watches them over and over again, stopping and rewinding the VHS tapes repeatedly to pore over a particular scene or phrase. His family indulges this to a point, working the VHS remote for him. Eventually, when Owen is able to do this repetitive work, he is left to direct it himself. Over time, Owen begins to mimic the words of the characters on screen, first with the repeated use of the phrase "juicervose"[7] and eventually "bootylyzwitten."[8] Juicervose, the family learns, is from a key song in *The Little Mermaid*, in which Ursula, the evil tentacled underseas witch, barters with the heroine, Ariel, for Ariel's desired ability to go on land—which will cost her "just your voice." Owen becomes fixated on this phrase. He subjects his family to watching the musical scene repeatedly, ending, each time, with this phrase: "just your voice." How could this child, who lost his voice before the age of three, not be trying to communicate with this attempt at facilitated mimicry? The Suskinds are momentarily excited—Owen has found a way to communicate, albeit mediated through film and the precise use of VHS technology—until they are told by their psychiatrist that Owen's behavior is mere echolalia, a meaningless repetition of sounds. But then it happens again with "bootylyzwitten," which the family comes to realize derives from *Beauty and the Beast*, and which is the lesson of the movie: Belle, the titular beauty, comes to love the Beast through her realization—and his—that "beauty lies within." Again, how could this not index some otherwise inaccessible and intentional meaning making of Owen's? How could he not be trying to communicate his interior experience to those around him?

With "juicervose," "bootylyzwitten," and a handful of other more complex interactions as indications that Owen has a means to communicate, however nonnormatively, Ron sets about staging an intervention. While Owen is resting in bed, looking at a book, Ron puts on a puppet of Iago, the parrot sidekick of the nefarious Jafar from Disney's

Aladdin,[9] and positions himself so that Owen can see the puppet but Ron remains invisible. Speaking as Iago, Ron begins an experimental conversation with Owen:

> "So, Owen, how ya' doin'?" I say, doing my best Gilbert Gottfried. "I mean, how does it feel to be you!?"
> Through the crease [in Owen's bedsheet], I can see him turn toward Iago. It's like he was bumping into an old friend.
> "I'm not happy. I don't have friends. I can't understand what people say."
> I have not heard this voice, natural and easy, with the traditional rhythm of common speech, since he was two.
> I'm talking to my son for the first time in five years. Or Iago is.

The Suskinds discover that Owen can communicate, but it only occurs through the scripts, characters, and interactions provided by Disney films. Ron can initiate an interaction by affecting a particular accent and performing a line from a Disney film as if he were a specific character, and Owen will respond in kind by adopting the affectations of the appropriate character from the film to perform the next line—and eventually whole scenes. With their intimate knowledge of the films, Ron can usually find a scene to reenact that is appropriate for a given situation. When Owen has a hard day at school, Ron adopts the role of Merlin from *The Sword in the Stone*, provoking Owen to adopt the role of a young Arthur. In this way, Ron can produce a socially meaningful interaction with Owen. Even if it might appear to be mere performance of a Disney scene, it still provides Ron with a mechanism to communicate with Owen and access his subjective experience. The Suskinds come to accept that Owen is able to find some kind of intimacy and connection through the narratives, characters, contexts, and relationships enabled by his repetitive consumption of Disney films. They go to great lengths to provide Owen with a steadily growing library of films to memorize and mine for social interactions to imitate. Over time, through mimicry, Owen is able to extrapolate from a character or narrative to improvise both as characters from the Disney stories, and increasingly to find a version of himself that is not a reenactment of a character from a Disney film but something more. Ron explains, "At bedtime, Cornelia talks about Dumbo sleeping in his tree. She just has to throw out one line, like Timothy Q. Mouse saying, 'Come on, Dumbo, you can do it,' and Owen slips into context, integrates the tree references, and hurries off to bed. . . . Though all of our words are scripted by others, we are literally communicating through these words and the stories they tell."[10] Owen enrolls his family in a complex play of mimicry and interpretation, creating what is fundamentally his own modular framework for the interpretation of his communicative acts. This is entirely enabled by the facilitating technologies—the VHS device, the films, his parents, psychiatrists, and teachers—who see the Disney films as a legitimate way for Owen to communicate and upon which to found his sense of self.

The problem that the Suskinds face is what they see as the artificiality of Owen's communicative practices. Is there something wrong with his relying on a fictional universe of characters and situations to communicate with real people, his family, classmates, and caregivers? This question comes to the fore during a family vacation to Walt Disney World, an experiment on the Suskinds' part to see how Owen will interact with the characters who had become so dear to him through his media consumption. By this point, Owen had begun to carefully index in his memory all of the voice actors of the Disney characters, building an enormous database of social connections and metatextual relationships, and Owen takes advantage of his time with the living characters to discuss these behind-the-scenes connections they share. In response to Owen's observations about these connections, a Disney World Pooh "nods and shrugs, and Owen embraces him."[11] From afar, Ron ruminates: "Our eyes begin to adjust, to see what he sees. These characters are part of a family. His family. He's grown up with them, relied on them, learned from them. This is his chance to tease out their relationships to one another, discover what binds them to one another."[12] In reflecting on Owen's relationships with the Disney characters, Ron suggests to Cornelia that the emotions he experiences are not the same as "real emotions with actual people. . . . He has to know, deep down, that these characters—that they're not real."[13] If Ron is staking a position that there is a profound difference between relationships with real and artificial people, Cornelia's response is more equivocal. Ron reports her as responding, "Look, kids believe in Santa Claus long after they suspect there may be some logistical issues. Belief and nonbelief can hang together for quite a while."[14] The important thing, they agree, is not the reality of the relationship but the effects that the relationships have on Owen. They note that thanks to his relationships with the Disney characters, he has become "calm, self-possessed, and sure of himself."[15] The Disney universe has provided Owen with a model of society and relationships, and the model is real even if the relationships are unidirectional. The Disney characters have no feelings about Owen, no reciprocal relationship with him. The question for the Suskinds increasingly becomes whether Owen can transpose those emotional feelings about fictional persons onto the real world, with its relationships that are more complex than the unidirectional investment Owen has developed with the Disney characters.

Owen is enrolled in a school for students with learning disabilities, the Lab School in the Washington, D.C., area, and as his confidence and fluency with the Disney films grows, he advances to enrolling others in his scripted interactions. This culminates most successfully in his staging of the Disney film *The Song of the South* as a play at the Lab School when he is eight years old.[16] *The Song of the South* is a largely forgotten mixed-medium Disney film, combining live-action actors with animated characters, and it tells, among other stories, the tale of Br'er Rabbit and the Tar Baby, a folktale of the American South. Because Owen knows the film so well—all of the lines, all of the intonations, all of the gestures and affectations—he is promoted to the lead role of Br'er Rabbit. Owen's idiosyncratic sociality becomes the animating basis for an ongoing class project that pulls everyone together. Leading up to the performance, his classmates begin rehearsing, fashioning costumes, and building sets. Owen's performance is perfect, an imitation exact in its reproduction. Ron writes that Owen is

> immediately in character. Of course, he's in character all the
> time. That means knowing his lines is not a problem, talking
> to the pot of tar—"What's the matter with you? I said,
> 'Howdy!'"—as he gets one arm stuck, then the other, then his

legs, and finally his head, talking all the while and drawing laughs and nods from the audience. . . . It's exactly the way it is in the movie, every movement and syllable.[17]

The other students do well enough to get through the performance, Ron noting that they, unlike Owen, occasionally seek out their parents in the audience, aware of the social work they are doing in their performance. Owen, meanwhile, is locked into the play, rendering the performance as precisely as he can. When his fellow actors stray from the script, Owen does as well, but helps to get the characters back on track. He can improvise when needed to ensure that the play stays on track. Ron reflects, "Cornelia and I realize that . . . all we really want: for him just to be in the mix."[18] The Suskinds take Owen's performance as an indication that Owen is on his way to integrating the Disney content into his educational experiences, if not his everyday life more generally.

Over the following summer, this integration of the films into everyday life leads him to the staging of the Disney adaptation of Roald Dahl's *James and the Giant Peach* with a cast composed of his brother and cousins at a family reunion.[19] Counter to everyone's expectations, rather than play the protagonist of the story, James, Owen is more interested in portraying the lowly Earthworm, one of James's many sidekicks. Lacking the classroom time to prepare for the play, Cornelia works with Owen to simply costume each of the players, choosing an item or two that iconographically represents the character's personality for the audience. Rather than have a whole script to memorize, Ron and Cornelia provide each of the children with loose summaries of the scenes to remind them of the main character and plot points. Ron then asks each of the children to step forth and introduce their character. When it comes to Owen, he explains his choice of being the Earthworm: "The Earthworm . . . is scared sometimes and confused. . . . He's jealous of the Grasshopper and Centipede and characters who can do things that he can't. And that's why I'm the Earthworm."[20] The performance of *James and the Giant Peach* comes off more shambolically than the more prepared *Song of the South*, but it serves its purpose, namely, catalyzing Owen's growing interest in the figure of the sidekick. This turn to the sidekick hints at Owen's identification with sidekicks more generally, as he comes to see himself not as the main protagonist of his life but rather as the second-order character in someone else's life—the lives of his family members. For a child who is really at the center of his family member's lives, with them shuttling him from home to school to doctor's offices as they care for him through his daily routines, this turn toward the role of the sidekick seems paradoxical. But that Owen knows himself through an explicit engagement and reenactment of media might offer a clearer basis for understanding his place as a sidekick: Owen exists alongside dominant means of communicating, like a sidekick alongside a protagonist.

Beyond his literal reenactment of the Disney films, eventually Owen comes to rely on his deep knowledge of the Disney films, their characters, and the characters' motivations to extrapolate a sense of interiority and selfhood to his own life. In the following, Owen uses his knowledge of a film to provide advice to a boy "like him," at his psychiatrist's urging. His psychiatrist is attempting to get Owen to think about his own situation, but in the third person, because Owen seems unable to think of, or resistant to thinking about, himself in direct terms. But in answering the prompt, Owen extrapolates from the film at hand, surprising his father and psychiatrist both.

> "All right, Owen," [Owen's psychiatrist] Dr. Griffin says, leaning forward, his hand framing the air before his face. "Let's say, there's a boy like you, different from lots of other boys, who's fearful of the future, of growing up, and wants to start going back to being a little kid." He pauses. "What would Rafiki [a wise, old monkey from Disney's *The Lion King*] tell him?"
>
> Without missing a beat, Owen says matter-of-factly, "I'd prefer Merlin [from Disney's *The Sword in the Stone*]."
>
> Dan stammers. "Umm. Okay, then. Merlin!"
>
> "Listen, my boy, knowledge and wisdom are the real power!" Owen exclaims as Merlin, in the voice of Karl Swensen. And then he keeps going. "Now, remember, lad, I turned you into a fish. Well, you have to think of that water like the future. It's unknown until you swim in it. And the more you swim, the more you know. About both the deep waters and about yourself. So swim, boy, swim."

Dan looks at me, eyes wide. He's watched the movie plenty of times—but can't place the second part. I shake my head. Not in there. Yes, there's a scene where Merlin turns himself and Arthur into fish. That seemed to be Owen's trigger to update those lines. But where are the words coming from?[21]

In his ability to move from the film at hand to his everyday life, Owen invokes the shadow of society in his references to "the deep waters." Although Owen is having troubles in his relationships with other people and in self-motivation, he is able to act as a sidekick-cum-mentor to himself—or a boy "like [him]." In so doing, he encourages himself to engage with society, to come to "know" himself as a subject, society as a set of reciprocal animations, and himself as part of that society. The films become more than a way for Owen to interact with his family. They become the basis for Owen's relationship to society, they animate his relationships with other people and his environment, and they serve as a mechanism to conceptualize himself as a social actor.

ANIMATING FAMILIES, COMMUNITIES, AND SUBJECTIVITIES

Over time, Owen's interest in sidekicks develops into a project bringing together his favorite sidekicks from Disney movies into the plot of his own film. A central plot device in Owen's film is the relationship between animation and reality, between the artificial and the real. The central character is Timothy, a version of Owen, who is lost in a dark and foreboding wood and who finds allies in the sidekicks that find their home there. Together, they overcome a series of threats and come to realize the importance of their collectivity but also their individual capacity to overcome adversity—the hero inside each of them that transcends their role as sidekick. In preparing for their battle against the final villain of the film, it becomes important for Timothy to know "the first moment I opened my eyes," and Merlin casts a spell allowing just that: "He sees himself taking shape on the animator's drafting table and he sees a mirror."[22] Timothy and his companions find the mirror, and in the final battle, Timothy looks into the mirror: "The boy opens his eyes and for the first time, sees himself. It's his face—not animated, but real. As he truly is."[23] Timothy has a female counterpart, Abigail, who also looks into the mirror and sees her real, nonanimated self, and they come to realize their love for one another—a love so strong that it dissolves Goretezzle, the final villain, into his composite computer code. Computer animation being less real than hand-drawn animation, and that in turn less real than flesh and blood, Goretezzle is dissolved in the face of Timothy and Abigail's true love. The animated sidekicks dissolve as well, revealing that they are actually Timothy's family and friends. In answer to Timothy's question, "Has it been you all along?," the characters respond, "But it's been you, too. It's you who helped to create us. To animate our lives with a special love."[24] Animation, for Owen, is a fundamental principle of life. Yet there are degrees or kinds of animation, with some being closer to real than others. The film serves a social purpose: the plot provides Owen with a way to think through his social situations and his role in the lives of others. He comes to realize that even sidekicks have complex lives, however dependent on others they may be, and that real relationships are more important than artificial ones.

The Suskinds come to think of Owen's relationship with the Disney movies—and the Suskinds as a family and their collective relationship with the Disney movies—as a kind of affinity therapy.[25] Ron explains: "Our son has turned his affinity for animated movies . . . into a language to shape his identity and access emotions that are untouchable and unmanageable for most teenagers, and even adults."[26] This stands in opposition to some behavioralist theories, which seek to deny or restrict access to the things that children like Owen love most in an effort to establish them as rewards for good behavior so that children might be rewarded with a viewing of a beloved film for having completed chores and homework. Instead, the Suskinds adopt a full immersion approach: Owen watches as much television as he likes, and he spends his other time drawing Disney characters and plotting his film about sidekicks. Moreover, the Suskinds as a family are fully immersed, especially once they realize the therapeutic potential of Owen's fixation. Only through their full immersion are they able to recreate the scenes that are most appropriate to a specific situation, thereby communicating with Owen. Over time, they come to realize that Disney films serve a similar purpose for other children and families, and while Owen is enrolled at Riverview,[27] a college designed for young adults diagnosed with autism, he starts what he refers to as Disney Club. Each week the members convene to watch a Disney film and use it as the basis to reflect on their lives. They interrupt the watching of the film to discuss the events of specific scenes, using the action in the film to think about the interior lives of characters and the complexity of social situations—and to use these scenes to conceptualize their everyday lives. As Ron explains, "The club members are 'talking Disney' to each other as a way of talking about themselves and their deepest feelings. There are heartfelt testimonies . . .—beyond anything most folks think these kids could manage—and singing. They all sing the songs, every lyric, like their lives depend on it."[28] Affinity for the Disney films, the Suskinds realize, extends beyond their family. Like their family, others seem to have taken a similar approach to raising their children, and as a result, the affinity between viewer and media extends to exist between viewer and viewer. The Disney Club becomes society in miniature, showing how animation through facilitation creates the basis for subjectivity.

As Owen ages, one of the looming questions that the Suskinds face is the nature of his future. What kind of family will Owen be able to have, to facilitate and be facilitated by? This becomes especially important as he begins to develop a romantic relationship with a young woman. Turning to the contacts that they have made with parents of other children diagnosed with autism, the Suskinds are faced with bleak reports that force them to address the frustrating possibilities Owen might confront as he continues to live his life in a society where he is seen as disabled. Other parents report the need to frustrate the reproductive desires that Owen might face, forcing the Suskinds to address Owen's possibilities for having a biological family of his own, as well as his recognition by the state: "The parents of a couple we had met at Riverview, and had each just turned thirty, told us about sterilizing them both (because who would raise their children if they had them) and how their 'wedding' was a small religious ceremony, because they'd lose federal disability benefits if they were legally married."[29] Normative family structures, based on biological and legal kinship, are thwarted for Owen—or at least made more complicated. Ron and Cornelia accept that if Owen chooses to have children as an adult, his parents, brother, or another family or institution will need to help care for the children, if not care for them entirely. This does not make biological reproduction impossible, but it does require Owen to accept the reality that any family he starts will be nonnormative by American standards. The difficulty here is that the Suskinds have also been warned against a multigenerational household, with other parents telling them that what is best for Owen—and for themselves—is to foster independence, or at least the facilitated illusion of independence. Ron reports that "others talked about their kids being in group homes, sometimes lonely and full of yearning, and many of them unemployable. The message, nonetheless, was 'moving back home is not good for them or for you,' as one parent said, but be prepared to be involved in their lives forever, even if it may not be the lives you want or they want."[30] These realities—of sterilization or foster care, of no state recognition of marriage, of facilitated independence—expose the limits of Owen's animated family and make clear how the history of eugenics in the United States continues to shape possibilities for individuals like Owen and his peers.[31] The Disney universe makes Owen's increasingly normative subjectivity and relations possible, but it cannot mediate these social challenges. The Disney universe can provide Owen with order, but it cannot overcome the disorder in his relationship to society at large, the state, and normative expectations of American kinship.

By the end of *Life, Animated*, Owen is in his early twenties, has graduated from Riverview, and is living—at least part time—away from his parents in a shared home with other young men his age who have also been diagnosed as autistic. While visiting with his parents, Owen reflects on his experience of losing his abilities to understand language and communicating with others—and the critical role that the Disney films played in his ability to regain these capacities. Ron writes,

> [Owen] recounted our first days in Washington in 1993, when the autism hit full force and this whole apparatus began to form. He said he couldn't understand anything we were saying—it was all "blabbering," he said—and couldn't tell us what he wanted. Cornelia asked if this was scary and frustrating. He seemed to turn inward. Living minute to minute as they do, autistic folks

can sometimes go back to an instant and live it over. It was "weird," he said, haltingly, and "also worrisome." And that the only things that remained the same before and after the terrifying change were the Disney movies. With his auditory processing gone haywire, I asked him if he could understand any of the dialogue in the movies. He said he could over time, because the movies were "exaggerating" everything. Then he reeled off his dozen favorite animated films. Without those movies, "there would never have been me," he said, and "I would have never talked a lot."[32]

Whatever doubts might have been expressed by the educators and psychiatrists that the Suskinds interacted with over Owen's early life, by the Suskinds' reckoning, Owen's Disney affinity therapy worked. It provided the Suskinds with a mechanism to communicate with Owen in the therapy's earliest stages, as well as a means for him to communicate with other children, first in rather indirect ways and then, at Riverview, in ways that make evident his understandings of himself and others. It also provided a mechanism for Owen to conceptualize himself as a person and subject. If there is a problem with this therapy, it is that it depends on the fluency of others in the worlds of the Disney films. Unlike everyday, shared language, which has an inbuilt capacity for generalization and abstraction, the language that Owen uses, predicated as it is on his affinity for Disney films, is highly specific. To be able to relate to his fellow members of the Disney Club, Owen depends on their knowledge of the Disney films, the characters, and situations. Through this highly specific knowledge, Owen and his fellow Disney lovers are able to develop social relationships, animated by their shared affinity. Like other therapies, this depends on the steady consumption of Disney films. As new ones are released, those who depend on them for a shared language need to continue to watch each of the films, because not knowing the contents of a film might lead to a failure in one's ability to communicate with others. This is not just the language of fans who share a common love but a means of interaction that Owen depends on for the basis of self-knowledge, social relationships, and his ability to navigate the world and its complexities.

Regardless of these potential drawbacks, in their acceptance of this animating basis for social connectivity, the Suskinds show how the family serves as a necessary point of mimesis for children, a mechanism for socialization, which if it fails might produce disorderly forms of communication and social relations, but when it succeeds serves as a bridge to society at large.

The Televised Man

CONNECTIVITY WITHOUT ANIMATION

David Karasik depends on mass media for his social interactions. He grew up without the luxury of being able to repetitively rewind and replay media. Instead, he depended on reruns and highly serial media, with each episode generically like the episodes before it. Born in the 1950s, David depends on reruns of *The Adventures of Superman* and the weekend ritual of *Meet the Press*, as well as other highly repetitive television shows that are regularly broadcast. As his sister, Judy, explains in their family memoir, *The Ride Together*,[33] which alternates between prose chapters written by Judy and comic strips drawn and written by his younger brother, Paul,

> Throughout our childhoods, David would walk from room to room in our house, being different people, talking in different voices, a squeaky one for Doberman of *Sergeant Bilko* or Jimmy Olsen of *The Adventures of Superman*, a self-assured, slippery voice for Bilko or for Bud Abbott when he did an Abbott and Costello movie, holding his body in different ways to represent the different characters, breaking for advertisements and announcing different products. . . . These are not word-for-word re-creations, but condensed versions, featuring the pivotal moments of each scene, drawing on the language that drives the plot, like a storyboard of a show, or a series of friezes telling the familiar story of a holy figure moving through his destiny.[34]

David does not have access to the kind of reproductive media technologies that would give him the fine-grained knowledge of the TV shows he would need to memorize the texts completely. Instead, he comes to know the characters—Superman, Jimmy Olsen, Gorilla Watson, Sergeant Bilko and his crew, and, maybe not entirely surprisingly, political figures, who can be counted on to say similar things repetitively. David learns gestures, comportment, lines of dialogue, and stories; he weaves this generic content into narratives that he can play through repetitively. His shows structure the day in two ways. First, he watches them when they air, providing touchstones for the organization of his day, and second, he schedules the performance of his own shows, providing himself with reliable events in his everyday life. In both cases, David is animated by his media, but his family is not animated in the same way. Unlike the Suskinds, the Karasiks largely leave David to his animating media, thereby not fully connecting with him or facilitating a fully recognizable subjectivity made possible through shared animation.

David is the oldest of four children born to Monroe and Joan Karasik, followed by Michael, Judy, and Paul. Their lives in Maryland during the 1950s are comfortably upper middle class. Monroe works out of the home, and Joan takes care of the children with the help of an in-house maid and nanny. The family lives in an affluent white neighborhood, and their care provider is a black woman, Dorothy, who bonds closely with the children and cares for them throughout their lives. Each of the children is schooled in public schools, and by the Karasiks' account, David spends time in institutions that his parents pay for or that receive state funding, including both residential facilities and day treatment institutions. However, throughout most of his life, David never seems to fit in well with the institutions he is sent to, or the institutions he is sent to are insufficient in their ability to care for him, so he spends most of his life living with his parents and siblings in their suburban home. The Karasiks do not become invested in David's relationship with his most-liked media. They might pose the occasional question, or, as Paul recounts, tease David for his mispronunciation of key words from theme songs, but the Karasiks never adopt roles provided by the media. They therefore never make the media into a therapeutic bridge to society, they never animate the texts, and they do not allow the texts to animate their family. Instead, David is left without a full means to communicate with his family and society. Over time, his family comes to be able to infer the meaning of his citational speech, but it is an imprecise project. Family members can tell when he is upset or playful, but his speech acts are often oblique. David's communication limits his engagements with the world, and in his later years, he is institutionalized in a series of residential facilities. *The Ride Together* uses a parallel structure, following the Karasiks' broader engagement with the care of others, particularly the care of Joan's father, Henry Pascal, and her sister, Cornelia, generally referred to as Sister, alongside their care for David. After Joan's mother's death, Grandpa and Sister move into the Karasiks' home, so as to facilitate their care. As Judy recounts, by the point they moved in, Grandpa had broken both hips, had nerve damage related to a shingles outbreak, and was mostly blind as a result of this nerve damage. He was nearly immobile at the age of ninety-five and required constant support in the house. At the age of forty-seven, Sister used a wheelchair and required constant caregiving. As Judy reports, "When she was born she suffered a massive cerebral hemorrhage that caused multiple, severe handicaps."[35] Sister never walked, could not speak, had poor hearing, and lacked fine motor control. She spent her days in a wheelchair and would be moved from room to room to catch the sunlight or to be on the edge of social activity. Sister experienced noticeable pleasure; she had favorite perfumes and enjoyed social engagement. As the Karasik children were growing up and David was enrolled in a day treatment program, the family caregiver, Dorothy, took primary responsibility for the care of Grandpa Henry and Sister. With the children in their teens and twenties, the Karasiks enjoyed greater flexibility in how they spent their time, and it was in the midst of a family vacation that Judy experiences a profound lesson in the care for others.

Returning home from a family vacation by herself to take a driver's education course, Judy rejoins Grandpa and Sister in the Karasiks' home, along with Dorothy and an overnight nurse hired expressly for the task of taking care of Grandpa and Sister while the family was on vacation. Coming downstairs in the evening, on the same floor as Grandpa's bedroom and the family room, Judy finds the night nurse impassively watching television while Grandpa moans and calls for help from his bedroom. She asks the nurse to check in on her grandfather but is told, "He'll quiet down. . . . He gets like this."[36] Judy quickly realizes that this neglect has been going on all week, and that the nurse has been callously disregarding her charge as caregiver for Grandpa. Henry continues to call for help and eventually starts screaming, which lasts for five minutes. Judy feels trapped: "If I went in [to Henry's room], I would only do the wrong thing, and everything would get worse. [The nurse] wouldn't help if everything got worse. I would end up killing him."[37] Judy takes this as a lesson that care can only be provided by those who understand the family and its dynamics, which leads her to call Dorothy. Dorothy's long-term knowledge of the family, and the people in it, provides her with an intimate understanding of their needs and the workings of the family as an animating, facilitating network. And Dorothy has the ability to displace the nurse.

Dorothy arrives and enters Henry's room. Judy writes, "I heard my grandfather sigh. Then he spoke. He did not moan; he spoke."[38] Henry was uncomfortable in bed, unable to move himself. He simply needed to be readjusted, making the night nurse's negligence all the more glaring to Judy. What Judy takes away from this event is the need to know how to care for others in order to be independent herself. Judy writes, "It wouldn't be until years later that I would learn how to lift someone, how to change a bed underneath someone, how to feed a grown person who ate only soft food. But that night I learned that a person needs to know these things, to be independent."[39] For Judy, care for others becomes inextricable from the care for the self. To be independent in the United States, one cannot be beholden to others— not for one's care or for the care of kin. The family provides a network of care that facilitates the independent experience for each individual through shared interdependence based in intimacy. The network can be extended—as in the case of Dorothy—and it becomes extended through shared intimacy that is predicted on animating connections. The night nurse shares none of this intimacy with the family; she never becomes part of the network. The night nurse's refusal to care for Grandpa in his time of need does not indicate her independence; rather, her refusal to engage in this play of intimacy building is a refusal to animate and be animated through shared connections. She is not part of the family, nor will she ever be.

A few years after this incident, Grandpa Henry dies. The Karasiks flirt with the idea of institutionalizing Sister, but Dorothy will not accept the idea. She offers to take Sister into her home, caring for her full time, with the support of her husband, Eddie, and her cousin, Flowree, blind because of complications of diabetes. Eddie and Dorothy refinish their sunroom into a bedroom for Sister and take her in, a move that is enabled by Joan's understanding of Sister's personhood: "She herself would care for Sister as someone who needed to be taken care of, but [Dorothy's family] the Whites would care for Sister as a member of the family."[40] Sister lives with Dorothy, Eddie, and Flowree for nearly six years. What brings this arrangement to an end is a fire caused by an electrical short in the television next to Sister's bed. Sister dies from smoke inhalation, rescued too late by Eddie, who is burned across his body as he attempts to carry Sister from the fire. Flowree also dies from smoke inhalation, having attempted to recover a lockbox filled with money for their church from the fire. At Flowree's wake, Judy and Joan have a conversation about Sister and the care she received over the course of her life, from 1920 through her death in the early 1970s. Judy asks, "Mom . . . do you think Sister would have had a different life if she'd been born forty or fifty years later?"

> Oh sure . . . Therapies have changed. The whole attitude toward people like her has changed. . . . I tried [physical therapy with Cornelia] once. I had her on the floor once. I was trying to see if she could crawl. . . . Grandpa stopped me. He didn't think it was right. . . . She wasn't a toy, she was a human being—that's how he would have put it. I was using a cookie or a carrot to see if she would try to move by herself. Anyway, I stopped. I never tried again.[41]

In Dorothy's and Joan's respective modes of care for Sister, Judy sees the interrelationship of personhood, care, and interdependence. Being dependent on one another facilitates independence, but independence also depends on the facilitation of an individual's personhood, of not being a toy, a mere object for the desires of others. This realization shapes Judy's understanding of David's own experiences in institutions and how he can be cared for by nonfamily.

INSTITUTIONAL FAILURES AND FAMILY CONNECTIONS

Amid David's reliance on day treatment programs, where he spends the better part of a day, returning home each night for dinner and bedtime with his family, he spends long periods of time at two residential institutions, Camphill Village and Brook Farm. Camphill Village, Judy writes, "really *was* a village, where everybody helped and had their part in supporting daily life."[42] Because David can read, he has a daily assignment of delivering baked goods from the bakery to other homes. But after nine months at Camphill, David leaves. The problem that the Karasiks identify is that it lacks enough structure for David. Monroe explains to the other children, "You kids know how David needs things to happen in an ordered way. The program is ordered at Camphill, but it isn't ordered like David." Camphill required residents to participate in "cultural and other activities," and as Joan and Monroe explain to Judy and her brothers, "David already has a lot going on in his head. He needs time to himself and he's not so flexible about that."[43] This situation leaves both David and the other residents of Camphill Village frustrated, and when David is frustrated, he can lash out at people. Judy explains that David typically "started by rapping and fiddling his fingers on his skull, as though he were revving an engine. If whatever was going on inside of him got worse, he attacked people—it didn't always make sense who. He could pull your head to his and grind his forehead against yours, repeating the names of people who didn't exist outside of television. It hurt."[44] Because Camphill was not organized as a residential hospital, with a variety of staff including security, David's physical outbreaks relied on the voluntary residents of Camphill to intervene to restrain him. David's violent behavior put other people at risk, and the Karasiks accepted that they needed to find a new situation for him, which at the time resulted in his moving back home.

Later in his adulthood, David would move to Brook Farm in Pennsylvania, located about two hours away from the Karasiks' Maryland home. Brook Farm, by Judy's account, was a rural setting, owned and run by a couple, Rudolph and Diane Zarek.[45] Rudolph was noted for his generosity, owning a small plane that he volunteered to help others with, and the Zareks developed the plan for Brook Farm out of an interest in gentle behavior modification. This seemed especially effective for David, and throughout his fourteen years at Brook Farm, his violent outbursts seemed to dramatically lessen.[46] At a twenty-year celebration for Brook Farm, things began to change. David had recently experienced an injury to his back, having tripped on the stairs—or so the Karasiks had been told. The Karasiks noticed that David was heavily drugged, dozing off throughout the celebration. They had been told that the drugs were meant to ease his back pain, but a few months later, David had a broken rib, and, on a separate occasion, a broken finger. Suspicions were cast on David's medication; was he being overmedicated? But then, a year after the ceremony, Judy received a message from her older brother, Michael: "Brook Farm is losing its license to operate, rampant reported cases of abuse both physical & sexual."[47] The residents of Brook Farm are immediately evacuated and placed in temporary housing while more permanent homes are found for them. But Judy takes the situation as an indictment in her care for her brother: "Doubtlessly I had met the person who hurt my brother; I had shaken the hand that had pulled back my brother's finger until the bone cracked. And I had smiled at the man and I had walked away and gotten in to the car and left my brother with him. . . . I left my brother alone."[48] In the investigation of Brook Farm, authorities find a locked box of complaints filed by employees against one another—complaints that had never been investigated by the Zareks or that had been quietly ignored. When a resident was admitted to a local emergency room, adult protective services began an investigation, later finding that in 1996 a client had died at the farm from a series of injuries and that a separate resident had been found to have been beaten for "two to three hours."[49] From idyllic and caring, Brook Farm had descended into an abusive institution that its residents could not communicate about to their families. The Zareks had lost control of their staff, who received less and less training and support while the Zareks were simply trying to make ends meet in a changing landscape of residential psychiatric care that had progressively lost state support.

By 2001, David had settled into a program for individuals diagnosed with autism located near the family's home. The program supported group living arrangements and community work. That a program like this could exist by 2001 had everything to do with the changing understandings of autism as a neurological disorder, and one that specific kinds of institutional arrangements could facilitate. David's inflexibility and its related frustrations could be managed institutionally in ways similar to how the Karasiks dealt with them, but it required accepting his inflexibility as part of his neurological capacities and recognizing that what might appear irrational to outside observers had an order all its own for David. The projects that David initiated created a sense of order for himself, as Judy sees in two of his seemingly inscrutable designs for everyday activity. Staying home with David while Monroe and Joan travel to Martha's Vineyard for vacation, Judy finds that "all the glass tumblers in the house, from the small juice glasses to the crystal highball set, had been filled with water and set in a long row on the sideboard. . . . I figured David had done this, but I didn't know why. I decided to leave it as it was for the time being."[50] What Judy observes over the course of her parents' vacation is that the content of the glasses is slowly being drunk at a rate of three each day. David had measured his parents' vacation in glasses of water that he would drink during his daily performances of his television shows, providing him with a clear measure of how much time was left before they returned.

If the glasses provided David with a visible countdown until his parents' return, then his papers provided him with daily structure. His papers were "covered with television show synopses, in his typical style, sprinkling uppercase letters within words, underlining a letter here or there, as though for emphasis, or according to some private code or some hidden rhythm."[51] David fastidiously collected paper from throughout the house for his collection, and part of Judy's caregiving responsibilities included ensuring that David did not use any papers—bills, correspondence, and so on—that belonged to someone else. Paper needed to be rationed to ensure that David was working on the right paper. Judy recounts being distracted by her work responsibilities while staying with David and forgetting to get him new paper, and one morning she finds him severely agitated, attacking himself. Judy rushes out to get him a pad of paper to work on, and he quickly settles into working on filling the paper with his writing. Judy explains, "The autism stopped battering my brother with the frustration and went back to its usual habit, which was fascinating David with the patterns and images and ideas inside his head."[52] David has a system or set of systems that he relies on, and as Judy observes, facilitating David's subjectivity and personhood means being intimate with these ordering structures. Facilitation requires intimacy with the dynamics of David and the Karasiks as a family and animating network.

David's presence in the family serves its own ordering purposes, clearly articulated in the event of Monroe's loss of a pair of glasses during the period that David is living at Camphill Village.[53] An increasingly frustrated Monroe dispatches the remaining children—Judy, Paul, and Michael—to scour the house for his glasses. When they finally find them at the bottom of a laundry basket, Joan remarks, "You know, if David was here, we wouldn't have to wonder if something got lost. We'd just blame him."[54] As chaotic as David's presence may sometimes be for the family, the dynamics of the family have evolved with David as an intimate part of its structure. As both Paul and Judy recount, this can lead to frustrations—for them as well as for David—but David also provides a way to explain things like lost eyeglasses. It is not that David actually causes these everyday disorders but that his presence provides a way to make sense of the otherwise inexplicable behaviors of individuals in the family.

Much later in their lives, Judy takes David for a short road trip during a period when she is spending all of her time traveling. During this short trip she confronts her "real brother" with the help of the recently released *Rain Man*. Raymond Babbit, the autistic character at the center of *Rain Man*, is portrayed as an orderly savant, able to count cards for his gambling brother, Charlie. Charlie uses Raymond's card-counting capacities in a gambling scheme, making Raymond—and his autism—the heroes of the film because they deliver Charlie from his financial distress. Judy confesses to having cried her way through the viewing when she saw the film in the theater, explaining that it seemed to be so much about David. When she rewatches it on television while on the road trip with David, who is sleeping in the same room as her, she finds herself afraid that David will awaken and see the film.[55] She comes to realize that her anxiety about David's seeing the film stems from what the film had done for her: *Rain Man* made autism look like a neat and tidy category of neurological disorder, able to explain away all the quirky and disorderly behaviors that David and their family experienced. But lying in that hotel room, Judy realizes that there is nothing neat and orderly about David, even with a medical category to explain his idiosyncratic behaviors and experiences. For Judy and her family, David is disorderly, and his chaos makes sense of him and the Karasiks as a family.

THE FAMILY AS PROCESS OF FACILITATION

During David's early years, the Karasiks, like many parents today, sought the expertise of a variety of physicians and psychologists, who eventually would diagnose David as autistic, but prior to that—and representative of how such conditions were thought about in the 1950s and 1960s—David was diagnosed as having aphasia, which Joan is told by their doctors is "possibly due to organic causes, possibly emotional causes. . . . They say that early lack of parental warmth can cause stress." Monroe replies, "Please! If anything you're too doting with that child and don't pay enough attention to your loving husband."[56] At least playfully, Monroe sees the family as a zero-sum affectional system: whatever affection is paid to David is not being paid to him or to the other children in the family. Moreover, Monroe sees that too much affection, like too little, can lead to the development of pathologies. This model of the family suggests that there is a homeostatic quality to the family, and by extension society. "Normal" individuals are those who receive neither too much nor too little affection, and they in turn require no excessive affection from caregivers and provide no excessive affection to their children; over time, the family reproduces itself within normative bounds, and thereby reproduces society as a whole. Where there is pathology, however, one can detect a failure in the system, a failure to "learn to love"—as psychologist Harry Harlow puts it in the title to his book—within appropriate norms. Monroe's joke points to the centrality of mothers—and the likelihood that they will bear the blame for any perceived disorder of their children. As Paul explains in one of his chapters, "Over the years doctors labeled David variously as minimally brain damaged, aphasic, trainably retarded, schizophrenic, and/or autistic. A contemporary diagnosis might call

David 'a nice guy who has mental retardation with distinct autistic behaviors and controlled epilepsy who is trying to get along in someone else's world.'"[57] David's summarized diagnostic history captures twentieth-century approaches to neurological disorders: the symptoms remain the same, but the categories change to capture David's particular mix of experiences. Paul is also acutely aware of "someone else's world" being fundamental to David's everyday experiences, pointing to how disorder is fundamental to the experience of communication for and with David because his modes of interaction do not meet social expectations of "normal" behavior.

It is not that Joan loves David too much—or that she loves Monroe or the other children too little—but rather that the Karasiks treat David's love of media as a fixation and not as a therapeutic medium for much of his life. Judy explains that David "has all of his shows on a careful schedule, his own schedule, which has nothing to do with what is on the television at that particular moment but everything to do with a system that we don't understand but which David does and feels strongly should be respected. He can get very angry if the schedule has to change."[58] David is taken by the family to be self-contained in his relationship with the media he consumes. Judy sees the power of David's media consumption to be largely organizational; he seems to use it to order his day, providing him with a regular unfolding of events that his family is peripheral to. When family members do interrupt him, or when his replaying of the narratives is shaped by events in the day beyond his control, as Judy notes, David becomes disorderly, attacking himself and at times his family members. This occurs in an event that Paul recounts wherein he needles David about his mispronunciation of a word in the opening announcement on *The Adventures of Superman.*[59]

Paul returns home from a busy day at school looking forward to eating a snack and reading comic books on the family room floor. When Paul comes home, he finds David in the midst of a weekly political news program reenactment that includes mention of a still-living John Kennedy, although Kennedy was dead at the time—a fact Paul corrects. David replies, "Fiddle-faddle! You're Wilbur the mischievous monkey!" Paul goes looking for a snack in the kitchen, only to find the cookie jar empty, which he blames on David. Consoling himself with graham crackers, he flops down on the family room floor to read superhero comics, only to be interrupted by David: "Yes, it's Superman, who can bend steel in his bare hands . . . change the course of bikey rivers." Already perturbed, Paul interjects, "That's 'mighty'! 'Change the course of mighty rivers!'"[60] David seems unflappable in his recounting of Superman's powers, but as the episode progresses, he steps on Paul's comics, leading to their seemingly inevitable physical conflict. The event leaves David agitated and Paul sequestered in his room. There, Paul finds solace in his favorite comic, "Tales of the Bizarro World," a recasting of Superman's universe where everything is inverted, where ugliness is celebrated and beauty is found revolting. As much as Paul and David find themselves in conflict, Paul realizes in rereading his comic book that "there's something comforting about predictability . . . me and Dave . . . we like reruns."[61] In making such a claim, Paul sees David not as impossibly different from him but as sharing in a key capacity that makes them similar: a love of predictability and repetition.

In this love of predictability and repetition, David and Paul offer a way into conceptualizing the role of media in the production of everyday language, communication, and subjectivity more generally. Whereas Joan—and by extension most of the Karasik family—sees David tuning out of social life by tuning into his favorite media, Paul sees David using the media as a means to shape his world. As Paul explains,

> Tuning-in meant tuning-out all that static. No disrespect to Mrs. [Karasik]. . . . but she got the analogy all screwy. ". . . For David, things arrive splintered . . ." It ain't splintered inside, it's splintered outside. Inside it's as tidy and rich as Fort Knox. But outside! All of them safecrackers with their tommyguns! It's enough to make the toughest yegg crack![62]

Society, relationships, interactions, obligations—these things compose the static that David seeks to calm through his engagement with media. Paul sees David's animating relationship with media as a way to balance David's internal desire for order with the disorderly world around him. David's experience of the world is inverted from those he interacts with, who see David as the disorderly one. David has a language with which he orders the world, but because of his family's inability to engage him through that language, he lacks the ability to communicate with them in recognizable ways. Symbolic conceptions of language hold that language is always a rerun; it depends on its framing and historicity, on its ability not to make epiphenomenal meaning but to cite the existence of a prior meaning. Modular communication does not depend on historicity, but it does depend on framing.[63] David could communicate with his family if they participated in his framed world, which is facilitated by a potentially shared media. What this form of communication requires is a disavowal of the historicity of language and the ability to allow language to be interpreted epiphenomenally—to allow language to be animating in its engagement with a shared world.

Take David's use of a character, Gorilla Watson, from *The Adventures of Superman*, a symbol that he uses as he ages to signify potential threats. Judy is able to understand David's framing usage of Gorilla Watson and thereby can communicate with him about his anxieties related to attending Paul and his new wife's wedding party. David discusses the wedding entirely in terms of Gorilla Watson, whom David has transformed over the years into a general but potent threat lurking outside the family network:

> "If Gorilla Watson comes to Paul and Marsha's wedding party, what will you do?" Dave asked me.
> I replied, "I'll call the police and have them drag away that thug!"
> "Who?" David asked.
> "Gorilla Watson," I replied.
> David smiled. "He's a real rotter," added my brother, pleasurably rolling the insult around on his tongue, "isn't he?"[64]

Language depends on significance, and communication depends on interpretation. Interpretation depends on facilitation and on the actions of others in actively ghostwriting for each other through modular interactions. Whatever problems might be entailed in the imprecision in everyday speech, one of the discrete actions in our acts of communication is arbitrating vagueness. Meaning is ascribed to others, and thus intention is assumed as well. These are the problems of shared significance. But epiphenomenal interpretation depends on no such history of meaning; instead, it offers in its moment of engagement a space for immanent meaning making. Consider Judy and David's use of Gorilla Watson as a sign of his unease. A strict reading of Gorilla Watson's significance would point to his appearance as a villain in *The Adventures of Superman*, and might draw on his criminal activities and intent. A playacting engagement with Watson might inspire David or Paul—who admits to playacting with David in this way from time to time—to embrace this element of Watson's character and perform his role from the television show. Gorilla Watson is no static sign, though. He needs to be animated in communicative practice to make sense. In turn, Gorilla Watson animates the communicators, with David or Paul acting the role. Knowing what to do with Gorilla Watson depends on knowing David and his means of communicating, a form of knowing that is made possible through the intimate connections that the Karasiks experience as a family, fostered by their mutual care for supporting independence through animating interdependence.

Harry Harlow and the Invention of the Family

EXPERIMENTING WITH THE FAMILY

The role of the family has long been remarked on by psychiatrists and neuroscientists to conceptualize the production of both pathology and normalcy. This is emblematized in the mid-twentieth-century work of Harry Harlow at the University of Wisconsin. Harlow is best known for his use of "wire mothers" to model the relationship between infants and their mothers. In decades of experiments on maternal attachment, Harlow's laboratory tested the effects of having animate and inanimate caregivers. Harlow's experiments—as dreadful as they are by contemporary standards, depending as they do on the social isolation and distress of generations of monkeys—point to the role that animation plays in subject formation. Inanimate material relationships do not make subjects, whether monkeys or humans. Inanimate material relations produce the inhuman and the inhumane. Harlow's experiments enact social relations through models that rely on the nuclear family—and, more intensely, infant–mother relations—thereby naturalizing certain social forms as the basis for human development. Over time, he develops a model of maturation that sees normative development moving from the dyadic relationship of infant and caregiver outward to society. The normative development of this set of relations depends on the bond established between infant and caregiver, and any perturbation in that relationship can lead to problems later in life, be they interior problems of the self or exterior problems in relationships with others. Harlow brings together materialist conceptions of physiology and the brain with symbolic understandings of social relationships. Most important, he attempts to model the social through inert, material proxies. In so doing, he shows how it is not matter alone that animates an individual into subjectivity. Animating interdependencies produce subjects. Making subjects of persons depends on being animated, and this animation depends in turn on play and intimacy to make connections between individuals in the development of a robust nervous system.

Harlow relies on a variety of bad mothers. Some are wire frames with a nursing bottle embedded in them with a nipple exposed for suckling; some are wire frames draped with fabric without nursing bottles; some are monsters. Harlow explains,

> One was a shaking mother which rocked so violently that the teeth and bones of the infant chattered in unison. The second was an air-blast mother which blew compressed air against the infant's face and body with such violence that the infant looked as if it would be denuded. The third had an embedded steel frame which, on schedule or demand, would fling forward and knock the infant monkey off the mother's body. The fourth monster mother, on schedule or demand, ejected brass spikes from her ventral surface, an abominable form of material tenderness and succor.[65]

Most of the monster mothers, Harlow goes on to explain, had comfortable cloth surfaces that the infants were drawn to cuddle with. The experiment's "ghoulish goal" was to create psychopathological behavior, but the sad conclusion that Harlow came to after observing the children find solace in these monster mothers was that "love, all kinds of love, is a mechanism . . . of almost unbelievable power."[66] A bad mother, in other words, is better than no mother at all. That the monster mothers move, that they are animated in a limited way, is no mistake: an animated mother, however abusive she might be, inspires attachment. There is life to her in a way that inert wire mothers do not possess. Animation seems to indicate intent to these young monkeys. Where there is intent, there may be choice. And where there is choice, there may be a way to inspire these monster mothers to behave differently.

Start with an easy experiment: Harlow takes a mother–infant pair and places them in an empty room. The room opens into another room, and in that other room are toys that tempt the infant to explore them. The infant will eventually go into the other room and play with the toys. Harlow then measures how long that "normal" child will spend time away from her or his mother before she or he goes back to check in with the mother. Once the baseline is established, the experiment is made more complex. Now when the child goes into the toy room, after a few minutes of play, there is a loud, startling noise. The infant runs back to the mother to seek comfort. Once calm, the infant goes back to explore the toys, and eventually there is another loud noise. The infant runs back to the mother to be consoled, summon courage, and head back into the toy room again. A well-bonded child, one who is secure in her or his independence and interdependence, will eventually be unperturbed by the loud noise, knowing that mother is only a short distance away in case any true threat reveals itself. Then the experiment gets repeated, this time with poorly bonded infants. These infants, raised by inanimate mothers, start in the empty room with their artificial mother, and the process of exploration and surprising noises is repeated. These children spend less time with their artificial mothers, check in with them less, and rely on them less than the well-bonded children. Depending on the kind of artificial mother they have, the children are even less likely to rely on her for anything, knowing that an abusive or metal mother is no comfort at all. Instead, they rely on themselves—or are maybe entirely unaware that they may be in danger, having been so poorly socialized that they do not recognize environmental threats as threats to their bodies. Inanimate mothers may be persons, but they fail to make robust subjects of their children.

Communication is important for Harlow, and he sees the ability to interact in communicative ways as central to the mother–infant relationship, and eventually to all social relations. Humans especially are seen as being dependent on communication in the form of verbal language and "abstract symbols," which, he suggests, is "possible only because of the evolution of specialized neural processes."[67] For Harlow, communication relies on capacities that are biologically given rather than socially created. When children are impaired in their ability to communicate, Harlow sees this impinging on the mother–infant love period, leading to disorderly relations between the mother and infant, and eventually between the infant and society. This explains how neurological disorders that find expression in communication can fundamentally skew an individual's social development. To make this point, he draws on ideas of normative development that he sees in the laboratory between mother–infant pairs of monkeys and extrapolates to human experiences of autism, drawing a conclusion that biologically derived affect disorders are compounded by maternal responses:

> The basic variables producing maternal acceptance are the developing "feedback" mechanisms of the infants themselves. When these infants begin to smile at and with the mothers, they promote a mutual feeling of pleasantness and warmth. The normal development of maternal affection to her infant offers insight into the nature of the human autistic child. The autistic child is an infant toward whom the human mother has difficulty in developing affection in spite of the fact that this same mother has established normal maternal relationships with older or younger children. The infant cannot . . . communicate or interact with the mother but goes its own autistic way, leaving the mother's affection no place to go.[68]

For Harlow, autistic children are independent, but because they never fully participate in the reciprocal mother–infant relationship, they will never be able to be interdependent. Because of this foundational communication disconnection—this lack of feedback—Harlow sees autistic children, and by extension other children with neurological disorders, as never able to fully embrace mother–infant love, so they are lastingly socially impaired. As Harlow explains, "When both incoming and outgoing messages from communication through gestures, eyes, touch, and sounds are eliminated, communication ceases to exist, and loving, learning, and living are affected for an indefinite rest of the lifetime."[69] Communication, he suggests, occurs between persons through their mutual facilitation of each other, thereby making subjects of persons.

It is hard to read Harlow now. It is hard to see the merit in the generations of children and parents—even if they are monkeys, not humans—that he and his laboratory staff systematically abused in the name of science, especially in relation to findings that seem so obvious now. It stands to reason that a child raised by an artificial mother in the absence of any social connection with another living thing would develop poorly, would be socially anxious and noncommunicative, and would experience affect disorders. How many variations of an experiment are necessary to show this definitively? How many generations of children, begat from forced impregnation of poorly socialized mothers, are necessary to make it clear that attachment to a living caregiver is necessary for individuals to develop the capacity to make socially meaningful attachments to others, including their own children? Harlow is writing against dominant psychological science of the time that conceptualizes subjectivity as being primarily internally derived. In this model, pathology is not the result of social interactions but rather some inborn degeneracy. Instead, following Sigmund Freud and the psychoanalytically inspired social psychologists of the mid-twentieth century, Harlow is trying to show how social interactions—or the lack thereof—are determinative of individual pathologies. Such a view accords with the then-growing group of cyberneticists, who began to develop theories of feedback as generating subjectivity through social dynamics.[70] Harlow hopes to definitively show that pathology, particularly in the form of affect disorders like autism and schizophrenia, is the result of poor social relations, and especially bad attachments with parents, specifically mothers, but in a manner dependent on neurophysiology. At its worst, Harlow's work was taken to impugn mothers for the neurological disorders of their children; at its best, Harlow offers a model for the development of subjectivity through interdependence—an animated and animating subject formation. Harlow's emphasis on inborn capacities shaped by social interactions continues to haunt neuroscience, as is evident in discussions of hereditary illness and epigenetics.

MAKING DISORDERLY SUBJECTS

Here are Harlow's experiments at their worst, what he refers to as experiments in partial and total social isolation. "Partial social isolation" is the "raising of infants from birth onward in bare wire cages without companions."[71] Monkeys in partial social isolation could see other monkeys—similarly raised in cages—but they could not physically interact with them; there was no possibility to play or to comfort one another. These monkeys could also see laboratory staff as they went about their daily activities. Despite not being able to interact with other individuals, the knowledge that other creatures exist in the world ensured that they were not as "disturbed" as those raised in total social isolation. Over time, Harlow notes of the partially isolated monkeys that

> the subjects were not only devoid of heterosexual behavior at maturity but showed exaggerated oral activities, self-clutching, and rocking movements early in life, then apathy and indifference to external stimulation. . . . An animal might sit in the front of its cage staring aimlessly into space. Occasionally one arm would slowly rise as if it were not connected to the body, and wrist and fingers would contract tightly—a pattern amazingly similar to the waxy flexibility characteristic of some human catatonic schizophrenics. The monkey would then look at the arm, jump away in fear, and subsequently attack the offending object.[72]

Beginning life in partial isolation results in these monkeys' being both detached from other monkeys but also impassive in relation to their environment—and, for some extreme cases, it means a detachment from their own bodies. Those raised in total social isolation fare worse. The ability to raise monkeys in total social isolation was a complicated procedure that required technological experimentation. Over time, what was developed was an opaque cage with walls on each side, except for a one-way mirror that allowed the researchers to observe the monkey.[73] The monkey's only knowledge of the outside world was the appearance of a laboratory assistant's hand, which helped the baby feed during the first fifteen days of life. Harlow writes, "Monkeys reared in total social isolation for 90 days were enormously disturbed when admitted to the great wide world of wonder, and two of them actually died of self-induced anorexia before we recognized the syndrome and instituted forced-feeding."[74] For those monkeys who were raised in total social isolation for just three months and were force-fed through their first month of social introduction, they would eventually become "normal for all measurable purposes."[75] For those raised in total social isolation for six months, this was not the case:

> Monkeys subjected to 6 months of total social isolation from birth and then allowed to interact with agemates were very adversely affected for the rest of their lives. They spent their time primarily engrossed in autistic-like self-clasping, self-mouthing, and rocking and huddling. The isolates never interacted successfully with normal peers over an 8-month period, although pairs of isolate monkeys did show limited recovery in terms of exploration and even play with each other.[76]

Total social isolation would seem to prove Harlow's overarching point that a lack of even the barest social contact profoundly affects an individual's ability to interact in the most rudimentary ways. Somehow, though, the knowledge of other individuals existing, as is the case for the partially socially isolated monkeys, allows monkeys to overcome the initial shock of the "wide world of wonder" and eventually form social bonds with other monkeys. Damaged monkeys may be able to play with one another—their shared early life of total social isolation makes them more similar to one another than to other, "normal" monkeys— but they never fully socially recover. That too proves another of Harlow's points, namely that societies can exist that are fundamentally socially askew in their structures of attachment and emotional connection. This skewed sociality is then reproduced even if biological drives would ideally assert a bonding environment that would lead to normative modes of connection.

Extrapolating from the monkey models to humans is a challenge for Harlow, in no small part because of the artificiality of both partial and total social isolation protocols. No human child could be found to have survived if abandoned at birth, thereby modeling total social isolation, although, as Harlow's colleagues who studied children in orphanages after World War II document, there were cases that approximated partial social isolation. What researchers found was that children entered a period of "despair," which included "dejection, stupor, retardation of development, retardation of reaction to stimuli, marked decrease in activity, and withdrawal from the environment."[77] For young children, reuniting with one's mother seemed to restore normal development, but for older children, there was a period of what John Bowlby referred to as detachment, which was marked by hostility toward the mother after their reunion. Bowlby's conclusion was that the anxiety produced by the separation of the child from the mother was so profound as to interfere with the basic biological functioning of the child—a systemic interruption of physical and emotional development. Harlow notes that human-based research on isolation always has to be accidental, in no small part due to "ethical considerations,"[78] but also because "the attitudes of all caretakers, parents, hospital and orphanage personnel may influence the investigations allowed the experimenter."[79] The "wide world of wonders" is too complex for humans to be controlled by scientists, unlike the world of monkeys, which can be technologically and ethically shaped to ensure their partial or total social isolation. Because the few humans followed by Bowlby could eventually overcome their despair and detachment, it may be difficult to accept that what Harlow perceived in monkey social relations could be easily extrapolated to human emotional development. But the power of Harlow's model is its abstract potential in seeing bonding through reciprocal animation as the basis for all social relations.

FROM THE MONSTER MOTHERS TO THE ANIMATING FAMILY

Over time, Harlow recognized that play is critical in social relations, between children and their environment, between parents and children, and between children and their peers. Harlow sees play developing along a normative line, from play with inanimate—or seemingly inanimate—objects to parent–infant play, to peer play. Drawing a distinction between the animate and inanimate, Harlow sees the potential in human infants for play as unmatched in the animal kingdom: "Human children have presocial play capabilities unmatched by any other animal. The child drops his spoon on the floor and the mother replaces it religiously and relentlessly, again and again. . . . From the child's point of view this is not social play, but asocial play. The mother is merely an inanimate object with marvelous cooperative capabilities."[80] Play precedes mutual recognition; there is no "theory of mind" operating at the presocial level,[81] as children play with the objects in their environment, even if these objects are steadily replaced by parents who are facilitating the play. Animation precedes personhood.

What comes next are forms of play that rely on social interaction: "Play with inanimate objects precedes social play of comparable complexity. For example, the tiny tot plays with his dangling mobile and musical bells before he is six months old, whereas the social-partner games of peek-a-boo and patty-cake develop some months later."[82] In these later games, theory of mind begins to play a role, as children begin to anticipate the actions of others and attempt to understand the motives of others, as expressed in communicative acts of surprise and suspense. In modeling these affective responses, play opens up possibilities of mimicry, which lays the basis for more expansive social interactions in life. As Harlow notes, "One of the primary functions of peer play is the discovery and utilization of social and cultural patterns. Play acquaints the child with the existence of social rules and regulations and their positive as well as negative consequences."[83] Social isolation is especially debilitating because of its suppression of this capacity for play, which is profoundly realized in Harlow's experiments. Harlow explains, "We also discovered that 12 months of total social isolation from birth had even more drastic effects than 6 months on behavior in the playroom. Exploration and even simple play were nonexistent. Torn by fear and anxiety, aggression was obliterated in these monkeys, and even the simple pleasure of onanism was curtailed. They sat huddled alone in the corners or against the walls of the room."[84] Isolation leads to the inability to play with others and even with oneself. The inability to play results in a kind of social inanimacy, an inability to be moved by others and to move others. As Harlow notes, even "aggression was obliterated," and the totally socially isolated monkeys experience an inability to engage with their peers in any way. For Harlow, this is more proof that a bad mother is better than no mother at all—or, rather, an abnormal family is better than no family at all.

At its worst, Harlow's research was taken to support the idea that mothers are to blame for any emotional or developmental irregularities in their children, an idea that is echoed in the Karasiks' early discussions of David's development. Harlow's earliest research does focus on the mother–infant relationship, and his model of development embraces that formative relationship. Over time, Harlow begins to accept the presence of fathers as being as important as mothers, if often only as a substitute for the mother.[85] He also begins to experiment with multifamily arrangements, where infants can be cared for by adults and older children who are not their biological relations.[86] In accepting these revisions to the mother–infant dyad, Harlow begins to accept, if only tacitly, how human families and societies are actually arranged, with multiple vectors of attachment and caregiving made possible through kinship and social connections. Throughout his research, Harlow is experimenting with the family as a social form, first the mother–infant dyad, then the mother–infant–father triad, and eventually the multifamily network. In so doing, he accepts that the family—whatever its form, whether it be nuclear or multihousehold and multigenerational—provides society in miniature. However it is composed, the family is also where the fundamental capacities of social life are modeled, learned, reinforced, and facilitated through reciprocation. Each family is a metonymic enactment of society. The family serves as the site for the establishment of relationships, the understanding of what relationships are, and the development of particular capacities that are intended to help produce and maintain social and environmental relationships. The capacities developed in the family then become the basis for the development of relationships with other nonkin in society.

Problems occur, however, when there is a mismatch between the capacities instilled in an individual in the family context and those capacities expected by society. The capacity for love that Harlow sees as essential to the development of healthy subjects depends on social recognition of particular kinds of love as normal. Yet because society becomes the meeting ground for individuals each raised by a potentially idiosyncratic family, there are profound possibilities for disorder to arise, as each minisociety is not a strict metonymic representation of dominant social norms. Each family is a site of mimicry, and individuals learn to love through the enactment of behaviors that are rewarded by one's parents, one's peers, and eventually one's romantic partners. By extension, the family is the site for the development of appropriate behaviors. The family is not simply a system of cause and effect but rather a system that reifies behaviors into norms through institutionalized mimicry that depends on, and is reinforced through, facilitation that recognizes certain kinds of persons.

By highlighting the role of animation in his experiments, it becomes clear that facilitation is the key to subject formation, not institutional recognition. This is apparent in the oblique corners of Harlow's research. That socially isolated monkeys can become social despite their total deprivation of physical contact with other monkeys and humans may be due to their recognition of social actors and persons in their environments—including monkeys in remote cages that they are barred from interacting with, or the human hands delivering food and water. That monkeys raised by monster mothers can form social attachments to other monkeys—and that totally socially isolated monkeys can bond with other totally socially isolated monkeys—points to the necessity not of recognition but of dual facilitation, of reciprocal animation. Who knows what those baby monkeys think of their monstrous mothers? But that their mothers act on them—unlike the wire and cloth mothers, who are merely inert—seems to inspire in the infant monkeys a potential to socially attach. Harlow writes glibly, "Mother love is not obtained by putting a quarter in a vending machine. Both mother love for the baby and baby love for the mother result from many variables promoting mutual reaction between the mother and child."[87] What is key in this formulation is the "mutual reaction" that he posits as being the basis of the reciprocal mother–infant bonding predicated not on subjectivity but on ascribed personhood. The mother and infant animate each other, if only indirectly, as the monster mothers demonstrate. There is no intent in the monster mothers' behaviors, yet their children treat them as animating persons. However harmful the monster mothers' actions are, the young monkeys are undeterred. They hold on while air compressors blow their fur nearly off; they wait until a mother's spikes retract. The infants might see their mothers as reacting to them, and in their potential to react, they are facilitated in their subjection, however nonnormatively. What Harlow, the Suskinds, and the Karasiks show is that becoming animated in this way, through mutual reaction, is the basis of connectivity and intimacy. The family can serve this purpose, however it might be configured; it need not be the obligatory, heteronormative American family of the middle twentieth century. Further, the family as a network is the gateway into society and social relationships more broadly. As children move into new relations, they carry with them the animacies that have facilitated their earlier connections, not unlike Owen Suskind's Disney Club. The challenge becomes conceptualizing the connections between individuals in the family as the basis of social connectivity more generally, and how the facilitation of a person in the context of the family can inspire transformations in society's facilitation of nonnormative subjectivities through the development of animating, modular, facilitating nervous systems.

How to Build a Nervous System

INVERTING THE NERVOUS SYSTEM

Family therapist Mony Elkaïm tells the story of cyberneticists Humberto Maturana and Francisco Varela telling the story of biologist L. S. Stone's experiments with amphibian vision. Stone surgically removes the eye of a tadpole, then reattaches it rotated 180 degrees from the position it started in. The tadpole grows to maturity. When it is a frog, the experiment really begins. When Stone covers the rotated eye, the frog lashes its tongue out at prey as normal. But when he covers the normal eye, the frog's tongue strikes 180 degrees from its intended target.[88] Maturana and Varela tell the story again and again[89] because it demonstrates something elegant for them, namely that the nervous system is a self-contained structure. They demonstrate the same claim in their own research on color vision, showing that input from the retina is not transmitted to the cortex along "an incoming telephone line"[90] but rather shaped by other nervous impulses contained in the body that shape incoming stimuli. The eye is a source of input, but its input is shaped by the structure of the body, meaning for Maturana and Varela that retinal cells are agitated by light waves, and what the cells convey to the brain is not information contained in the light waves but in the cells. For Maturana and Varela, the implication of this is that the nervous system is a closed system. The nervous system is not a reliable conduit for understanding a material, objective reality outside of the body. Color blindness can be explained as a differential response to light waves in the cells of the eye rather than as some misapprehension of reality, meaning that rather than being a disability based on social norms, color blindness is an impairment located in the body of the individual. Or on the other end of the spectrum, a society that does not recognize a particular color would be seen as shaping the interpretation of a cellular reaction, not denying the existence of a color that others can perceive. As Elkaïm explains, glossing Varela,

> Perception . . . cannot exist without an interaction between the organism and visible light waves. But the process triggered by light waves when they perturb the organism's visual receptor cells is open to many possibilities. For each organism it is the structure of the nervous system, and consequently the history of the organism that has led to this structure, that determines what happens. Color discrimination cannot exist without interaction; nevertheless, color does not reside in the wavelengths of light.[91]

How Maturana and Varela—and Elkaïm—explain the experience of the world for any organism is through a structural coupling that occurs between an individual and its environment. There is the structure of the organism and the structure of the environment. Bodies and environments are able to interact because in some fundamental ways, they are able to act on one another. The frog has eyes that see visible spectrums of light that help it track the movement of prey; it has feet that act on solid ground and in water; it has skin that conveys heat to keep its body warm. For Elkaïm, this is important because there are only structural couplings and because "it is impossible to describe any therapeutic situation without including oneself, and what happens is always circular."[92] The family as a network is not a self-contained system but rather a structure that binds individuals together and links them with other individuals, society, and their environment. The individual structurally couples with other members of the family, and the family structurally couples with the family therapist. In these couplings, what was once perceived as an isolated, individuated person is revealed to be intimately tied to other actors in the individual's social environment through interdependence. Maturana and Varela see the frog as cut off from its environment, but it is equally possible to see that the environment—the couplings that the frog is animated through—make the frog a frog, just as a human person is made a person through the facilitating technologies that aid its being in the world. The individual has a material experience, but it is only through interdependence that the individual becomes a thing in the world—first a person, then a cybernetic subject.

The cybernetic subject is an animated one. In its earliest configurations, cybernetics, as developed in the social sciences from the 1930s through the 1960s, laid emphasis on the reciprocal function of feedback. Stimuli in an environment caused reactions in actors in that environment, and the actions of actors shaped reactions in other actors and in the environment. The guiding principle in early cybernetics was that these systems maintained homeostasis, both at the level of individuals in their behavior and at the level of society. The work of Gregory Bateson is fundamental here: "The behavior of any one individual in any one context is, in some sense, cognitively consistent with the behavior of all the other individuals in all other contexts. . . . We may say that the patterns of thought of the individuals are so standardized that their behavior appears to them *logical*."[93] Bateson uses cognition and "patterns of thought" to conceptualize how "behavior" comes to make sense to a subject, suggesting that "the whole body of behavior [is] a concerted mechanism oriented toward affective satisfaction and dissatisfaction of the individuals."[94] Each society is arranged differently than others, but it still produces affective experiences for individuals that individuals accept as being satisfactory and as aligning with the expectations that they have for the behavior of both themselves and others.

The challenges that Bateson lays out are twofold. First, behavior and its interpretation are logical. They abide by dominant common sense, which reinforces the existence of behaviors that might produce effects that would be unacceptable in other societies. Second, communication is integral to the promotion and maintenance of patterns of thought at both the level of interpersonal inactions and society. In the case of social patterns, this leads to the preservation of social norms, and in the case of individual patterns, this can be seen in the choices that parents and teachers make in shaping the behavior of children in particularly mimetic ways. What follows from these suppositions is an attempt to conceptualize disorder as arising from a failure in communicative practice—what Bateson refers to as a double bind. Whereas for Bateson the double bind is an isolated social fact, for Elkaïm, who conceptualizes the interdependence of family members as the basis of subjectivity, the double bind is the basis of all social relations.

The double bind was an early attempt on Bateson's part to explain the cause of schizophrenia, a condition he saw as arising from the efforts on the part of children to act on conflicting messages from parents. Bateson explains that the double bind requires five elements: "Two or more persons . . . repeated experience . . . a primary negative injunction . . . a secondary injunction conflicting with the first at a more abstract level, and like the first enforced by punishments or signals which threaten survival . . . [and] a tertiary negative injunction prohibiting the victim from escaping the field."[95] "Escaping the field" could be as simple as being able to say that a double bind exists and that the subject is caught in a trap that disallows satisfactory action. Yet because of the existential threat that a subject experiences—a child dependent on a parent, a spouse dependent on a partner—the metacommunicative act that would expose the paradox embedded in the injunctions is impossible to express. As Bateson explains, "The ability to communicate about communication, to comment on the meaningful actions of oneself and others, is essential for successful social intercourse."[96] Elkaïm provides the example of a mother asking her child to sit on her lap. She does not actually want the child to sit on her lap, as indicated in her tone and gestural communication, which the child is aware of but cannot speak about. The child is trapped. If the child sits on his mother's lap, he abides by what Elkaïm refers to as her official program, but he contradicts her worldview. In Elkaïm's telling, the canny child would approach his or her mother affectionately but then become distracted by a pretty button or piece of jewelry on his or her mother. In this way, the child obeys the implicit injunction to show affection to his or her mother but does not actually sit on her lap. The less canny child, however, does sit on the mother's lap and is reprimanded in some way. In the double bind, there is no winning by following the official program. Instead, the worldview needs to be upheld so as to avoid any existential threat. As a theory of schizophrenia, the double bind has long been eclipsed by organic neurological explanations for the disease, but as a general social phenomenon, Elkaïm sees the double bind as leading to the continuance of functional dysfunctionality. Despite a dysfunction—as diagnosed by a therapist—the family continues to function, abiding by its own internal logic and order, however pathological it might seem to outsiders.

Bateson's view of the cybernetic subject brings together the cognitive and noncognitive in what he refers to as habits. In the context of the double bind, he explains that "individuals must comprise *two* contrasting psychological mechanisms. The first is a mechanism of adaptation to demands of the personal environment; and the second, a process or mechanism whereby the individual becomes either briefly or enduringly committed to the adaptations which the first process discovered. . . . [an] *immanent state of action.*"[97] In this configuration of the individual, Bateson sees the first demand of interaction as being one of learning. What a child is doing in an interaction is learning what the appropriate response is to a situation. In the first instance, the child is learning how to respond to the official program of the parent or other social actors. In time, the child becomes invested in the response he or she has learned, and so doing installs that response as a fundamental habit. Thus, what was once a cognitive act of learning becomes a noncognitive response that maintains relations between individuals, and between an individual and his or her environment. Taken together, these cognitive and noncognitive processes lay the foundation for the cybernetic subject, what Bateson conceptualizes as the externally defined person and the internally defined self:

> What is a person? What do I mean when I say "I"? Perhaps what each of us means by "self" is in fact an aggregate of habits of perception and adaptive action *plus*, from moment to moment, our "immanent states of action." If somebody attacks ... the very habits and immanent states which have been called into being as part of my relationship to them at that moment—they are negating me.[98]

The subject can be threatened existentially through metacommunicative acts: the exposure of a double bind or any suppressed interdependence can call into question the status of the individual as an individual. Similarly, the interruption of a material interdependency, as in the caregiving connections between individuals, can unravel the self-conception of an individual as an individuated person.

FACILITATING THE CYBERNETIC SUBJECT

The cybernetic model that Bateson provides troubles the boundaries that are usually applied to the individual. The skin is not the container of the individual but is instead merely one of many sensory organs that mediates the individual's relationship with the environment. The skin—and the senses more generally—are the facilitating technologies that individuals are born with, although they may vary in their capacities across individuals and societies. To make this point, Bateson provides an example that relies on sensory impairment, which I used to open this book's preface:

> Consider a blind man with a stick. Where does the blind man's self begin? At the tip of the stick? At the handle of the stick? Or at some point halfway up the stick? These questions are nonsense, because the stick is a pathway along which differences are transmitted under transformation, so that to draw a delimiting line *across* this pathway is to cut off a part of the systemic circuit which determines the blind man's locomotion.[99]

Our sensory organs are implicitly accepted as parts of our selves. We are born with them, and they determine our capacities in a material way. They can be shaped, and actively are shaped, through the patterns of thought and the logical organization of satisfaction in a society for individuals. This leads, fundamentally in Bateson's view, to conceptual drift between the material world and subjective—and social—experiences of it. Bateson suggests in his example of the use of a cane for a blind person that the naturalness that is afforded to sensory organs should be extended to all of the technologies that humans use to know the world, explicit or implicit. The walking cane is an explicit technology: it is wielded by the body to extend the body's sensory capacities. Taking the cane away from the blind man entails a limitation of his sensory capacities, and it shrinks his nervous system to be contained within the boundaries of his body. As Bateson explains elsewhere, "The network is not bounded by the skin but includes all external pathways along which information can travel. It also includes those effective differences which are immanent in the 'objects' of such information. It includes the pathways of sound and light along which travel transforms of differences originally immanent in things and other people—and especially *in our own actions*."[100] Human sensory apparatuses detect "differences which make a difference,"[101] but only some differences are recognizable as differences. This recognition is dependent on the technologies that are used to detect them. If this makes it sound as if the only important extensions of the nervous system are explicit technologies, Bateson—and Elkaïm—emphasize that this recognition of difference is a function of what Mataruna and Varela conceptualize as structural coupling: the meeting of two actors, or an actor and an environment, through which animation can occur. This animation is not strictly cognitive but can also be a function of habitual interaction. The blind walker who detects an incline changes his or her comportment appropriately without thinking about it, a capacity for response honed through immanent states of action.

For Bateson, parents and societies make the children that they need. Putting an individual into a double bind situation is not an intentionally sadistic choice on the part of a parent or society but more often the result of injunctions that have been handed down from generation to generation. This would seem to explain how a disease that is primarily social in its effects could be seen as necessarily hereditary: the children of schizophrenics will raise schizophrenics themselves because of their parenting, not their genes. Or, in Elkaïm's family systems therapy, a child who is raised to believe that asking for help is a sign of weakness will grow into an adult who finds satisfaction in a family situation where he or she is always experiencing incapacitating injuries and being put into a position where he or she must receive help from others without needing to ask for it. The other members of that family will similarly reinforce the idea that asking for help is undesirable, but will be satisfied by providing help to those in need. The result, as Elkaïm sees it, are families deeply invested in their symptoms and organized around a functional dysfunction. In this model of family interactions, the double bind is a facilitating technology, albeit a potentially destructive one. The double bind produces particular kinds of subjects, but subjects that are only fully recognizable within a specific system. The size of that system, at least for Elkaïm, is rather circumspect in the form of the family. Yet because couples can come together in a diverse social field of subjects with different family backgrounds, there are resonances of experience across the social field. What might seem rather idiosyncratic in one person's family experience can be similar to another person's experience. These two individuals are able to negotiate a structural coupling that satisfies them both, although the experiences that led them to that point may be quite different. The implication of Elkaïm's more generalized understanding of the double bind as a means of facilitating persons and subjects is that rather than the very specific relationship Bateson conceived of, all of society exists within a manifold field of potential double binds awaiting activation through interpersonal interactions.

Organic impairments might seem to chafe against the conception of a double bind, but they fit into the functional organization of families and societies through the logics of satisfaction and dissatisfaction that Bateson suggests are the basis of cybernetic societies. Elkaïm would view the care of a person—and potentially even that person's diagnosis—as fitting into the system of the family. That the Suskinds seek out the kinds of professional help, educational opportunities, and social experiences that they do for Owen is based not solely on Owen's material experiences of the world but also in the various needs of the family members, who at times seek a return to normalcy and a potential cure for Owen. In the early years of Owen's life, the Suskinds might be seen as a family system that is far from homeostasis as they attempt different therapies, seek different schools and support networks, and reorganize themselves to support Owen as best they can—as the kind of person they hope to make of him. That the Suskinds eventually reach a point of homeostasis is predicated on their collective abilities to find satisfaction in a particular way of interacting with Owen, facilitated as it is through the world of Disney films and the development of an idiosyncratic, modular nervous system. Similarly, the Karasiks' early years of seeking a diagnosis, treatment, and support for David positions them as far from homeostatic. Over time, they reach a point of being able to accommodate David's needs alongside those of other family members, reaching some point of satisfaction, even if it might be quite different from what the Suskinds experience. One approach to care is not intrinsically better or worse than another. In both families, some level of satisfaction is reached for all of the family members. The challenge that Elkaïm would point to, however, is that subjects raised in these families may carry with them unspoken and uncommunicable expectations about social relationships that may make relationships difficult or impossible with people and in social organizations that differ significantly from their natal families. Moreover, subjects may also seek to reproduce particular kinds of conditions that facilitate their need for specific forms of social relations that were found in their natal families.

DISRUPTING THE NERVOUS SYSTEM

Elkaïm's systemic view of the double bind explains why families, communities, and whole societies can be functionally dysfunctional. Old social scientific views of functionalism posited that each feature of a society served a particular function, and the functional whole was reproduced generation by generation so as to maintain the order of society.[102] These theories have been largely discredited, in no small part because they fail to account for change over time and posit, much like early cybernetics, homeostasis as the aim of social organization. But Elkaïm's family systems therapy suggests that subjects and families—and whole societies—are invested in their symptoms. What in one society is an unremarked-on variation of experience is the basis of a social epidemic in another society. Schizophrenia and autism are two conditions that are recognized as neurological disorders in the United States but that in many other countries are considered part of normative human experience, so families and institutions are organized to care for persons in ways that do not pathologize these nonnormative experiences.[103] Yet in the United States autism is increasingly seen as a growing and inexplicable epidemic, and schizophrenia is continually considered a debilitating disorder.[104] A systemic view of the care for individuals with these conditions would ask what, if anything, individuals, families, organizations, and society at large find satisfying in the conceptualization of these conditions as disorders in the way that they are currently conceived of. What is the function of treating neurological disorders as disabilities?

This is not to minimize the experience of persons or families who experience neurological disorders but rather to work to conceptualize how neurological disorders as such work to create the terrain of the neurological and reify particular ways of being and facilitating persons. The history of the care for individuals with neurological disorders over the twentieth century relied on institutionalization, generally in the form of residential hospitals and care facilities when children did not live with families. For many families, and the Greenfelds are an example of this, the independence of the family from the disabled individual was facilitated through institutionalization; Noah's eventual institutionalization allows his parents and brother to engage with him as they desire. But over the latter half of the twentieth century, partly because of deinstitutionalization efforts,[105] individuals were more likely to stay with their families, much like the experience of the Suskinds, Karasiks, and Goddards, and receive support through day treatment programs. This shift from state-supported removal of an individual from a family to the facilitated support of an individual remaining with the family is predicated on American expectations about what family relations should look like and what independence through interdependence entails. In both cases, the organization of the family is predicated on institutionalized support, but contemporary approaches to this support place more emphasis on the continued interaction of the family as a whole unit. On the one hand, this transformation in the support of families has to do with reductions in funding for state-based institutional care as a function of neoliberalism. On the other hand, this transformation in social arrangement supports ideologies of the family, namely that the responsibility of care for individuals is not that of the state but that of kin. Intentionally or not, this return to the family upholds cybernetic conceptions of subjectivity, seeing the interaction of individuals in a family context as integral to care and person making. Care for an individual with a neurological disorder requires the transformation of his or her caregivers, as they adjust to the changing expectations they have of their family member, as well as their expectations of themselves. The Suskinds are an exquisite example of this kind of transformation, as they adjust their expectations of Owen to meet his capacities for communication and social interaction as animated by the Disney films. They also change their family communication patterns and what they find satisfying, which eventually accords with Owen's experiences with other young adults who similarly find facilitation through the Disney films. Yet these interactions change the family system over time. Potentially they may also change society over time, family by family, leading to an emergent nervous system of reciprocally animating facilitators.

The classical cybernetic view of these potential pressures for change would point to the need for homeostasis in the system, that society would seek to preserve its worldview despite a change in the official program. Whatever changes might have been wrought by deinstitutionalization movements in the United States, other changes occurred in tandem in order to support the same system of satisfaction in society. One coextensive shift with changes in institutionalization was the movement in understanding disorders like schizophrenia and autism as caused by social relations, as embedded in the double bind or Harlow's modeled mothers, toward organic, material conditions that are the result of genetics or other "natural" causes. The sociopsychological was displaced in favor of the neurological. Such a shift moves the causal explanation for any individual's disorder away from family interactions and toward inevitable biological destiny. In these neurological and materialist frameworks, disorder lies in the genes, or at most in a genetic–environmental interaction that may have been influenced by the actions of parents. The neurological is self-contained, circumscribed by the body, and isomorphic with the individual as a discrete object, not unlike Maturana and Varela's reading of Stone's frog. Symbolic–psychological interaction, as Bateson and Elkaïm make clear, is a process that shapes each participant, whether at the level of the individual or society. Cybernetic models have the potential to bring the neurological and the symbolic together, as they conceptualize the material and the symbolic as necessarily interrelated and dynamically changing over time.

As Bateson conceived of change occurring, changes in the environment or in the actions of an individual would be responded to in ways that ensure that these changes were mitigated for the preservation of the system as a system. Homeostasis at the level of the individual and society are primary concerns, even if they are unspoken ones. Too disruptive a change or actions on the part of individuals would lead a system away from homeostasis or near-homeostasis and could potentially induce a crisis in the system. Change could be accounted for through enormous disruptions—in Bateson's examples, largely related to culture contact facilitated by colonialism—but change could also be accounted for through the gradual permutation of a system through interference or noise in the system of feedback. The localization of disorder into a family system, and particularly in the mother–infant dyad, as Harlow's work models, was taken as indicating that norms disrupt the possibility of a systemic change in society. The movement toward the neurological as an organic explanation for individual disorder sequesters the possibility for change even further, at least insofar as organic explanations for disorder render them the inevitable product of an individual's biology. What the neurological as an explanation fails to account for, however, is how neurological disorders are treated by society and how they become the basis for interactional relationships between individuals—within a family as well as in society more generally—and how they depend on the internalization of the nervous system. The nervous system is not something that is bounded by the body but is facilitated by social formations; it is not interior to the body but is made possible through networks of facilitation that reside outside of the individual. In one society, where facilitation of a particular set of capacities fails to render individuals into persons, the nervous system of individuals is abrupt and curtailed. In another society, where facilitating technologies are sought to solve an identified disability—the Lightwriter for nonverbal communicators like Peyton Goddard, hearing aids for CeCe Bell, animated interactions as in the case of Owen Suskind and David Karasik—nervous systems extend in more open ways. The counterexamples of the Greenfelds and Henry Kisor point to how, when a nervous system is curtailed, individual possibilities are curtailed as well. They might be managed with success, as Kisor does, but they may also lead to family and individual hardship, as in the case of the Greenfelds. Expansive nervous systems make more possibilities possible, and Elkaïm takes this as the mission of contemporary psychotherapy.

Elkaïm proposes a set of tools for the refashioning of social relations, which he refers to as assemblages, singularities, amplification, and resonances. The purpose of a cybernetically informed psychotherapy is to make more possibilities possible, and Elkaïm sees the ethical role of the therapist as being the facilitator of these possibilities, which can occur through the therapist's "chance" interventions. Always careful to recognize the singular nature of the relationship between individuals, as well as the ways that the therapist is brought into these already existing sets of relations, Elkaïm is not prescriptive in what will change a family system—or a system generally—but instead places emphasis on the assemblages that resonate between therapist and client. For one family, water plays a variety of specific symbolic roles, and Elkaïm latches on to their use of water to amplify it in his consultation with that particular family. Water's role in how the family conceptualizes death, and particularly the death of the family's matriarch, provides a way for Elkaïm to initiate metacommunicative acts between himself and the family. In another family, competence plays a central role in the family's continued functional dysfunction, and it is through Elkaïm's performance of incompetence that he is able to open the family's awareness of the importance of competence and incompetence in their continued plights. These amplifications are only possible because of the shared animation that Elkaïm has with the family members he treats. Another therapist might pick entirely different assemblages to make resonate between the family and therapist. In each case, the importance is in making the implicit explicit, in making the world-view of the participants explicitly articulated in its paradoxical form alongside the official program that subjects profess to value. The individual, the brain, the neurological, and communication might all be considered assemblages in Elkaïm's way of thinking, and to change the system whereby neurological disorders are taken as being indicative of less than full human personhood, they might usefully be amplified to expose the underlying, paradoxical assumptions that reify individuals as divorced from an interdependent relationship with their sociotechnical environment, the actors in it, and the facilitating technologies that make connection possible. Intensifying these taken-for-granted neuroscientific categories helps destabilize these concepts as objects and unravels the knitting that holds the brain together as an epistemic, causal object.

FIVE

Facilitated Subjectivity, Affective Bioethics, and the Nervous System

*I*f personhood and subjectivity are separable, then what are the ethical implications of treating individuals as nonpersons despite individuals recognizing themselves or others as subjects? Or treating persons as nonsubjects? In answering these questions, I turn to the lives of two families, the Ackerman–Wests and the Schiavos. The Ackerman–Wests struggle with Paul West's loss of language, the result of a stroke. This loss affects his ability to communicate with others and to interpret what others are trying to communicate to him. As a professional writer, this is a particularly difficult experience for him, and he works to return to language with his wife—writer Diane Ackerman—and caregivers. Through their efforts, he accomplishes this return slowly and fitfully. Over a yearslong process, Paul writes a memoir of his aphasia, which runs in parallel to Diane's own memoir of caring for him during the same period. Paul's loss of communicative capacities affects how he comes to conceptualize himself as a subject; it shapes how people treat him as less than a full person. Paul sees himself teetering on the human/nonhuman divide, feeling that his access to language is what makes him human. It is through the connections that Paul has with the world that are facilitated by those who care for him that he is eventually able to regain his communicative capacities. Paul provides a clear example of the affective, cybernetic basis of subject formation through the interaction of physiological, symbolic, and material forces, mediated by animating relations and made possible through modular institutions of care.

If Paul's loss of and eventual return to language tarry at the threshold of humanness, personhood, and subjectivity, Terri Schiavo's persistent vegetative state challenges the limit of the categories of the human, personhood, and subjectivity in the United States as based in neurological capacities and supported by medicine, science, and the law. Cared for principally by her husband and hospice staff, Terri's life is subject to ongoing legal challenges from her parents and kin, which Michael, her husband, sees as attempts to cynically wrest Terri's estate from his control. Terri is kept alive with a feeding tube for fifteen years, during which time Michael grieves the loss of his wife while continuing to care for her body. If she was once unquestionably a person, then Michael comes to see her as less of one through his encounters with U.S. law, medicine, and neuroscience. The various tests that are performed to assess Terri's brain activity confirm that she has lost not just her abilities to communicate but also her capacity for personhood altogether, as defined by American forms of scientific and legal expertise. As a result, Michael comes to terms with allowing Terri to die. This erosion of Terri's personhood is possible in no small part as a result of the centrality of the brain in assessing capacities of personhood. In models of persons who do not depend on communication or on the existence of the brain or cognition, Terri could still be counted as a person. Michael and Terri's shared experience points to the challenges of neurological reductionism and its relationship to personhood, subjectivity, and the category of the human. Embracing an affective and cybernetic conception of the nervous system helps focus attention on the importance of developing robust facilitating networks of modular animation as the basis of connection and ethical obligation.

I conclude this chapter with a discussion of bioethics in the United States, particularly as it is influenced by biopolitical thinking that focuses on the value of human life through the discourse of quality of life. Assessing the value of individual lives is harmful both to individuals and to bioethics as a system of thought. Instead, we should use bioethics as a way to conceptualize the connections and capacities made possible in individuals through the diverse facilitating networks that make up our worlds. If value is displaced from an internal, inherent quality to an external, facilitated capacity, we must face bioethical questions: Are we doing enough to make lives livable? What will we lose in our disavowal of the obligations of reciprocation? What kinds of nervous systems are we making? In answering these questions, I turn in the epilogue to reflect on living and dying in the nervous system by considering the lives and deaths of people close to me and how grief—as an affective register but also as an index of connection—might serve as the basis for an affective bioethics that builds livable worlds for a greater variety of human experience. I close with an incitement to consider subjunctive grief—anticipatory grief of future loss—as a way to ground conceptualizing the bioethical obligations incurred by affective subjectivity.

The Couple Who Couldn't Communicate

FROM SUBJECT TO OBJECT

Paul West was a writer by trade, writing some fifty books throughout his life. He spent his career at Penn State University in State College, Pennsylvania, but in retirement, he and his wife, Diane Ackerman, moved to Ithaca, New York. There they wrote books, enjoyed the Finger Lakes, and participated in the local community, largely built around Cornell University and Ithaca College. At the age of seventy-three, in 2003, Paul experienced a stroke. In addition to paralyzing his right side—his dominant side for writing and other daily activities—it left him with profound aphasia. For a man who had built his sense of self on his wordsmithing and his ability to communicate in artful and playful ways, the aphasia was profoundly debilitating. For a couple that had built their relationship on wordplay and communicative jousting, the aphasia was deeply troubling for both of them. First Paul and then Diane write memoirs of their experiences of Paul's stroke and recovery, Paul's memoir detailing the stroke and his aphasia as he experienced it and Diane's recounting the changes in their lives as they adapted to Paul's new state. Taken together, their memoirs offer a rich, complementary account of Paul's experience and changes, as well as Diane's adaptations to Paul's aphasia. In so doing, they provide a parallel account of a debilitating neurological disorder and the individual and collaborative labor that goes into the recovery process.

The memoirs also provide a robust account of how a life without communicative capacities is experienced and how it shapes individual and collaborative worlds.

While in the hospital, during his earliest speech therapy sessions, Paul begins to recover some speech functions. This follows intensive work on the parts of his speech therapists to shape his mouth in old ways to make familiar sounds and words. But Paul's experience of aphasia—which Diane refers to as a psychic cramp—means that even when he can make a sound, the sound lacks meaning to him. He can repeat a requested sound, but his interpretive abilities are impaired. Similarly, in his efforts to make his feelings known and desires expressed, he has difficulties summoning sounds that are meaningful for other people. Added to this mix of communication challenges, Paul is awash in anxiety. His inability to communicate—and to understand the stroke and aphasia as conditions—leaves him in a state of near-constant distress. Over time, however, he does begin to recover language, as Diane recounts:

> As his besieged brain began to quiet down, Paul said his first
> intelligible words, uttered in frustration while yet struggling
> to make himself understood. . . . "Stir the nevis! Stir the nevis!
> Mem, mem, mem!" he kept insisting. "You gad clottal to stir
> the nevis!!!". . . . It took several days, and Paul flicking the light
> switch on and off repeatedly, while pointing at me with his free
> hand, to figure out that what he wanted me to do was pay the
> electric bill.[1]

Paul's anxiety leads him to want to communicate to Diane about these mundane stressors, which have an immediacy that he feels compelled to convey. They also have a domestic edge to them, pointing to Paul's conception of his role in their family and the tasks that depend on his full presence. He worries not so much about the bill as what the effect will be of not paying the bill for their family. From these immediate communicational needs, Paul eventually begins to develop a repertoire of phrases that he can use with Diane and the hospital staff members whom he encounters throughout the day. As he explains:

I had graduated, by now, from "Mem. Mem. Mem," which was nearly language, to "Men. Men. Men," which was language right and proper. There followed on these nonsensical exaggerations not exactly a host of words but a series of reminders. "No" would not shake the timbers of an old man's dream, but "It's simple, stupid," might disturb any person looking for a topic.[2]

Paul's language returns to him in uneven and unexpected ways. It is not that he attempts to recall a specific phrase so much as a phrase comes to him fully formed; it may not be the most appropriate thing for a situation, but it is said nonetheless. And as words and phrases are added to his vocabulary in this way, they tend to stick, although this sometimes depends on the prompting of those around him. It is in this context that Diane decides to propose the idea of writing his memoir of aphasia, *The Shadow Factory*.

The stroke occurred while Paul was hospitalized for a severe infection related to kidney stones he was unable to pass. During his recovery in the hospital, while Diane was visiting, he excused himself to go to the bathroom. He recounts his experience of the stroke like this:

> Just as I finished drying my face, with hands still wet, was like a bolt of beautiful lightning, which seemed to muddle my face in a variety of contortions. For a moment, I felt there had been an electrical surge of neon lamp or something. But the lamp stayed on, and I realized something had gone wrong with my face, including the head, the mucous membranes, and the jaw that was sealed up beyond all repair, because I tried to speak and call out, without result.[3]

Paul loses all of his communicative capacities, experiencing what his physicians diagnose as global aphasia. He both cannot speak and cannot fully understand what is being communicated to him. Moreover, all symbolic reference is lost to him. As Diane explains, "Aphasia doesn't just cripple one's use of words, but the use of any symbols, including the obvious ones: numbers, arrows, semaphore, sign language, Morse code. But also the lightning bolt that spells electrical danger, the three triangles that warn of radiation, the intersecting arcs that announce a biohazard . . . even the paper-doll man and woman on restroom doors."[4] After his stroke, Paul could not make himself understood or understand those around him. Nor could he comprehend the symbolic content of things in his environment, including the signs in the hospital, the symbols on a television remote control, or the numbers on a telephone. He was suddenly and thoroughly without language. And without language, the world he had created for himself—with Diane—began to unravel, as did his claim to neurological subjecthood. But with the careful facilitation that Diane and Paul's caregivers provide him, he overcomes his feelings of being less than human and develops an emergent subjectivity through his new communicative capacities.

Before Paul's stroke, he and Diane had lived the lives of professional writers. They were not tied down to a specific place for work but rather were home together for long periods of writing and editing, then away on research trips and book tours. During these periods apart, they would stay in daily contact through the telephone, leading to what Diane refers to as "telegamy" or "marriage at a distance."[5] When they were together, they were together, and when they were apart, they stayed together through the telephone. Their marriage was therefore one facilitated by technology, which allowed them intimacy but also the solitude they each desired in order to do their work. They each cared for themselves, and cared about each other. With Paul's stroke, however, Diane was suddenly put into the position of Paul's primary caregiver. She ruminates on the possibility of Paul's institutionalization, realizing that it offers her one path to freedom from his daily caregiving: "I could see why stroke victims were often entrusted to nursing homes; [the stroke] was like a divorce from someone you nonetheless loved, wanted to help, and were fated to look after."[6] Especially in the earliest days after Paul's stroke, he is so fundamentally changed in his temperament—frustrated and angry at being unable to make himself understood—and so disrupted in his communication that Diane's experience is one of profound estrangement. He is the man she has loved for decades, yet he has lost the communicative aspects through which she relates to him, and upon which they founded their marriage. Recognizing this impact on Diane as well as the devastating effects the loss of communication cause for him, Paul is moved to express his desires for his own death. After months of unsuccessful recovery, Diane reports: "'Dead,' he pronounced in a leaden tone. 'You're *feeling* dead?' He stared at me hard. I sat down on the bed beside him and cradled his limp hand. 'You wish you were dead?' He nodded yes, this time with a look so desolate raw it chilled me. . . . I know that, in Paul's eyes, in losing his words he had already died, all that remained was killing the empty husk."[7] Diane is unwilling to allow Paul's death, which he might have engineered through self-starvation; nor does she institutionalize him. Instead, she accepts the changes in her life that his caregiving will bring, replacing their telegamy with what she sees as a gendered experience of caring for Paul.

Diane and Paul's interdependence and independence, facilitated through the telephone, radically changes to the domestic space of the house after Paul's stroke, with Diane first deciding to move Paul back into their shared home after he is discharged from the hospital, then adopting a role that she describes as maternal.[8] She explains that moving Paul back into their shared home *"felt* right, but I knew there was no way I could manage his care all by myself. Or rather I could, but it would cost me *my* independence. Our lives had changed forever, but I didn't want to vanish into his illness—and it was hard not to."[9] In conceptualizing what the care for Paul entails, she recognizes that "our lives" changed, and that she was the one who would "vanish into his illness." Paul may be impaired by his stroke and the aphasia, radically changed in who he is, but he will persist as a person for Diane. Diane, however, sees her subjectivity threatened by the caregiving responsibilities she has adopted. In working through the responsibilities of caregiving for Paul, Diane conceptualizes her work as twofold. First is the actual bodily care of Paul; second is the auxiliary role she plays as part of his bodily apparatus—as part of his nervous system. Acknowledging both the somatic experiences of care as well as its intersubjective aspects, Diane notes, "Caregiving offers many fringe benefits, including the sheer sensory delight of nourishing and grooming, sharing, and playing. . . . But caregiving does buttonhole you; you're stitched in one place. With children, this labor is an investment in their future, and they sponge up lessons. With a stroke victim it's a relic of the past. . . .

Paul wasn't on a learning curve but seemed trapped in a circle."[10] It may be the haptic aspects of care that regiment Diane's experience of Paul's recovery in a daily and weekly way, but the intersubjective aspects of his ongoing facilitation expose how interdependent Paul and Diane are and how affective their connection is. Anyone could manage Paul's grooming and feeding, but only Diane can facilitate the lost communicative capacities that Paul has experienced. Only Diane can replace them, even if it means that she loses her apparent independence in exchange.

The Ackerman–Wests see the ironic tragedy in global aphasia happening to Paul, a man who had built his life and his relationships through erudite and playful language. Language for Paul was not only his means of everyday communication with other people but also the basis of his work. As a writer, without language, he would also lose all of his access to labor. As Diane writes, conceptualizing the implications of Paul's aphasia, "If he couldn't read or work, what would he do all day? Probably want me to keep him company—and that was understandable—though devastating to my work, my freedom."[11] The curtailment of Paul's labor potential also means intensifying demands on Diane's time, as if the independence Paul once found through his writing could be substituted for by a newfound caregiving dependence on Diane. She sees in his loss of language the inevitability of Paul's seriality, one day following the next with no differences, just brute repetition of base everyday experiences, as if he were institutionalized by the aphasia itself. Diane's impression of Paul's loss of language lingers. She explains, "Words had been his pastime, solace, and obsession for so many decades. How on earth would he now pass the time? . . . Surely his days now held more hours than before, idle hours alone and with no words as windup toys."[12] For Paul, the aphasia renders him isolated in a variety of ways. He is isolated from his old friends and colleagues, whom he can no longer communicate with; the hospital staff, who cannot understand him; Diane, whom he struggles to convey his concerns and desires to; and from himself as a subject. Language no longer provides him with a means to conceptualize the world around him or to engage in the communicative acts others attempt to enroll him in. Most devastatingly to Paul, it no longer provides him with a means to know himself; he can no longer work with words. As Paul later writes of this period,

> It is hard to persuade anyone that the life of man can be so bald and unproductive for weeks on end, but the truth is that a large number of us spend much of our time getting nowhere at all and fattening up our internal systems with fat nothings. . . . So one who entertains the vision of all points mustering to one final electric point can be disappointed again and again, for it does not happen. And many of these people go on to think less and less until one day they conclude operations in the final wave of blank inattention.[13]

There is no cure on the horizon for Paul—something he is intimately aware of, as is Diane. There is no full restoration of Paul to his pre-stroke condition. Paul is irrevocably changed, as is Diane. He may find new communicative capacities; he may find a way forward and out of the crushing seriality that his aphasia has imposed on him. But if he is to recover at all, it depends on overcoming the neurological disorder that he faces, which can only occur through the facilitation provided by the hospital staff, Diane, and his caregivers that leads them to build a new nervous system.

RETURNING TO COMMUNICATION THROUGH FACILITATION

In the weeks that follow Paul's stroke, he slowly develops the ability to pronounce a single, nonsensical syllable: "Mem." This is the result of great exertion on his part, but it results only in frustration because no one can understand what he means. He supplements his monosyllabic communication with gestures, attempting to convey his meaning through the waving of his good arm and the drawing of shapes in the air. Communicating with writing is impossible because his handwriting is illegible, and the symbolic interface of computers and typewriters is nonsensical to him. In attempting to convey what the experience of speaking was like, he writes, "What passed for a word in my neck of the woods usually formed three or four. For instance, the sample would run: the letter *I*, the letter *M*, the letters *EJ*, and possibly the letters *AFFB*. With such a workload it would be impossible to complete anything."[14] Writing about the same period in Paul's recovery, Diane notes, "Although he was able to make some of his feelings known through facial expressions and gestures, he was frustrated and furious that no one could understand his gibberish when it clearly made sense to *him*. He didn't know his own name or mine, and kept gesturing wildly that he wanted to go home."[15] To make matters worse, what Paul is attempting to convey is usually simple yet of profound importance to him, as in the case of expressing his desire to go home after months of living in the hospital. Language is slow for Paul, with every sound depending on his coordination of seemingly implacable facial muscles, as well as a cognitive struggle to ascertain what is being communicated to him by other people—including their interpretations of what he is saying. It is not simply a failure to be able to speak that Paul experiences but also an inability to interpret what is being communicated to him. Paul experiences an inability to both mimic and interpret. The remedies for this situation are occupational and speech therapy, which are arranged for Paul during his extended hospital stay and which seek to restore—at least in some limited fashion—his ability to move the right side of his body, his face, and his speech.

Paul spends days in the hospital's occupational therapy clinic and with speech therapists. One of the concerns of everyone involved is that Paul will aspirate food or drink, the result of his being unable to feel because of the stroke. This aspirating could result in his developing pneumonia and dying. The immediate result is that Thick-It is added to thicken all of his food to the consistency of pudding, including the liquids he consumes. He is also trained in new forms of bodily comportment; for example, he is trained to sit up straight while eating to ensure that the food passes straight down his throat into his stomach. Neither the Thick-It nor the change in posture is agreeable to Paul, and combined with the fear of aspiration, Paul loses forty pounds during his hospitalization and during the early weeks of returning home.

Once he is discharged into Diane's care, he begins to work with a series of four in-home speech therapists, each of whom stresses small enunciation practices, attempting to rekindle Paul's fluency with everyday words and sounds. These seem to be Paul's greatest challenges, and Diane hypothesizes that the earliest words that Paul learned in his life were located in the parts of his brain most thoroughly damaged. He has no problem recalling a word like "eldritch" to describe the fog in their yard, but naming an apple defies him. In order to circumvent the problems that Paul is experiencing in his ability to enunciate words, one therapist provides him with a keyboard that speaks what he writes. But Paul's aphasia is too profound: "I was too daunted by the presence of the computer and still prey to helpless laughter when I considered the enormous minified array of its keyboard. . . . I could not see the numbers and letters. The orthography was not even in the accustomed order but was a ramble away from my trained eye."[16] After dismissing each of the speech therapists for one reason or another, Diane and Paul finally decide to welcome into their house one of the nurses Paul had worked with during his time at the hospital, Liz, who was the one member of the nursing staff whom Paul and Diane had made a sincere connection with during Paul's hospitalization. Liz impressed them by not being pedantic with Paul and being willing to experiment with Paul's treatment and recovery.

Each day, for hours at a stretch, Paul sits down with Liz to dictate the next section of *The Shadow Factory* to her. Liz dutifully writes down each word Paul struggles to speak. The following day, Paul sits down to edit the text. Slowly, over months, the text begins to emerge into a narrative. Unlike Ackerman's memoir of the stroke and their recovery, which follows a linear timeline from the event of Paul's stroke through treatment and recovery, *The Shadow Factory* is loose with time and language. Paul chose this to actively make the reading of his experience of aphasia an estranging one, with a lack of clear referents in his sentences, confusion in the sequencing of the events that he experiences, including his stroke and recovery. The stroke occurs halfway through the memoir, forcing readers to question what they have been reading for the last several chapters. But this confusion is integral to Paul's experience of his stroke and the resultant aphasia. He has become unmoored from his sense of personal history; he is now afloat in language and time that now seem meaningless. Like Paul's early weeks of recovery, readers are without a frame for the interpretation of the language and events that are being described, and only slowly do they emerge into the event that strikes Paul speechless and impairs his movement.

The Shadow Factory is thus a mimetic text; it seeks to create in its audience the experience of the author. It poetically attempts to unravel language and time, making readers aware of their own language and their reliance on the temporal ordering of experience. Paul seeks to make disorder contagious, extending its reach beyond his experience of aphasia and into the society of his readers. In this contagion, his disorder may come to be accepted less as a disorder of his brain and communicative capacities and more as a function of society and the widespread inability to facilitate the lived experiences of people like Paul.

PERSONHOOD WITHOUT COMMUNICATION

Throughout his experience, Paul is influenced by his viewing of David Lynch's *The Elephant Man*, finding in Lynch's portrayal of Joseph Merrick's life a parallel to his own disorder. During speech therapy, when asked to name one of his books, Paul struggles, then exclaims, "I am an individual!" Diane writes, "That took my breath away. It was an allusion to a film we had seen, *The Elephant Man*, about a severely deformed nineteenth-century man who begins mute and is coached to speak. In one scene, cornered by an angry mob, he cries out: 'I am not an animal! I am a man!'"[17] The figure of the Elephant Man had been with Paul since the stroke, it seems, as he recounts his experience with his body's changing physiological responses as akin to Merrick's experience of his body. In reflecting on the importance of Merrick to his own self-conception, Paul writes: "Still, my mouth continued to slacken, and my impression of the whole superstructure was that it was actually getting bigger through growing outward, which seemed to promise an Elephant Man who could eventually speak in his impeded way."[18] Merrick—or at least Lynch's depiction of Merrick—offers some hope for Paul as he compares his experience of controlling his body and his ability to speak to Merrick's parallel difficulties. He also sees Merrick's social isolation and eroded claims to personhood as inevitably similar to the experience he will face in his new altered state. In voicing the thoughts of nameless others whom he will encounter in the world, Paul writes, "Who is this, they would utter, who once was so demure and now is dreadful? Is he human at all with his crossbow eyes and his elephantine stance? Is he deserving of pity or some other outlandish emotion, or should we pass him by? Not exactly an Elephant Man, he goes some small way to being one. What is wrong with him?"[19] Paul maps his physical experience—and communication difficulties—onto the world that he used to inhabit. He can no longer be seen as the urbane and erudite writer that he once was, regardless of the projects he undertakes with Diane's and Liz's help; he will always only be a minor Elephant Man. Like Merrick, Paul sees how his inner experience does not map on to his social experience and the experiences that others have with him. He will always inspire the question, "What is wrong with him?" and be unable to answer fully.

Paul uses the language of deafness—despite his sensory capacities remaining intact, although altered by his stroke—to describe his experience of aphasia, and by extension the social isolation he begins to experience as a result. In so doing, Paul captures the experience of social exclusion that those with communicative disorders often experience. He may be able to communicate in the limited environment of his home with a circumscribed community, but in the larger world, he is deaf. He writes of himself, "You are deaf in the broadest sense imaginable. You are deaf and they cannot hear you. So what is all the fuss about? They can pass you by without hating you, but fortunately many do not, trying to make sense of your silence."[20] For Paul, no tools can replace his lost capacities. The speaking keyboard he is given makes no orthographic sense to him, and there are no hearing aids of any sort that will translate the sounds that he hears into meaningful language for him. Paul's deafness is not solely an organic problem; it is not something that resides in the disordered parts of his brain. Rather, it is an effect expressed throughout his social relations and his interactions with his environment. These include his inability to eat, shave, and clean himself; his occluded vision; his slurred speech; his changes in temperament; and the changes in the structure of his and Diane's intimacy, including their loss of telegamy and domesticated caregiving. The term "deaf," like Paul's invocation of the Elephant Man, is meant to convey the disabling aspects of the stroke and aphasia that Paul experiences as an individual, but it also captures the social consequences of disability. He sees himself as less than a full member of society, unable to contribute to society in a way that is recognized as meaningful and valuable. The path forward for Paul relies on his willingness to acknowledge his interdependence on Diane and his other caregivers—and his ability to reshape his dependence on language as a means for knowing others and himself as a subject.

Throughout *One Hundred Names for Love*, Diane falls back on her understanding of the brain's inherent plasticity, that in the aftermath of Paul's stroke, through exercise, he will be able to recover his capacity for communication by allocating communicative functions to areas of the brain that might have other primary functions. She explains this as a possible result of the interaction between social opportunities afforded to Paul through his care and the biological building blocks of Paul's neurons: "From daily pressure and exposure, Paul's brain might change itself, probably by reassigning some lost language skills to surviving neurons. How long would that continue, I wondered, and, more importantly, how much ground could he regain?"[21] In the immediate aftermath of Paul's stroke, Diane sees the road to recovery as being individual. Something inside Paul will be "regained" through "daily pressure and exposure," whether that is through exercise or merely being in the world. But, over time, Diane admits, "I felt oddly like I was taking over some of Paul's higher brain functions (decision-making, interpreting, memory storage), shouldering the mental burden and adding it to my own. One brain laboring for two."[22] Paul may have experienced some recuperative plasticity, may have had functions restored through the therapy he was involved in as well as his everyday facilitation. But more important, through their intimate interdependence, Diane takes on the powers of cognition that are often ascribed to individual brains. In lieu of a technology that can overcome Paul's "deafness," Diane becomes that technology; she becomes an organ in his nervous system. Diane's transformation is most apparent in her account of her experiences with Paul after his injury, which are not discussed in Paul's memoir. Similarly, Paul is able to write *The Shadow Factory* through the ghostwriting facilitation provided by their caregiver, Liz. Yet her contributions to *The Shadow Factory* are only knowable through Diane's account of the process; neither Paul nor his publisher acknowledge Liz's contribution to the text. Taken together, *The Shadow Factory* and *One Hundred Names for Love* demonstrate how neurological disorders are not restricted to the brain. They are not simply material conditions to be overcome through technological remedy but social disorders that can only be overcome through the enrollment of individuals and institutions in creating new networks of facilitation, new models of communication and interdependence. It is not that Diane replaces Paul's impaired cognitive functions but that Paul's external nervous system needs to be refashioned in the wake of his stroke to make his connections to the world socially meaningful to others and himself in an emergent, modular way.

Years after Paul's stroke, he undergoes another brain scan. In looking at the results, the attending neurologist is shocked to see the extent of the damage in Paul's brain. He tells Diane, "I'd assume this man has been in a vegetative state." Diane replies, "Far from it. Would you believe he's written several books since then? That he's been aphasic but communicative, swimming a lot, living a much more limited life, but a happy and relatively normal one?" Despite the severe neurological damage Paul has experienced, he and Diane are able to forge a new life together as well as create new ways to collaboratively communicate. Diane describes to the neurologist all of the work they have done together and with the help of Liz. The neurologist responds, "I'm so glad you told me this about him. . . . It's important to know what's possible."[23] Not every person with aphasia can recover as Paul did, and Paul's recovery is largely mysterious—to medical professionals as well as Paul and Diane. At the very least, Paul and Diane's experiences would seem to argue against localization in favor of facilitated plasticity. Diane attributes Paul's return to language as an effect of their experimenting with caregiving. The four speech therapists they employed were not able to affect any change in Paul; instead, they needed to develop a modular therapeutic strategy that was tailored to Paul and his individual history and capacities. This meant Diane taking what she knew of Paul and creating language games that could engage him and help him develop the areas of communication he lost through his stroke. By clinical standards, Paul does make a profound recovery despite the extent of the injury he experiences, in no small part due to the individualized care that Diane and Liz are able to provide him with through his writing of an aphasic memoir. The same kind of facilitation is not available to everyone, as is clear in Diane's invocation of the specter of institutionalization.

Caring for Paul changes Diane. It also entails the transformation of their home and relationship. But for Diane, Paul's institutionalization would mean the end of their marriage as such—and presumably the end of Paul as well. It is easy to imagine Diane institutionalizing Paul while he was in his most vulnerable, least communicative state; if that had happened, he would never have recovered language in the way that he did. Paul may have been able to resist this outcome, or the institutional actors he worked with may have uncovered his latent communicative capacities. But the possibility remains that people may be lost not simply because of their disorders but because of the lack of facilitation provided to them as a result of the institutional logics of neurological disorder and care that rely on reductive neurological and symbolic models of subjectivity.

The Woman Who Wasn't a Subject

PERSONHOOD WITHOUT SUBJECTIVITY

You probably know about Terri Schiavo, or at least about her death. Terri was the subject of a multiyear political campaign and series of legal battles about her right to die, which finally happened in 2005, when she was forty-one. Her husband, Michael, had the power of attorney for her, and after several years of keeping her alive on life support, he finally decided to let Terri die by removing her feeding tube. Terri's parents and her siblings, the Schindlers, fought Michael's decision, arguing that Terri was not in a persistent vegetative state but was minimally conscious. Over time, awareness of the judicial fight between Michael and Terri's family drew media attention, and through the media, it eventually became a cause of religious conservatives in the United States, as well as their allies, most notably the then-governor of Florida, Jeb Bush, and his brother, who was then the president of the United States, George W. Bush. Fifteen years after the event that had debilitated Terri happened, and twelve years after Michael had decided to remove life support, Terri died in the hospice where she had spent nearly a third of her life. Terri had experienced a cardiac arrest at the age of twenty-six, largely as a result of an undiagnosed eating disorder. When her heart stopped, she subsequently experienced brain damage, the result of a lack of oxygen reaching her brain. When she was resuscitated, she never regained full consciousness. She was insensate, unable to communicate or care for herself. She was no longer a subject but rather a person-as-object caught in a web of relations that exceeded her. In her neurological disorder, Terri exposes the fundamental relationship between personhood and subjectivity as based in conceptions of the brain as the basis of neurological subjectivity. With her severe injury, Terri can be treated as a person, but she is not treated as a subject with an ongoing reciprocal relationship with her world. This occurs first in medical interpretations of Terri's condition, which is then ratified by legal proceedings and eventually accepted by Michael. Without subjectivity, Terri is treated as incurable, and Michael is allowed to let her die by removing the technology that facilitates her continued personhood.

Over the course of the many legal battles fought between Michael and the Schindlers, she was examined several times by physicians and psychiatrists. Michael would pay well-respected leaders in their fields to examine Terri, and those experts would generally agree that she was in a persistent vegetative state with no hope of recovery. The Schindlers would pay a less respected medical expert to examine Terri and return a finding of her being in a minimally conscious state. The court would order examinations, and those experts would agree with Michael's experts. In one representative case, an examination by neurologist Jeffrey Karp finds that

> the patient has evidence of profound brain injury. She apparently had this as a result of anoxic cerebral damage, secondary to a cardiopulmonary arrest in 1990. There was some seizure activity initially, but this has not been present for many years. . . . her EEG did not show seizures but just showed slowing compatible with her encephalopathy. A CT scan showed significant atrophy of a generalized nature. Her examination does indicate that she is in a chronic vegetative state.
>
> She does not meet the criteria of being brain dead, but . . . the patient is in a persistent vegetative state. She has permanent

and irreversible condition. Despite her eyes being open, she does not appear to be aware or responsive to her environment. There is an absence of voluntary activity or cognitive behavior, and inability to communicate or interact purposefully with her environment.

In the absence of good total and skilled nursing care, this patient would be unable to survive.

Again, since this has been a long time since the incident, I feel that her chance of improvement to a functional level is essentially zero.[24]

Terri is capable of movement, but she moves in ways that are unsettling for her friends and family. She groans and moans; her eyes move, sometimes seemingly following a person in the room; she smiles. As Michael explains in his memoir:

> Patients in a vegetative state may manifest signs such as moaning, groaning, crying, laughing, and wincing, but these are "subcortical mechanisms." That means that, for example, a cry or moan that may be triggered by what doctors refer to as a "noxious stimulus," such as severe menstrual cramps, is a subcortical response in the deeper portions of the cerebral hemispheres of the brain, as opposed to the outer layer of the hemispheres, the cerebral cortex, where conscious pain and suffering reside.[25]

Terri is not in her brain anymore. If she has personhood, it exists only in ascribed status, even if the Schindlers and their supporters try desperately to put Terri back into her brain and its capacities through appeals to various experts. Her personhood might exist in those—like her parents and family, their paid medical examiners, the invested conservative religious communities, and the Bush brothers—who attempt to facilitate it, who try and make Terri into a person despite the scientific and legal forces arrayed against them. Terri's nervous system comes to be made up of family, activists, state legislatures, governors, the president of the United States, and all of the media that bound them to her. She has no way of knowing it, but she is animating hundreds, thousands, maybe millions of people in various ways, although they exist in a nonreciprocal relationship with her. While these actors may treat her as a person, neuroscience—the very ally they seek to enroll in their fight—views her as without subjectivity, and potentially without personhood as well.

This is how Michael reports the event that led to Terri's eventual brain damage:

> Sometime after 5:30 A.M. I woke up because I needed to go to the bathroom. . . . As I started to get out of bed, it didn't even register that Terri wasn't there. And then I heard a thud. I threw off the sheet, got up, and ran out into the hall. The bathroom lights were on and I could see Terri on the floor. . . . She had one arm by her side and the other arm over her head—almost in a ballerina's pose. I got down on my knees, rolled her over so that she was facing me, and scooped her into my arm. "Terri, Terri, are you all right? What happened? What's going on?"[26]

Terri never recovers from the heart attack she has that morning, but her body does change over time because first she is in a coma, which she eventually awakens from. It is likely that this regaining of partial sentience compels the actions that follow over the next fifteen years, as various people see in Terri something that neuroscientists and physicians claim is not there—and Michael is the first person to experience this. Writing of an early visit to Terri's hospital room, Michael explains:

> For a week, maybe a little longer, Terri's eyes were completely closed. Then, one day, she opened them. I had just walked into her room and the nurse was there. She looked up as I came in, and seeing that I'd spotted Terri's eyes, she said, "Yeah, she just opened them." My reaction was predictable. I thought *This is great*, and I began talking to Terri, thinking, *She's awake!* But all I got in response was the moan that we would become so accustomed to over time. I was still looking for signs of progress, however, and if I'd seen her hand move, or see her move an arm or leg, even a toe, or her head would turn, I'd get excited. But the doctors said that these movements weren't significant.[27]

It is easy to see Michael's plight. On the one hand, he wants his wife to return to full consciousness, and every behavior he observes would seem to indicate that some kind of return is possible. On the other hand, the physicians and nurses whom he and Terri are surrounded by indicate that these possibilities are unrealistic; her brain is, they confirm, beyond recovery. Michael, however, is undeterred throughout the first years of Terri's persistent vegetative state. He seeks out novel treatments, dedicates himself to Terri's care, eventually becomes a certified nurse, and serves as her constant advocate in the hospital, nursing home, and eventually hospice. Nothing works to restore Terri to her previous fully conscious state, but she persists in her vegetative state, making the same subcortical movements and noises that others take to be indications of meaningful behavior and interactions—and that compel Michael's care for her through the first three years of Terri's persistent vegetative state.

NEGOTIATING PERSONHOOD IN MEDICINE AND LAW

It is during these first three years that Michael sues for malpractice two physicians whom Terri had seen in the years leading up to her collapse. Terri had been struggling with getting pregnant, a situation that was in retrospect a side effect of her eating disorder. The basis of Michael's lawsuit is that both doctors had had the opportunity to diagnose Terri's eating disorder, and had either collected data that could have pointed them to that diagnosis or had failed to ask for relevant information that would have led them to an eating disorder diagnosis. As Gary Fox, Michael's malpractice attorney, explains, "The long and short of Dr. Igel's testimony is that Terri Schiavo was showing signs and symptoms of an easily diagnosable condition. He did not diagnose or treat her problem, and, as a result, Terri Schiavo suffered a heart attack and will remain in a coma for the rest of her life."[28] Michael settles with one of the doctors for a small sum and wins his lawsuit against the other doctor, which results in a multimillion-dollar settlement. After legal fees, most of the funds that Michael receives are dedicated to Terri's continuing care, but as he tells it, the monetary awards are the beginning of the frictions between him and the Schindlers. Michael sees Terri's father in particular as feeling that he is entitled to some of the settlement money, claiming that he and his wife are equally emotionally affected by Terri's collapse and thus have a legal claim as her parents. Under Florida law, they do not have such a claim, so they begin to file a variety of legal challenges to Michael's guardianship. Michael pledges to donate his monetary awards to charity, and over time, he rescinds his status as guardian in place of a guardian ad litem appointed by the court. The Schindlers contest the findings of the court that Terri is beyond neurological recovery, insisting that they be appointed guardians of Terri, but they never succeed.

What is uncontested at the time of the malpractice trial is the jury's finding that Terri is beyond recovery. Gary Fox, Michael's malpractice attorney, explains that the jury was "convinced that she was not feeling any pain or suffering, that she had no cognition, and that she was truly in a deep, vegetative state from which she would never recover. Even the mainstream media never picked up on it. This issue was thoroughly analyzed, litigated, contested. We argued to the contrary, that she was feeling things, or at least we couldn't be sure she wasn't, and the jury decided no."[29] From the time of the earliest trial, Terri is accepted by the court as being beyond neurological recovery. Michael—and by extension Terri's family and friends—could choose to keep her on life support, but fundamentally, she is seen as being subject to others' manipulations rather than potentially able to recover her full personhood and subjectivity. This is later corroborated by Dr. Peter Bambakidis, who summarizes his findings:

> The preponderance of data and my clinical examination reveal no evidence of awareness of self, environment, or ability to interact with others. More precisely, there is no evidence of sustained, reproducible, purposeful voluntary behavioral responses to visual, auditory, tactile or noxious stimuli. Mrs. Schiavo exhibits no evidence of language comprehension or expression. Given the fact that her current neurologic status has remained essentially unchanged for at least ten years, I would state that her chances of meaningful neurologic recovery to be virtually nonexistent.[30]

Terri, legally and medically, is recognized as a nonsubject as grounded in neurological, symbolic, and materialist models of subjectivity. She has no "awareness," no "purposeful, voluntary" behavior, no "comprehension or expression," all capacities attributed to the brain and its normal functioning. Her family and their supporters may want to make a subject of her, but according to neurological and legal measures of her subjectivity, she lacks the fundamental capacities that will make her a subject. She can be animated, but she will not purposefully animate others in turn; there is no reciprocation in her relations, making her fundamentally inert by American standards of subjectivity.

During the early years of tension between Michael and the Schindlers, Michael takes Terri to see neurologist Dr. Thomas Harrison, who, after a technician conducts an EEG test, consults with Michael. Michael writes that Harrison concentrates "on the EEG graph, glancing over at Terri, and then looking up at me with this very calm but questioning look on his face. And then he smacked me with the medical equivalent of a two-by-four: 'Why do you let her live? She died three years ago. . . . I'm looking at the EEG and it's flat. There are portions where there's some electrical activity, but there's nothing cortically. Nothing, no cortical, top functioning.'"[31] Again, medical science steps in to check Michael's hopes. Terri is not getting better, nor is anything meaningful happening inside Terri's head. Terri, for all intents and purposes by neurological standards, died three years previously— that is to say, at least the subject who was Terri died then. Her body, however, lives on, aided by medical technologies to stay alive in the most rudimentary form, making her a person without subjectivity. This pushes Michael toward a conclusion: he will let Terri die.

In thinking through the findings of Dr. Harrison, he writes, "Now I'm sitting in a doctor's office and he's asking me, *Why do I let my wife live?* Can you imagine how it feels to get asked that question? It says you have the power of life and death over the person who is closest to you in the whole world."[32] Harrison, attempting to ameliorate the shock that Michael experiences as a result of his blunt assessment, explains, "Her top functioning, her knowing, her feeling, her awareness of who she is and who's around her—all of that is gone."[33] Harrison makes a distinction that places subjecthood, all "knowing," "feeling," and "awareness," in a part of the brain that Terri no longer has access to through her neurological disorder. Michael is forced to confront the fact that there is a split in the material being of Terri—her body and its behaviors—and Terri as a person. Whatever subjectivity Terri once had no longer exists. She is just a body, and all of her behaviors can be explained, neuroscientifically, as subcortical—as, effectively, meaningless and beyond the ability to convey meaning to or from Terri. Coming to terms with this, and with knowledge gained by his training as a nurse, Michael decides to let Terri die.

But the Schindlers insist on keeping Terri alive, arguing that she is in a minimally conscious state and that they have a continued reciprocal connection with her. During a much later legal hearing, Bobby Schindler says, "It is not speculative to say if Terri knew it was bringing my parents an ounce of joy in [their] life she would want to be like this."[34] The Schindlers argue that Terri's value to them is in her presence itself, and that what that presence consists of is less important than her state of being. During an early deposition, the Schindlers suggest that they would go to great lengths to keep Terri alive, assenting to both the possibility of assisted respiration as well as amputation in the case of her developing gangrene. Their reasoning is based in part on religious beliefs that they ascribe to the family's Catholicism. On the basis of that claim, during an early trial, Michael's lawyer asks a Catholic priest, Father Murphy, what his understanding of the Catholic perspective on Terri's situation and her parents' decision-making would be. Michael's lawyer asks:

> Do you recall in the deposition of Theresa's brother his testimony that he believes his parents [believe] that Terri is aware of their presence, and he testified that Terri's continued life is a joy to him? A joy to him and his family to keep Terri alive in this condition? He was even asked if Terri needed a respirator to keep her alive, would it still give you joy to have her alive on a respirator? And he said yes. He was asked if her limb had to be amputated would it give you joy to have her alive in this condition? And he said yes.

Father Murphy responds, "Keeping someone around strictly for your own pleasure strikes me as very antigospel. Sounds more like using someone than loving someone."[35] Later in the same trial, Terri's family members take the stand and attest to their continuing beliefs in the matter, despite Father Murphy's expert opinion. In listening to their testimony, Michael is deeply affected:

> Can you imagine what it was like for me to hear him talking about cutting Terri's arms and legs off? I knew it was coming, but I still went white. I wanted to vomit right there. I was thinking, *Oh my god, do you realize what you're saying? How could you possibly* consider cutting *your daughter's arms and legs off, when she couldn't even think or communicate, just to keep her alive? Are you that horrible? That hateful?* It made me very ill just hearing it.[36]

The conflict between Michael and the Schindlers is set up as a difference in the affective experiences they have with Terri and the values that they derive from them, and Michael places these affective differences into an ethical register. His invocation of "hateful" and "horrible" indicate a failure on the part of the Schindlers and their commitments to Terri's personhood that privilege their feelings of "joy" against Terri's stated wishes. If it is an affective connection, Michael sees it as self-serving, one-sided, and ultimately empty.

THE CONSEQUENCES OF CONTESTED PERSONHOOD

The Schindlers' attachment to Terri is paradoxical to Michael. Michael's understanding of Terri's eating disorder is that it developed in relation to verbal abuse perpetuated by her father throughout her youth. This is corroborated when Terri's brother, Bobby, reports during a deposition:

> There was a time when Terri was in her adolescence or late adolescence when she was very, very heavy. When they were in a busy shopping center near where they lived, there was a young black gentleman walking with a rather obese, obviously overweight, white young lady, and it was reported to me that Terri's father said to her "Terri, you see there, if you don't lose weight, you're going to end up just like that girl with a guy just like that"—or words less politically correct to that effect . . . actually, he used the "N" word.[37]

Michael takes Bobby's reporting of this incident as emblematic of the kind of abuse that Terri was subjected to throughout her youth, when she was seen by her family as "very, very heavy." That Terri's father would subject her to such verbal treatment at a young age appears to motivate Terri to manage her weight through binging and purging over the next decade of her life. Her bulimia seems to intensify as her marriage to Michael nears, and she precipitously loses a significant amount of weight. She maintains her bulimia throughout the early years of her marriage with Michael, which leads him to repeatedly remark on her loss of weight. Thinking that she is merely dieting, Michael is not alarmed; only in retrospect does he come to realize that her management of her weight is self-destructive. In learning of Terri's verbal abuse by her father—and what would appear to be a family milieu that supports such treatment—Michael realizes that she developed bulimia as an adaptation to an environment that breeds a dysfunctional understanding of Terri's body, its role in her self-conception, and her place in society. To Michael, it is apparent that Terri's family did not care about her as a person in her youth. Similarly, as she persists in her vegetative state, they continue to treat her more as an object than as a person, despite their attempts to legally have her recognized as exhibiting socially motivated behaviors.

The Schindlers' behavior toward Terri—the early abuses they subjected her to, their willingness to amputate her limbs—is counterpoised to Michael's ethical attachments to her, which are motivated by and crystallized in their marriage vows. During his testimony in the malpractice trial, Michael is asked by his attorney, "How do you feel about being married to Terri now?" He responds, "I feel wonderful. She's my life and I wouldn't trade her for the world. I believe in my wedding vows . . . through sickness, in health, for richer or poorer. I married my wife because I love her and I want to spend the rest of my life with her. I'm going to do that."[38] In the earliest years of Terri's persistent vegetative state, Michael is her near-constant companion, caring for her as much as his work—and eventually school—schedule allows. When he cannot be at the nursing home, he calls to check on her. When he is present, he insists on a level of care for Terri that results in him being referred to as a "nightmare" by the management and staff at the facility. Michael's care for Terri begins with his expectation that she will return to full consciousness, and as the realization that she will not sets in, he continues to care for her. This care is mandated by his vows to her, but it is motivated by his continued love for her as a person. The rhythm of Terri's daily needs animates Michael's life, and caring for her provides him with an ongoing project that organizes his life, including motivating him to get a degree in nursing and pursuing a career as a full-time nurse. In his career, Michael is often put into the position of needing to work with families who are making decisions about the end of a loved one's life—a situation that he develops a deep sensitivity to and that inspires him to befriend these grieving families. Through these relationships, he lives through death again and again, seeing other families make the decision to disconnect family members from life support or not treat infections, and the grief that inevitably follows. Yet because of the ongoing legal battles with the Schindlers, he is unable to grieve himself.

By 2005, fifteen years after Terri's collapse and twelve years after Michael had committed to allowing her to die, the legal challenges on the part of the Schindlers are exhausted. Moreover, the attempts of legislators in Florida and the U.S. Congress likewise are legally brought to an end. Finally, Terri is allowed to die. Michael has her feeding tube removed, and as her body begins to shut down, Terri begins the two-week process of dying. Protestors surround the hospice where Terri is living, and Michael is sequestered in a nearby apartment so he can visit her during these last weeks without fear of interactions with an increasingly hostile group of supporters of the Schindlers, some of whom publicly threaten Michael's life on the Internet. The Schindlers come to visit Terri in her final days, briefly and surrounded by journalists and supporters. Meanwhile, Michael visits frequently: "I didn't want Terri to die. But I also didn't want her to be in the position she was in. I never doubted that I was doing what she wanted, but that didn't provide much comfort as I sat and held her or stroked her arm. She was still my wife. She was a part of me. Terri was the first person who made me realize what love was all about."[39] Michael might be sentimental, but he is also speaking to an intimacy that is unsettling for others: how can he both profess his love for Terri and be willing to cut his connection from her through facilitating her death? In the moment of her death, Michael reports experiencing "an emotional upheaval. It's difficult to put this into words that truly convey the awfulness of the situation. Alone. Sad. Empty. It creates a numbing pain deep inside. An aching feeling in my heart. I looked at Terri and knew that the end wasn't far away. I realized we used to be a couple, and now we weren't going to be one anymore. Half of that was going away."[40] Michael's connection with Terri comes to an end, their years of intimacy ended by her death. The media attention continues, however, as does the use of Terri's death as a case for bioethics, legal actions, and conservative activism.

In her afterlife, Terri has continued to be animated in a ghostly fashion, used by others to think through what is at stake in living and dying as a noncommunicative person without subjectivity. Terri and Michael's experience exposes how neurological disorder and abnormal forms of neurological being in the world trouble American ideas about personhood and subjectivity, especially when they are grounded in reductive conceptions of the brain, and of the individual as a bounded entity. The connections that Terri enables show how personhood, facilitation, animation, and subjectivity work together with conceptions of the brain to render some decisions ethical and others "monstrous" and "hateful." For Michael, Terri's connections had atrophied to the point where she had become merely an object for most of the people who claimed that she was a person. Her continued existence as an object was more harmful—to her, to Michael, to U.S. society—than her death. Michael may not have been right in the decision that he made, but given how personhood and subjectivity are constructed in the United States, he had few choices available to him.

Connecting with the Nervous System

ARTICULATING AFFECTIVE BIOETHICS

Life is never singular. Life is not so much a state as a process, one that enrolls diverse actors in knowing and unknowing ways, through intentional and unintentional mechanisms. Across the many families discussed in this book, there is no singular life, no individual, who can be divorced from social and environmental contexts. They are all made through and facilitated by those nervous systems—systems full of other people, institutions, technologies, and nonhumans—that make their lives livable. Isolating the individual allows for pathologization and the ascription of disorder to the brain of a delimited individual, but this is only one way of seeing the brain and its effects. The neurological model of the brain as determinative of the person and subject ignores the many influences that make life possible and that undergird the bringing into being of personhood as an affective state and basis for relationships between people. But subjectivity is less an affective state than an affective process. It is the function of intimate investments in reciprocal bonds between persons, however those persons, human or nonhuman, are composed, and whatever form those bonds take, whether through spoken communication or some other form of modular animation and facilitation. Conceptualizing living and dying in the nervous system, comprising recognizable and unrecognizable actors who participate in old and emerging forms of interaction, forces one to address how connections are made, how they are sustained, and what they facilitate. Living and dying in the nervous system forces questions about what kinds of life are desirable and how they might be facilitated.

Whether it is deafness as a result of encephalitis or the seeming loss of communicative capacities as a result of a change in brain development related to autism, or whether it is the sudden loss of language associated with a stroke or the permanent loss of consciousness, many of the families in this book experience what they accept as a form of regression. Something that seems inevitable and given, something innately human, erodes or suddenly disappears. These losses motivate searches for cures and attempts to recover what has been lost. But in each case, there is no cure for what has been changed; there is no return to the original life a person had. These searches lead families from medical expert to medical expert, from one model of education to another, from dietary experiments to alternative healers, all in a search for what has been lost. In each case, families come to terms with that loss in terms that they can accept, whether in the form of institutionalized care for a loved one, intimate reorganization of family life to support an individual in the home, or long-standing legal battles to assert one's wishes. There is no going back in the context of neurological disorders. Although the lure of the brain's plasticity beckons and proves seductive for many, it can also become a trap, encouraging people to seek in the brain something that can never be restored. In confronting this reality, the material foundation of the brain serves as the boundaries against which discourses of plasticity and recovery found themselves, as if the only form of recovery is one that relies on the brain itself.

What the cases of the families in this book demonstrate, however, is that recovery is only possible through social reformation. Families can be remade, institutions can be remade, models of social participation can be remade, and anthropological evidence provides ways for reconceptualizing what families can be and how they can serve as means of connection to a larger world. In doing so, the connections of family members with neurological disorders and their human and nonhuman kin are remade as well. The Ackerman–West family's adoption of idiosyncratic speech therapy and memoir as recovery, the Suskind family's integration of Disney films into its communicative repertoire—these modes of therapy necessitate facilitating nonnormative subjectivity. They rely on knowing an individual and that individual's capacities, and they rely on facilitating them in an animating environment rife with intimate connections. Normative institutions that seek recovery and cures—or that maintain individuals in perpetual stasis—are unable to make the kinds of interventions that are needed. They substitute transcendent medical searches for cures for pragmatic therapy or resigned homeostasis for novel attempts at facilitation. Recovery is possible in reconfiguration, but this necessitates reconceptualizing the basis for connection, personhood, and subjectivity as beyond normative forms of communication and reductive models of being in the world.

Communication seems so given. It seems inevitable that any baby will grow into language. The inscrutable interior world of an infant will eventually come to be expressed, first in a word or two, garbled yet profound, and eventually in protosentences, then fully realized language. That communication has this inevitable quality is a function of its role in the concept of the person in the North Atlantic, and in the United States particularly. Communication is accepted as a transparent expression of the self, of interior worlds that can only be expressed through language. Communication is how feelings, thoughts, and intent are known to others, and the language of emotions, cognition, and intention are taken as superior to acts, as if self-expression in language is somehow more sincere, more transparent, than acts themselves. The ability to communicate in transparent, socially recognized ways is accepted as the basis for participation in society; that one can mimic communication styles and linguistic content is a marker of one's ability to interpret and be interpreted by others. These capacities are necessary to participate in the economic basis of everyday life; they are necessities for being recognized as able workers, competent citizens, and potential parents and partners. Lacking language, and lacking access to normative ways of communicating, disbars individuals from these fundamental aspects of social engagement, marking them as disabled and in need of treatment or containment.

In the families and institutions discussed in this book, alternative forms of care come into focus. They may not work for every individual and every family, but a more modular society that offers a variety of institutional forms and models for social engagement and connection makes more forms of life possible and enables connections across kinds of experience and modes of communication. The dominant communicative forms that are enshrined as the basis for everyday life in the United States are not the only ones possible. Only by acknowledging that they do not work for everyone, and that they do not facilitate equal and universal participation—if such a thing is possible—can they be disrupted. If a politics of life and affective bioethics motivates the inclusive politics that must come in the wake of displacing the brain as a site of reductivism, then they necessarily depend on articulating forms of intimacy and facilitation that will disrupt existing norms—and be deeply unsettling to some who have strictly defined notions of the person, subjectivity, and their relationships to language and communication.

Stressing the epiphenomenal aspect of social interactions and facilitation focuses attention on the ordinary ethics of everyday interactions,[41] particularly as they are predicated on the immediate emotional connection between persons. Anthropologists have grown increasingly interested in how the ethical is enacted in everyday interactions, often with reliance on cultural norms about the good.[42] This attention to ethics and morality in ethnographic contexts obscures how emotion is socially constructed yet deeply felt.[43] Affective bioethics places emphasis on feeling and connection as opposed to the morally right or the good, both of which rely on cognitive registers that occlude visceral intimacies and everyday facilitation. Basing personhood and subjectivity on interdependent affective capacities and the ability to facilitate them in others moves away from cognitivist prejudices in conceptualizing the person and subject as embedded in neurological, symbolic, and material models of subjectivity—and reified in discourses of neurological disorder—and toward cybernetic copresence as captured in the haptic relations that make up the facilitating networks that persons exist within in their everyday lives. Ethical obligations in the epiphenomenal moment are in making lives livable and in facilitating affective connections between persons. This may mean weighing the kinds of affective connections that are being facilitated, but it is in the adjudication of these connections that the ethical emerges. Some connections may be privileged over others as based on cultural norms of emotionality as a marker of affective connection, but in moving away from the seemingly intrinsic value of individuals to the connective relations between individuals, regardless of their apparent cognitive capacities, a new regime of personhood and subjectivity might be developed to allow for more nonnormative ways of being in the world. In the United States, the emotions at the forefront of importance are love and grief, both of which draw attention to the interdependence individuals have on one another. Putting them at the center of an affective bioethics provides a means to sidestep neoliberal conceptions of value and quality of life and to emphasize interdependence and connection.

The fault of a bioethics focused on quality of life is that it places value as an intrinsic quality within individuals, which in turn is based on their capacities or lack thereof. Affective bioethics renders the question of quality of life extrinsic to the individual. What are the connections that are facilitated by and through the animation of an individual as a person and subject? In considering the Schiavo case, Adrienne Asch, a bioethicist who came out of the disability rights movement, suggests that intersubjective reciprocity is the standard by which decisions about life and death should be measured. She argues,

The typical advanced directive or living will does not ask the right questions. It asks what sort of medical intervention we want or don't want. The questions that we ought to be asked is what am I experiencing? What will make me feel that I have something to live for? What is enough? . . . As long as the people who know me believe that I recognize them and can differentiate them from strangers, I want to be alive.[44]

Compare Asch's guidelines to the findings of neurologist and bioethicist Dr. Ronald Cranford, who, on examining Terri, explains that

She didn't have consistent visual pursuit. She had a random movement at that time, or what we call a "primitive visual orienting reflex," where she could actually follow for a short period of time, but, first of all, that's not the same as visual pursuit, and second, the primitive visual orientating reflex is a brain stem mediated reflex. If that were in any way indicative of consciousness, then she would've done it much more repetitively and it would have been much more constant and reproducible.

Michael understands this as, "Terri's *eyes* were capable of seeing, even tracking an object briefly and inconsistently, but her brain was unable to understand what her eyes were seeing."[45] Terri can no longer recognize those in her social world. She can be connected with, but she cannot connect herself to others.

There is no normative standard to judge whether a person has robust connections, generative intimacies, and reciprocal relations with the persons who people their world; nor should there be. But the reliance on value as a marker of personhood and social belonging reifies the individual as the base unit of bioethical consideration, and doing so supports regimes that implicitly, and sometimes explicitly, rely on metrics of value for eugenic policies. Focus on the brain allows this sort of decision making: the brain's capacities are claimed to be measurable through emerging medical technologies as well as old tests of intelligence, sensory engagement, and social fluency and appropriateness. These metrics change over time, and if history is any indication, they are influenced less by objective knowledge about the brain and its capacities than by dominant social norms about kinds of people and modes of being in the world.[46] A more anthropological approach to bioethics provides a means to redevelop personhood and subjectivity as processes that are a function of reciprocal bonds and interactions between people, and also between individuals and their environments. Subjectivity might be seen as a wild, emergent process that depends less on the material capacities of an individual body and more on the interactive potentials individuals have with the world they exist within. This focuses bioethics on the world, not the individual, and provides a foundation for conceptualizing how personhood and subjectivity can be made differently through emergent forms of interpersonal and intermaterial connections and dependencies.

One avenue for this intervention is in reconceptualizing what composes the American family as a network. American social norms have long stressed the constitution of kinship through blood and custom, through hereditary and legal recognition.[47] Over the late twentieth century, anthropologists pointed to the elective forms of kinship that individuals have developed, largely as an effect of a sense of belonging to nonnormative communities.[48] Anthropologists have also pointed to the fraying traditional forms of custom in the face of normative forms of American kinship, particularly in the face of immigrant communities acceding to social norms in the United States.[49] Across this varied work, what becomes apparent is that kinship and the American family are arbitrary institutions. Biological ties are important in the United States, as are the institutional recognitions that make up contemporary society, but families are more than everyday human influences. American families might also be taken to include the varied technologies that comprise the web of everyday facilitations that enable social and environmental connections. American kinship is predicated on the histories of invention in the sciences, medicine, and engineering that have built ideas about human capacities into everyday technologies, including communication and entertainment technologies, the food Americans eat, the pharmaceuticals Americans consume, and the prosthetics that enable "normal" sensory and mobility capacities. Conceptualizing the family in this way expands obligations beyond immediate connections of blood and custom, toward the vast network of lives that are facilitated by the technologies that people invent, use, and naturalize as necessary for participation in everyday life in the United States. This more cybernetic view of the family helps draw attention to the historical indebtedness technologies have—how normative ideas about human capacities disable individuals and find remedies in prosthetic technologies, and how science and medicine have come to depend on neurological disorder as situated in the individual, all in an effort to reify the individual as a separable object of pathology, blame, and intervention. Affective bioethics, with its attention to the intimate connections that make and sustain life, offers an opportunity to consider the embedded ghostwriting that facilitating technologies—not just relations to kin and the law—depend on, and how they make some lives livable while disabling others. Simultaneous to this historical perspective is an emphasis on the immediacy of existing in the world together.

Subjunctive grief denotes the loss we will feel in the future,[50] an attempt to capture the sadness and mourning that comes with death. Future grief is inevitable. That grief may be the basis for a politics of care to come, a way into adjudicating what kinds of nervous systems are desirable to be a part of, of connecting with, and of making. It is in this context that I return to where this book began, with Bateson:

> Consider a blind man with a stick. Where does the blind man's self begin? At the tip of the stick? At the handle of the stick? Or at some point halfway up the stick? These questions are nonsense, because the stick is a pathway along which differences are transmitted under transformation, so that to draw a delimiting line *across* this pathway is to cut off a part of the systemic circuit which determines the blind man's locomotion.[51]

Connection, Bateson suggests, is only partially intentional; we are subject to the forces outside of us, the histories we are born into, the relationships that are given to us, and the ghostwritten technologies and interactions that facilitate us. If I have focused most of my attention on the first part of Bateson's remarks, it is worth considering closely what Bateson means by "draw[ing] a delimiting line *across* this pathway . . . to cut off a part of the systemic circuit." That line, that cut, is not merely ideological obfuscation. It is also potentially an act of destruction that renders a form of life difficult or impossible. To conceptualize our lives as systemic circuits made up of the wild connections that we choose and those that we do not helps put into perspective how complex our nervous systems are and what the stakes might be in losing something—a connection, a relationship, a person. Working with a future-oriented grief that imagines possibilities and seeks to enable worldly engagements helps us move beyond the world as it has been given and toward worlds of facilitation, animation, and connection.

Living and Dying in the Nervous System

*M*y father, Robert, died about a year and a half into my working on this project. He developed Alzheimer disease sometime in his seventies. It was always unclear to us as he was progressing into dementia whether it was hearing loss or senility, and, being a physician, the last thing he was about to do was seek the advice of another doctor. Instead, he slowly changed over the years, first full of raging outbursts, then eventually calmed by an uncomplicated appreciation for his everyday life. We had been functionally estranged for years leading up to his death; I lived far from home throughout my graduate studies and then throughout my early career, with only a year spent in nearby Detroit. Over the years we would have brief telephone conversations, largely mediated by my mother, usually consisting of updates in my progress on one project or another, discussions of the weather—cold in Minneapolis, warm in Santa Cruz—and the price of gas. When he would come to visit—usually once a year, sometimes less—it was always with my mother and for a short time: a long weekend to see what my life consisted of wherever I was living. By the time my partner and I had our first child, he could not really travel anymore; it was too difficult for my mother to manage him in airports and on airplanes. For me, his death was slow, then abrupt. His last years were spent in a residential facility, arranged by my half-siblings against my mother's wishes, and my last memories of him are sad and difficult.

The last time he had come with my mother to visit in California, we took a day trip to San Francisco from our home near Santa Cruz, a little over an hour in the car each way through the rolling hills that skirt Silicon Valley before descending to the Pacific Ocean. We spent the early afternoon at Fisherman's Wharf, having lunch and watching the ships moving through the bay. Not far off, and visible thanks to a clear summer sky, was Alcatraz, and we recalled a family trip to San Francisco when I was a young teenager and we spent days on the highway driving to Seattle, reading *To Kill a Mockingbird*. On the way back to Santa Cruz, my father sat next to me as I drove, slack-jawed and vacant in a way that he never had been in his earlier years, letting my conversation with my mother wash over him as we sped through the sun-bleached hills of Woodside and Palo Alto. That vacancy was crushing, in no small part because with it came the deep realization that there was no recovery for him, only a slow and steady descent into dementia, which, by the next time I saw him, had eclipsed whomever he had been.

I visited him one last time while he was living in a residential facility in Michigan; I had come home to visit my family in the cold winter months, bringing a coat I never wore in California. The facility was fine, if inconveniently located for my mother, who would drive to visit him multiple times each week, spending a couple hours with him and chatting with the staff who took care of him. By then he had no recognition of who I was, or likely my mother as well. He was gladdened to see us, to have visitors, to talk; he was always a social creature, which was a large part of his interest in practicing medicine. Yet we could have been anyone. He smiled and joked, ate a lunch he never would have previously, and seemed unperturbed when we left. How sad it felt to see him unbothered by the world he now inhabited, a man who, before the dementia had fully set in, had escaped multiple times from another residential facility. He was no longer the man I had grown up with, yet there was an underlying affability that was familiar and enduring. He died from complications related to pneumonia. My mother buried his ashes at the foot of a tree he had always liked, a silent, ghostly tribute that haunts her yard.

During these years, my partner and I raised our first child and then our second. What a joy to watch these little people—and their friends—emerge into themselves, come into language and communication. How estranging to be surrounded by life and death in such an intimate way. Children come into language so fitfully, learning a word at a time, blabbering the rest of what they are trying to communicate, sure that they make sense to the people around them, resolute in their use of protolanguage. And then they actually learn to communicate, to engage with their parents, friends, and strangers, and suddenly the world becomes a different place for everyone involved. But there are those children for whom language does not come easily; nor do the social norms associated with communication.

I will always think about two children in my first son's preschool, a little boy diagnosed with cerebral palsy and a little girl diagnosed with autism. The little boy had trouble communicating with the kids around him—kids he so wanted to connect with. His frustration would lead to outbursts, the kinds accepted for two- or three-year-olds but not for older children or adults. After being misunderstood or ignored, he would lash out with a fist or a classroom object. But when someone was on his level, making eye contact, listening, he could communicate with gestures, if not with words. The little girl was the opposite. She had difficulties listening to others, driven by some internal motor that was unapparent to those around her. When it was time to pick up the kids who spent a half day at school, I would sit with her at lunchtime, talking and looking at books together. She needed patient engagement, quiet and subtle facilitation, to emerge into playfulness. But it was never the playfulness of her truck-pushing, screaming peers on the playground. It was something that needed to be deliberately crafted, a game of words and pictures. Communication does not come in one form; nor is it an index of an individual's claim to personhood. Facilitating communication depends on recognizing that development into language is not a unitary, inevitable path but one that must be built for everyone who is treated as a person throughout the life course.

My father was forcibly placed in a residential care facility by my half-siblings in no small part because he was losing language, losing memory, and, by their account, losing his mind. It was not that he was becoming difficult to manage—he surely would have become so in one way or another—but rather that they preferred he be cared for in a facility rather than by my mother. How graceless to shuffle our elderly off to an institution when they lose language, yet we find endearing the communicative blunders and adventures of our children. Loss and the impossibility of return is hard to witness and to live with, but the promise of something emerging—something like a person—is enthralling. Another person to welcome into the social fold, to connect with, to care for and facilitate, to imagine a future with—what could be more alluring? Losing connections, becoming estranged through distance and death, is saddening, yet it is that grief that should motivate an affective bioethics. Acknowledging that lives are made together means accepting that there is no outside of connectivity, only its denial. Denying that connectivity, denying the necessary animation and facilitation that make persons of individuals and subjects of persons, is a false protection from the inevitable losses of living and dying in the nervous system we are all a part of.

Looming over the network of connections and intimacies each of us is facilitated through in our nervous systems are the sudden and subtle potentials for change. Some of these happen to us; others we bring into being. I dwell on this sense of contingency often, particularly in my relationship with my children. Iggy, now three and a half, has grown alongside this book and has influenced it in ways neither he nor I can fully imagine or realize. His speech has changed dramatically over the years, but is still peppered with Iggyisms like "hey day day" when he is seeking to fill a sentence with words that he does not know or cannot pronounce. My partner and I worry about the future he might have: the potential for bullying, the likelihood that he might have to be homeschooled as a result of institutional biases that disfavor his kind of impairment, the chance that he might have as yet unknown comorbidities. But we commit ourselves daily to his facilitation, to a means of animating each other and our family, and to making a robust nervous system of care providers, games, technologies, foods, and play that move us beyond conceptualizing Iggy's speech as disabled and the effect of an unruly brain. His brain may have some influence on his physiological experience, but to reduce his experience of self and the world to his brain is to draw a delimiting line and to ignore the social, symbolic, and material forces that shape him and us. That delimiting line might also serve the ideological function of protecting us from grief, of being able to reduce the experiences individuals have as merely the effect of biologically predetermined capacities and inter-actions with the world. But to do so is to ignore the complicity we all have in making and maintaining the world we exist within. The nervous system is open, full of potential, waiting to be explored, teeming with animacies. Grief may restrain us from making and acknowledging the connections that we have to the world, but it might also motivate engagements with a modular world of possibility.

ACKNOWLEDGMENTS

*I*n the course of writing this book, I have come to realize that some books are written in public while others are written in private. This is a private book. It gestated for years; it changed in unpredicted ways thanks to the many interventions people made along the way. Because so many of the interactions I have had around the content of this book have been through peer review of articles, grant applications, and the manuscript itself, I am indebted to a wide array of anonymous scholars who may always remain anonymous to me. I am grateful for their insights over the many forms this project has taken.

When I peeked out of my privacy, I benefited immensely from engaged audiences who contributed to my constant reworking of the materials and my arguments. My gratitude to audiences at the University of Minnesota's Institute for Advanced Study; the University of Washington's Cascadia Seminar; the Department of Anthropology, History, and Social Medicine at the University of California, San Francisco; the Center for Cultural Studies and the Ethnographic Engagements Workshop at the University of California, Santa Cruz; the University of Pennsylvania's Sorting Brains Out conference; the Department of Anthropology at Cornell University; the Dean's Speaker Series in the Department of Anthropology at Binghamton University; the Department of Anthropology at the University of Toronto; and the Neurological Imaginaries initiative at York University. The conversations that each of those presentations engendered were enormously beneficial to my continued work on *Unraveling* and its parts, and I regret being unable to name each and every audience member who raised a curious question or challenging point—but know that those questions live on in the text.

A special thanks to all of the friends and colleagues who took the time to engage with the book in whole or in part over its many years of incubation, in writing or based on presentations (some of whom may have forgotten doing so): Gretchen Bakke, Bruce Braun, Don Brenneis, Elana Buch, Nancy Chen, Jim Clifford, Samuel Collins, Nathaniel Dumas, Denielle Elliott, Michele Friedner, Jennifer Gunn, Susan Harding, Cassandra Hartblay, Jean Langford, Daniel Linger, Stephanie Lloyd, Paul Manning, John Marlovits, Seth Messinger, Matthew Moore, Eli Nadeau, Eugene Raikhel, Josh Reno, Lisa Rofel, Danilyn Rutherford, Todd Sanders, Karen-Sue Taussig, John Tresch, Nishita Trisal, Anna Tsing, and Ian Whitmarsh all raised the right questions at the right time. Throughout the research and writing process, I also benefited from the spirited engagement of many of my students, and the graduate students I have worked with at the University of California, Santa Cruz, and Binghamton University have been especially helpful. Foremost among them are Patricia Alvarez, Celina Callahan-Kapoor, Gabrielle Hanley-Mott, Elizabeth Hare, Laura Harrison, Katy Overstreet, and Samantha Turner.

Throughout the long journey that this book has taken, I have been buoyed by the support of the editorial team at the University of Minnesota Press, which enabled me to finish my first book and begin this book with a generous fellowship provided by the Mellon Foundation. Jason Weidemann deserves special acknowledgment for helping me navigate a sometimes tricky process of revision. The staff at the press all do amazing, careful work that I deeply appreciate. I couldn't ask for better support.

As always, I am indebted to my family, which provides the time and space to work things out as well as the everyday interactions that inspire me to want to work through the challenges that my work entails. During the research and writing of this book, I have watched my eldest son, Felix, grow into a spirited reader, making my writing of a book make a deeper sense to him (as I dropped him off at school today, he wished me a "good day sitting at my computer!"); meanwhile, his brother, Ignatius, has grown into a walking, talking, running, singing, dancing little chef. Both are lovely companions and reward careful parenting. No book about care would be complete without a thanks afforded to the many caregivers and teachers who cared for Felix and Iggy while I worked, and while I cannot thank them all by name, I appreciate all of their labor and dedication. I can, however, name our dedicated grandparents, Melanie Wolf and Deborah and Steve Martineau, who have all provided critical support of our family as we moved from west to east and resettled closer to our extended families.

My partner, Katherine, has been a constant source of encouragement and insight, and this book has taken the shape it has in no small part as a result of our conversations, mutual interests, and committed support to each other. My deepest gratitude extends to her and to the time and thought she has committed to helping me to make my work less private and more worldly.

NOTES

Preface

1. Merri Lisa Johnson and Robert McRuer, "Cripistemologies," *Journal of Literary and Cultural Disability Studies* 8, no. 2 (2014): 127–47.

2. Faye Ginsburg and Rayna Rapp, "Disability Worlds," *Annual Review of Anthropology* 42 (2013): 55.

Introduction

1. Nikolas Rose and Joelle Abi-Rached suggest that neuroscience as a unified field is a recent accomplishment, and that for most of the twentieth century there was a diverse field of actors who would later be seen as constructing an emergent neuroscience. Alongside this diversity in disciplinary approaches to neuroscience was the lack of a unified object of interest. The brain as an epistemic object was a late invention and depended on a variety of technological innovations to make it a concrete thing. *Neuro: The New Brain Sciences and the Management of the Mind* (Princeton, N.J.: Princeton University Press, 2013).

2. Psychiatry, psychology, and neuroscience are not fundamentally structuralist in the sense that they argue for transhistorical truths about humanity through recourse to myth or structures that make evident seemingly natural structures in the brain. Instead, following Mary Douglas, I am interested in how regimes of order and disorder are created in order to make sense of the abnormal through its categorization and efforts to act on it. *Purity and Danger* (1966; reprint, New York: Routledge, 2002).

3. The fundamental tenet of Spinoza's ethics is that there is one substance and that all perceivable phenomena are a mode of that substance. At its most theistic, that one substance is God, and all living and unliving things are expressions of the divine. A more secular reading, which Gilles Deleuze

offers, sees the one substance as the material stuff of the cosmos. In both cases, the ethical precept is to treat all things, both living and unliving, as extensions of oneself and as due the care and respect that one affords oneself. This inter-dependence contrasts with Cartesian assumptions that the body is merely a vessel for the mind, and that what happens to the body is less consequential than those actions that affect one's cognition. See Gilles Deleuze, *Spinoza: Practical Philosophy*, trans. Robert Hurley (San Francisco, Calif.: City Lights Books, 1988); Moira Gatens, *Imaginary Bodies: Ethics, Power and Corporeality* (New York: Routledge, 1996); Moira Gatens and Genevieve Lloyd, *Collective Imaginings: Spinoza, Past and Present* (New York: Routledge, 1999).

4. By bringing together the accounts of scientists—who are creating the categories of able-bodiedness, normalcy, and neurological order—with those of individuals and families diagnosed with neurological disorders, my goal is to treat these knowledge producers symmetrically, with neither having a claim to total knowledge. Instead, building on science and technology studies approaches to knowledge production, each is better understood as affected by the other, with doctors, scientists, and psychologists revising their theories in the face of individual and family experiences with disability, and individu-als and families viewing their experiences of neurological order and disorder through discourses provided to them by scientists, doctors, and psychologists. For discussions of symmetry in research design, see Barry Barnes, *Scientific Knowledge and Sociological Theory* (New York: Routledge, 1974); Bruno Latour, *We Have Never Been Modern*, trans. Catherine Porter (Cambridge, Mass.: Harvard University Press, 1993); Emily Martin, "Anthropology and the Cul-tural Study of Science: From Citadels to String Figures," in *Anthropologi-cal Locations: Boundaries and Grounds of a Field Science*, ed. Akhil Gupta and James Ferguson (Berkeley: University of California Press, 1997), 131–46.

5. For a comparative example that focuses on the overlapping and some-times contradictory approach to psychiatric personhood, see Tanya Luhr-mann, *Of Two Minds: An Anthropologist Looks at American Psychiatry* (New York: Vintage, 2000).

6. I use the term "disorder" rather than terms like "disease," "disability," "illness," and "sickness," each of which carries its own connotation. What is salient across these different ways of thinking about nonnormative experi-ences is that they are disruptive of ideas of order, both in the sense of an individual's fit into the expectations of others and in the sense of an individ-ual's self-conception. "Disability" is often construed as a lack of capacity—for example, a missing limb, or an inability to speak or hear. As disability studies scholars have established, these are lacks predicated on a social order that

normalizes some ways of being in the world and that marks other forms as pathological or abnormal, referred to as the "social model of disability," following Tom Shakespeare, "The Social Model of Disability," in *The Disability Studies Reader*, ed. Lennard Davis (New York: Routledge, 2010), 266–73.

Moreover, as Tobin Seibers has argued in *Disability Theory* (Ann Arbor: University of Michigan Press, 2008), "disability" has increasingly become a term used within rights-seeking social movements that are identitarian in their efforts to signal how dominant social orders produce particular experiences of the world as disabling and specific individuals as disabled. "Disease" assumes normal physiological development and homeostasis. At its worst, "disease" conceptualizes conditions like dwarfism as pathologies in need of medical intervention rather than part of human biological variation, a view critiqued by Georges Canguilhem in *The Normal and the Pathological*, trans. Carolyn R. Fawcett (New York: Zone Books, 1991). As much as they are words in popular use, "sickness" and "illness" are terms social scientists use to designate the societal effects of disease and its subjective experience, respectively; see Arthur Kleinman, *The Illness Narratives: Suffering, Healing, and the Human Condition* (New York: Basic Books, 1988); Nancy Scheper-Hughes and Margaret Lock, "The Mindful Body: A Prolegomenon to Future Work in Medical Anthropology," *Medical Anthropology Quarterly* 1, no. 1 (1987): 6–41; Allan Young, "The Anthropologies of Illness and Sickness," *Annual Review of Anthropology* 11 (1982): 257–85. Neurological disorders fit into all of these categories simultaneously, but their most important feature is that they are disorderly. This disorder is predicated on the behaviors that individuals exhibit: nonnormative modes of communicating or the inability to communicate altogether, lack of social awareness and etiquette, friction between institutional expectations and individual action, and misalignment of metrics of evaluation and the capacities of individuals. Disorder is multifarious and is predicated on the orders that have been created to govern individuals, their relationships, and the institutions of everyday life. On discipline and institutional order, see Michel Foucault, *Discipline and Punish: The Birth of the Prison*, trans. Alan Sheridan (New York: Vintage, 1995).

7. Over the past decade there has been a boom in social studies of autism, ranging across the social sciences and humanities. Although there is no consensus as to how autism is being approached by scholars, it is clear that the underlying politics of attending to autism in the present moment is motivated by an interest in demonstrating the complex social worlds that the category of autism has created for individuals diagnosed with autism, their caregivers and kin, and the scientists and physicians who have specialized in the

etiology, diagnosis, and treatment of autism and related concerns. See Anita Broderick and Ari Ne'eman, "Autism as Metaphor: Narrative and Counternarrative," *International Journal of Inclusive Education* 12 (2008): 459–76; Gil Eyal et al., *The Autism Matrix* (Malden, Mass.: Polity, 2010); Des Fitzgerald, *Tracing Autism: Uncertainty, Ambiguity, and the Affective Labor of Neuroscience* (Seattle: University of Washington Press, 2017); Roy Richard Grinker, *Unstrange Minds: Remapping the World of Autism* (New York: Basic Books, 2006); Brendan Hart, "Autism Parents and Neurodiversity: Radical Translation, Joint Embodiment and the Prosthetic Environment," *BioSocieties* 9, no. 3 (2014): 284–303; Anne McGuire, *War on Autism: On the Cultural Logic of Normative Violence* (Ann Arbor: University of Michigan Press, 2016); Chloe Silverman, *Understanding Autism: Parents, Doctors, and the History of a Disorder* (Princeton, N.J.: Princeton University Press, 2013); Jennifer Singh, *Multiple Autisms: Spectrums of Advocacy and Genomic Science* (Minneapolis: University of Minnesota Press, 2015); Melanie Yergeau, *Authoring Autism: On Rhetoric and Neurological Queerness* (Durham, N.C.: Duke University Press, 2017). Additionally, there has been a recent growth of interest in the social study of dementia and Alzheimer disease, in part driven by the experiences of care that scholars have had in supporting aging parents. See Lawrence Cohen, *No Aging in India: Alzheimer's, the Bad Family, and Other Modern Things* (Berkeley: University of California Press, 1998); Margaret Lock, *The Alzheimer Conundrum: Entanglements of Dementia and Aging* (Princeton, N.J.: Princeton University Press, 2015); Janelle Taylor, "On Recognition, Caring, and Dementia," *Medical Anthropology Quarterly* 22, no. 4 (2008): 313–35.

8. There is a robust body of scholarship focused on schizophrenia, hysteria, and depression, largely in the context of psychiatry in the United States. Across this literature, there has been a long-standing interest in demonstrating how these psychiatric categories are differentially applied along lines of class, race, ethnicity, gender, and sexuality, often compounding perceived differences among groups by associating women with anxiety and depression, black men with schizophrenia, and members of the lower classes with susceptibilities to mental illness that might be accounted for by attending to their lived environments and the effects it has on individuals, families, and communities. See David Healy, *Let Them Eat Prozac: The Unhealthy Relationship between the Pharmaceutical Industry and Depression* (New York: New York University Press, 2006); Emily Martin, *Bipolar Expeditions: Mania and Depression in American Culture* (Princeton, N.J.: Princeton University Press, 2007); Jonathan M. Metzl, *Prozac on the Couch: Prescribing Gender in the Era of Wonder Drugs* (Durham, N.C.: Duke University Press, 2003); Jonathan Metzl,

The Protest Psychosis: How Schizophrenia Became a Black Disease (Boston, Mass.: Beacon Press, 2011).

9. Walter Freeman and James Watts, *Psychosurgery* (Oxford: Charles C. Thomas, 1942); Jack Pressman, *Last Resort: Psychosurgery and the Limits of Medicine* (Cambridge: Cambridge University Press, 1998).

10. For a discussion of the diagnostic criteria of autism, with a particular focus on social meaning, see Simon Baron-Cohen, *Mindblindness: An Essay on Autism and Theory of Mind* (Cambridge, Mass.: MIT Press, 1997). For a comparative perspective from someone diagnosed with autism, see Temple Grandin and Sean Barron, *Unwritten Rules of Social Relationships: Decoding Social Mysteries through Autism's Unique Perspective*, ed. Veronica Zysk (Arlington, Tex.: Future Horizons, 2005).

11. Roman Jakobson, "Two Aspects of Language and Two Types of Aphasic Disturbances," in *On Language*, ed. Linda Waugh and Monique Monville-Burston (Cambridge, Mass.: Harvard University Press, 1995), 115–33.

12. The field of deaf studies has a long tradition. Many contributors to deaf studies have personal experiences with deafness, either being deaf themselves or being kin to deaf persons. Approaches have varied, but a consistent set of themes across the literature points to how alternative forms of communication, such as American Sign Language, provide members of the deaf community with a means of communication at least equivalent to spoken language. However, for aural communicators, nonauditory means of communication are derided, and deafness is a seen as a medical problem in need of treatment. For a variety of perspectives on deafness in the United States, see H-Dirksen Bauman and Joseph Murray, eds., *Deaf Gain: Raising the Stakes for Human Diversity* (Minneapolis: University of Minnesota Press, 2014); Brenda Brueggemann and Susan Burch, eds., *Double Visions: Women and Deafness* (Washington, D.C.: Gallaudet University Press, 2006); Lennard Davis, *Enforcing Normalcy: Disability, Deafness, and the Body* (New York: Verso, 1995).

13. Lennard Davis has argued that the origins of "normal" lie in the nineteenth century with the rise of statistical thinking and the ability to construct a norm based on the averaging of human experiences and capacities. He compares the rise of the norm to that of the ideal, which he suggests was a dominant mode of thinking before the rise of normalcy; with ideals, everyone falls short. But with norms, those who are unable to meet the standard expectations of normalcy are in danger of being perceived as disabled. With norms guiding medical practice, disabled bodies are provided with therapies, prosthetics, surgeries, or pharmaceuticals in an effort to make them normal. This view of disability is deeply influenced by Michel Foucault's conception

of disciplinary institutions and their basis in biopolitical governance, which is itself dependent on the rise of quantitative thinking in the eighteenth and nineteenth centuries. See Davis, *Enforcing Normalcy*; Michel Foucault, *Abnormal: Lectures at the Collège de France, 1974–1975*, trans. Graham Burchell (New York: Picador, 2003); Michel Foucault, *The History of Sexuality*, vol. 1, *The History of Sexuality*, trans. Robert Hurley (New York: Vintage, 1990).

14. Alessandro Duranti and Charles Goodwin, eds., *Rethinking Context: Language as an Interactive Phenomenon* (Cambridge: Cambridge University Press, 1992).

15. Dorothy Cheney and Robert Seyfarth, *Baboon Metaphysics: The Evolution of a Social Mind* (Chicago: University of Chicago Press, 2008); W. Tecumseh Fitch, "Unity and Diversity in Human Language," *Philosophical Transactions of the Royal Society B: Biological Sciences* 366, no. 1563 (2011): 376–88.

16. Susan Gal, "Language Ideologies Compared," *Journal of Linguistic Anthropology* 15, no. 1 (2005): 23–37; Susan Gal and Judith Irvine, "Language Ideology and Linguistic Differentiation," in *Regimes of Language*, ed. Paul Kroskrity (Santa Fe, N.M.: School for American Research, 2000), 35–84; Michael Silverstein, "Language Structure and Linguistic Ideology," in *The Elements: A Parasession on Linguistic Units and Levels*, ed. R. Cline, W. Hanks, and C. Hofbauer (Chicago: Chicago Linguistic Society, 1979), 193–247; Michael Silverstein and Greg Urban, eds., *Natural Histories of Discourse* (Chicago: University of Chicago Press, 1996).

17. Charles Goodwin, "A Competent Speaker Who Can't Speak: The Social Life of Aphasia," *Journal of Linguistic Anthropology* 14, no. 2 (2004): 151–70; E. Mara Green, "One Language, or Maybe Two: Direct Communication, Understanding, and Informal Interpreting in International Deaf Encounters," in *It's a Small World: International Deaf Spaces and Encounters*, ed. Michele Friedner and Annalies Kusters (Washington D.C.: Gallaudet University Press, 2015), 70–82; John B. Haviland, "(Mis)Understanding and Obtuseness: 'Ethnolinguistic Borders' in a Miniscule Speech Community," *Journal of Linguistic Anthropology* 23, no. 3 (2013): 160–91; Erika Hoffmann-Dilloway, *Signing and Belonging in Nepal* (Washington D.C.: Gallaudet University Press, 2016).

18. Gregory Bateson, *Steps to an Ecology of Mind: Collected Essays in Anthropology, Psychiatry, Evolution, and Epistemology* (Chicago: University of Chicago Press, 2000); Jurgen Ruesch and Gregory Bateson, *Communication: The Social Matrix of Psychology* (New Brunswick, N.J.: Transaction Publishers, 2008).

19. Alessandro Duranti, *The Anthropology of Intentions: Language in a World of Others* (Cambridge: Cambridge University Press, 2015).

20. Harold Garfinkel, *Studies in Ethnomethodology* (Malden, Mass.: Blackwell, 1984).

21. Anthropologists have long explored models of personhood that do not accord with North Atlantic traditions of the rational individual as enshrined in liberalism. Among anthropologists who have conducted fieldwork in South Asia and Melanesia, the idea of the corporeally bound individual did not seem to explain how persons were constituted. See McKim Marriott, "Hindu Transactions: Diversity without Dualism," in *Transaction and Meaning: Directions in the Anthropology of Exchange and Symbolic Behavior*, ed. Bruce Kapferer (Philadelphia, Pa.: Institute for the Study of Human Issues, 1976), 109–42; Marilyn Strathern, *Reproducing the Future: Anthropology, Kinship, and the New Reproductive Technologies* (New York: Routledge, 1992). As David Armstrong has argued in *A New History of Identity: A Sociology of Medical Knowledge* (New York: Palgrave, 2002), over the course of the eighteenth and nineteenth centuries, the individual was increasingly understood as bound by the skin as an effect of how medicine and science conceived of disease, with disease lying within a body. This leads to the widespread ideology of overcoming one's body-boundedness in romantic connections, losing a sense of self through the production of a new shared identity. But in South Asia and Melanesia, such boundedness was not readily apparent. Instead, individuals were seen as intimately connected and indissociable because of their connections through substances like shared food, blood, and semen. Marriott referred to this as "dividuality" in an attempt to draw attention to how the logic of personhood built on an idea of the body, but inverted the North Atlantic traditions of divisibility at birth, instead suggesting that the onus of creating individual personhood was something that motivated action through one's life. Separating from one's natal family depends on sharing substances with other possible kin networks and thereby creating distance and difference from one's natal family and alliances with new possible kin. In both frames—that of North Atlantic individuality and South Asian and Melanesian dividuality—personhood is ascribed by those in one's social world. Far from being an intrinsic capacity of the individual, personhood is something that is attained through cultural logics of value. In societies where infant mortality is high, personhood may rely on attaining a certain age, which may be possible only through recognition on the part of parents that a child will be able to thrive, as discussed by Nancy Scheper-Hughes, "Culture, Scarcity, and Maternal Thinking: Maternal Detachment and Infant Survival in a Brazilian Shantytown," *Ethos* 13, no. 4 (1985): 291–317. A child lacking in this perceived potential may have resources withdrawn, leaving the child to die or to prove a capacity to thrive,

and thereby to earn status as a person. In the U.S. context, personhood—as recognized by the state—has long been predicated on racial and gendered logics, with the Three-Fifths Compromise asserting that slaves counted as less than a full person, and suffrage and civil rights movements bestowing on women and black individuals state-recognized full personhood. At the level of interpersonal interaction, anthropologists have shown how dominant ideas about independence in the United States are fraught with attempts to deny the interdependence that makes American individualism possible, from the avoidance of conflict to the obscuring of caregiving for children and elders. These state-based and interpersonal systems of attributing personhood have consequences for social recognition and rights, and also for the development of identity and subjectivity. See Elana D. Buch, *Inequalities of Aging: Paradoxes of Independence in American Home Care* (New York: New York University Press, 2018); Carol Greenhouse, "Signs of Quality: Individualism and Hierarchy in American Culture," *American Ethnologist* 19, no. 2 (1992): 233–54.

22. Faye Ginsburg, *Contested Lives: The Abortion Debate in an American Community* (Berkeley: University of California Press, 1998); Rayna Rapp, *Testing Women, Testing the Fetus: A Social History of Amniocentesis in America* (New York: Routledge, 1999); Janelle Taylor, *The Public Life of the Fetal Sonogram: Technology, Consumption, and the Politics of Reproduction* (New Brunswick, N.J.: Rutgers University Press, 2008).

23. In her study of intellectual impairments and their role in political theory, Stacy Simplican argues that the liberal tradition has depended on the differentiation between those with full cognitive capacities and those with partial or impaired cognition. The implicit—and sometimes explicit—comparison between individuals with full capacities for deliberation and self-determination and those who are seen as lacking those qualities has provided the basis for the inclusion of some kinds of persons in the social contract and the disenfranchisement of others. Simplican, *The Capacity Contract: Intellectual Disability and the Question of Citizenship*.

24. Anthropologists have long been interested in the process of enculturation—that is, the way that children are brought into a cultural system of knowledge and practice. The guiding assumption of much of that literature is that a child will unproblematically be able to adapt to the social expectations of those in his or her social world and will slowly accommodate their desires. In cases where this transition to social norms does not occur, a child might be seen as disorderly in some culturally prescribed way. See Kathleen Barlow, "Attachment and Culture in Murik Society: Learning Autonomy and Interdependence through Kinship, Food, and Gender," in *Attachment Reconsidered:*

Cultural Perspectives on a Western Theory, ed. Naomi Quinn and Jeanette Marie Mageo (New York: Palgrave Macmillan, 2013), 165–88; Jean Briggs, *Never in Anger: Portrait of an Eskimo Family* (Cambridge, Mass.: Harvard University Press, 1971); Paul Riesman, *First Find Your Child a Good Mother: The Construction of Self in Two African Communities* (New Brunswick, N.J.: Rutgers University, 1992).

25. A Roschian approach to personhood might provide the basis for this kind of model. In Roschian prototype theory, which shares similarities with Lennard Davis's discussion of ideals, a prototype serves as the basis for judging the proximity of any thing to its category. For example, in the category "furniture," there are a wide variety of possible things; a chair more closely resembles the prototype of furniture than a stool, yet neither is the ideal form of furniture simply because there is no actual ideal. See Eleanor Rosch, "Cognitive Representations of Semantic Categories," *Journal of Experimental Psychology: General* 104, no. 3 (1975): 192–233. Adopting such an approach—with the caveat that there is the danger of a cisgendered, white, able-bodied man becoming the prototypic person—allows for the possibility of thinking of persons as always not being full persons. All persons strive to be ideal persons, but the ideal is perpetually elusive.

26. Emile Benveniste, "Subjectivity in Language," in *Problems in General Linguistics*, trans. Mary Elizabeth Meek (Coral Gables, Fla.: University of Miami Press, 1973), 223–30.

27. Lorna Rhodes, "Changing the Subject: Conversation in Supermax," *Cultural Anthropology* 20, no. 3 (2005): 388–411; Lorna A. Rhodes, *Total Confinement: Madness and Reason in the Maximum Security Prison* (Berkeley: University of California Press, 2004).

28. Donna Haraway postulates an ethics of touch in her consideration of interspecies relationships, in which the primary ethical call is for the obligation of copresence, of collective stewardship. Haraway, *When Species Meet* (Minneapolis: University of Minnesota Press, 2008).

29. Medicalization is the process whereby what was once taken to be natural is accepted as pathological and in need of medical intervention. Medicalization serves the capitalist interests of pharmaceutical industries and fee-collecting physicians, but it also serves as a means to control populations through medical surveillance and the view of resistance to medicalization as noncompliance. Scholars have nuanced this approach in conceptualizing biomedicalization, which has been driven by emergent technologies in and out of the laboratory, leading to an increased foothold of medical rationalities in conceiving individual and collective lives. See Adele Clarke et al., eds.,

Biomedicalization: Technoscience, Health, and Illness in the U.S. (Durham, N.C.: Duke University Press, 2010); Peter Conrad, *The Medicalization of Society: On the Transformation of Human Conditions into Treatable Disorders* (Baltimore, Md.: Johns Hopkins University Press, 2007).

30. Michel Foucault aligned the rise of disciplinary institutions—the hospital, the asylum, the factory, the barracks, the school, and the prison—with modernity in the North Atlantic, and particularly in France. For Foucault and scholars following in his way of thinking, institutions are guided by norms that are used to shape the behaviors of those who interact with them. If a student performs badly in school, he or she may be recommended for medical treatment to become "normal." If that treatment proves insufficient, then the student may find him- or herself imprisoned or conscripted by the army, all in an effort to recuperate the individual into the productive mainstream of society. Inasmuch as these institutions continue to shape the landscape of U.S. everyday life, the question persists as to whether they are guided by a singular, shared understanding of normal or whether there are emergent, sometimes conflicting expectations of what a person should be and how she or he should be treated. See Foucault, *History of Sexuality*; Michel Foucault, *The Birth of the Clinic: An Archaeology of Medical Perception*, trans. A. M. Sheridan Smith (New York: Vintage, 1994); Foucault, *Discipline and Punish*.

31. Following from Carol Gilligan's intervention into thinking about differences between how American men and women experience their relationships with social others, "care" has become a central concern for social scientists, particularly in relation to aging, child-rearing, health and illness, and disability. Berenice Fisher and Joan Tronto have suggested that "caring be viewed as a species activity that includes everything that we do to maintain, continue, and repair our 'world' so that we can live in it as well as possible. That world includes our bodies, our selves, and our environment, all of which we seek to interweave in a complex, life-sustaining web." Fisher and Tronto, "Toward a Feminist Theory of Caring," in *Circles of Care: Work and Identity in Women's Lives*, ed. Emily Abel and Margaret Nelson (Albany: State University of New York Press, 1990), 43. Tronto has extended this analysis to the study of institutions, arguing that the implicit features of the family be made explicit in institutions that seek to provide care. Tronto, "Creating Caring Institutions: Politics, Plurality, and Purpose," *Ethics and Social Welfare* 4, no. 2 (2010): 158–71. Recently anthropologists have become especially interested in thinking through how care operates differentially—and sometimes in unsettling fashion—between communities with dramatically varied expectations of what care looks like, who it is for, and how it lays the basis for social relations

within and between communities. Central to this literature is awareness that care networks are necessarily interdependent and that individuals mark their interdependence through their care relations. However, in some cases, care relations serve to obscure the interdependence between persons and those who care for them; this is especially the case in contexts where independence is idealized. See, e.g., Buch, *Inequalities of Aging*; Angela Garcia, *The Pastoral Clinic: Addiction and Dispossession along the Rio Grande* (Berkeley: University of California Press, 2010); Carol Gilligan, *In a Different Voice: Psychological Theory and Women's Development* (Cambridge, Mass.: Harvard University Press, 1983); Neely Myers, *Recovery's Edge: An Ethnography of Mental Health Care and Moral Agency* (Memphis, Tenn.: Vanderbilt University Press, 2015); Akemi Nishida, "Relating through Differences: Disability, Affective Relationality, and the U.S. Public Healthcare Assemblage," *Subjectivity* 10, no. 1 (2017): 89–103; Denise Spitzer, "In Visible Bodies: Minority Women, Nurses, Time, and the New Economy of Care," *Medical Anthropology Quarterly* 18, no. 4 (2004): 490–508.

32. Simplican, *Capacity Contract.*

33. Interdependence is central to many disability studies' critiques of U.S. society, often focusing on how the independent individual is the norm but is only possible through the existence of a broad network of other individuals who care in direct and indirect ways for that individual and provide her or him with an infrastructure of support through which independence can be realized. See Alison Kafer, *Feminist, Queer, Crip* (Bloomington: Indiana University Press, 2013); Eva Kittay, *Love's Labor: Essays on Women, Equality, and Dependency* (New York: Routledge, 1998); Mia Mingus, "Access Intimacy, Interdependence and Disability Justice," Leaving Evidence (blog), April 12, 2017, https://leavingevidence.wordpress.com/. One of the challenges with discussions of interdependence is recognizing the nature of the network of care, which can be built on systemic injustices and inequalities, depending on the care of some for others, often without recognition or through the naturalization of care work as a capacity of particular kinds of people—for example, mothers or women. On this, see Buch, *Inequalities of Aging*; Simplican, *Capacity Contract.*

34. For a discussion of facilitated communication, see Douglas Biklen and Donald Cardinal, eds., *Contested Words, Contested Science: Unraveling the Facilitated Communication Controversy* (New York: Teachers College Press, 1997); for a critique of facilitated communication, see Diane Twachtman-Cullen, *A Passion to Believe: Autism and the Facilitated Communication Phenomenon* (Boulder, Colo.: Westview Press, 1997).

35. Don Kulick and Jens Rydstrom, *Loneliness and Its Opposite: Sex, Disability, and the Ethics of Engagement* (Durham, N.C.: Duke University Press, 2015).

36. Deleuze, *Spinoza*; Gatens, *Imaginary Bodies*; Gatens and Lloyd, *Collective Imaginings*.

37. Marilyn Strathern, "Cutting the Network," *Journal of the Royal Anthropological Institute* 2, no. 3 (1996): 517–35.

38. For complementary theories of animation derived from video games, literature, and art, see Sianne Ngai, *Ugly Feelings* (Cambridge, Mass.: Harvard University Press, 2007); Teri Silvio, "Animation: The New Performance?," *Journal of Linguistic Anthropology* 20, no. 2 (2010): 422–38. Like Ngai and Silvio, I share an interest in the affective qualities of animation, and I similarly focus on media as the means through which individuals come to be animated. However, my focus is on the contextual quality of the theory, derived as it is from the experience of families that rely on media to form the basis for reciprocal relationships. Although potentially intensified in our hypermediated present, my conception of animation is a basis for all human sociality, suggesting that animating institutions and media are necessary corollaries for the ascription of personhood and development of subjectivity.

39. New materialism attempts to resituate ontological conceptions of the world in a robust materialism that draws from a diversity of philosophical and scientific approaches. A core tenet to these approaches is that the world is vibrant and has material effects on human life in seen and unseen ways; human misrecognition of the material determinants of agency and life obscures the powers that organic and inorganic matter have on human societies and knowledge practices. See Karen Barad, *Meeting the Universe Halfway: Quantum Physics and the Entanglement of Matter and Meaning* (Durham, N.C.: Duke University Press, 2007); Jane Bennett, *Vibrant Matter: A Political Ecology of Things* (Durham, N.C.: Duke University Press, 2010); Diana Coole and Samantha Frost, *New Materialisms: Ontology, Agency, and Politics* (Durham, N.C.: Duke University Press, 2010).

40. Reading Norbert Elias's *The Civilizing Process*, trans. Edmund Jephcott (Malden, Mass.: Blackwell, 2000), alongside Roger Caillois's "Mimicry and Legendary Psychesthenia," *October* 31 (1984): 17–32, points to the interplay between mimicry and socialization. For Elias, the process of socialization— whereby an individual comes to inhabit the social norms of a society—is one that is steadily reinforced through social pressure, both from peers and from those in power. In time, a child will limit antisocial activities and come to fit into society with little or no friction associated with the functional care of

the self. For Caillois, mimicry serves as a means of camouflage, particularly for nonhuman animals that are able to blend into their environment through formal qualities of their appearance. But socialization is a form of mimicry too, leading children to mimic their peers and elders to meet social norms, to camouflage themselves as "normal" within a given society. The inability to mimic in these ways can mark a child as aberrant and in need of discipline. For another approach to mimicry and its social function, see Michael Taussig, *Mimesis and Alterity: A Particular History of the Senses* (New York: Routledge, 1993).

41. At the heart of Judith Butler's understanding of subjectivity is the performance of the self, a process wherein individuals respond to the institutionalized expectations of identity and inhabit scripted roles. This performance can be subverted in deliberate and accidental ways in an effort to disrupt these expectations and scripts. But fundamentally this performative conception of subjectivity is based on a system of recognition whereby institutions and institutional actors legitimate claims to subjectivity—and by extension personhood—on the part of individuals who uphold expectations of the subject. This conception of subjectivity depends on a deliberate, cognitively "normal" individual who responds to institutional imperatives appropriately; such a view fails to include individuals for whom such performances are difficult or impossible. See *The Psychic Life of Power: Theories in Subjection* (Stanford, Calif.: Stanford University Press, 1997); *Gender Trouble: Feminism and the Subversion of Identity* (New York: Routledge, 1999); *Giving an Account of Oneself* (New York: Fordham University Press, 2005).

42. For discussion of the disability rights movements in the United States, see Sharon Barnartt and Richard Scotch, *Disability Protests: Contentious Politics, 1970–1999* (Washington, D.C.: Gallaudet University Press, 2001); Doris Z. Fleischer and Freida Zames, *The Disability Rights Movement: From Charity to Confrontation* (Philadelphia, Pa.: Temple University Press, 2011). Earlier waves of disability activism targeted accessibility, specifically making the shared built environment of sidewalks, buildings, and homes accessible to individuals with motor (and in some cases sensory) impairments. See Aimi Hamraie, *Building Access: Universal Design and the Politics of Disability* (Minneapolis: University of Minnesota Press, 2017). Over time, disability rights has come to focus more on nonnormative cognitive styles, sometimes under the banner of neurodiversity, in an effort to create more inclusive social policies and spaces for individuals seen as having a neurological disorder. See, e.g., Thomas Armstrong, *Neurodiversity: Exploring the Extraordinary Gifts of Autism, ADHD, Dyslexia, and Other Brain Differences* (Cambridge, Mass.: Da Capo, 2010); Steve Silberman,

Neurotribes: The Legacy of Autism and the Future of Neurodiversity (New York: Avery, 2015). For responses to neurodiversity by individuals who identify as autistic, see Julia Bascom, ed., *Loud Hands: Autistic People, Speaking* (Washington D.C.: Autistic Press, 2012).

43. In a pair of pieces on so-called control societies, Gilles Deleuze suggests that the normative disciplinary institutions of modernity have given way to more partial, disconnected, and localized societies that seek to control individuals through fragmentary conceptions of norms. A workplace may demand one norm, a family may demand another, a school yet a third. The individual is left to respond in each of those contexts with appropriate behaviors, and the failure to meet expectations can result in negative consequences. The result is that individuals are left to discern the demands placed on them and must respond appropriately or risk losing access to social connections. See Deleuze, *Negotiations*, trans. Martin Joughin (New York: Columbia University Press, 1995).

44. I discuss La Borde at length in chapter 2. L'Arche is an experimental community created by Jean Vanier that has homes around the world. Shared homes are composed of able-bodied and disabled individuals who support one another in an effort to sidestep the client–caregiver relationship and develop a more egalitarian and mutually reciprocal partnership. For a discussion from Vanier, see *From Brokenness to Community* (Mahwah, N.J.: Paulist Press, 1992). For a recent ethnographic approach to L'Arche, see Patrick McKearney, "Receiving the Gift of Cognitive Disability: Recognizing Agency in the Limits of the Rational Subject," *Cambridge Journal of Anthropology* 37, no. 1 (2018): 40–60.

45. I coined the term "multibiologism" in *The Slumbering Masses: Sleep, Medicine, and Modern American Life* (Minneapolis: University of Minnesota Press, 2012). Multibiologism was an attempt to conceptualize an ethics of inclusion that built on an understanding that some biological human variation could be accepted as difference without being treated as pathological and in need of medical intervention. In *The Slumbering Masses*, the motivating case was the diversity of human sleep, with biphasic sleep often being seen as a pathology (e.g., insomnia) and in need of pharmaceutical treatment. Instead, social arrangements could be made to allow for nonnormative sleep patterns, which would also disrupt the disciplinary and controlling nature of everyday institutions. Rather than see these variations of human experience as rooted in stable understandings of biology, human biology itself should be conceptualized as an immanent field subject to sociotechnical shaping. See also Matthew

Wolf-Meyer, "'Human Nature' and the Biology of Everyday Life," *American Anthropologist* 121, no. 2 (2019): 338–49.

46. David Harvey has argued that the neoliberalization of the economy and property occurred alongside the Thatcher and Reagan governments in the United Kingdom and the United States in his *Brief History of Neoliberalism* (Oxford: Oxford University Press, 2005). For Harvey, neoliberalism serves as an economic principle as well as a cultural dominant in the North Atlantic, from which it begins to circulate globally. Because of the long-standing cultural emphasis on the individual and individuality in the United Kingdom and the United States, neoliberalism develops in locally specific ways that favor the interests of corporations and the wealthy. As neoliberal discourses and practices enter other geographic spaces, however, its logics are subject to local traditions of politics, economics, and culture. See Jean Comaroff and John L. Comaroff, eds., *Millennial Capitalism and the Culture of Neoliberalism* (Durham, N.C.: Duke University Press, 2001).

47. The neoliberalism literature is diverse when it comes to how neoliberal discourses affect processes of subjectivity, but its approach to the individual shares a conception of self-interest and market calculations as being the fundamental change in subjectivity as a result of transformations in the management of the global, national, and local economies that favor privatization and financialization over earlier models of liberalism. See Ilana Gershon, "Un-friend My Heart: Facebook, Promiscuity, and Heartbreak in a Neoliberal Age," *Anthropological Quarterly* 84, no. 4 (2011): 865–94; Emily Martin, *Flexible Bodies: Tracking Immunity in American Culture—From the Days of Polio to the Age of AIDS* (Boston, Mass.: Beacon Press, 1994); Nikolas Rose, *The Politics of Life Itself: Biomedicine, Power, and Subjectivity in the Twenty-First Century* (Princeton, N.J.: Princeton University Press, 2006).

48. Liberalism in genomics and neuroscience can be seen in the ways that pathologies are ascribed to individual bodies through the metonymic relationship between one's body and one's medical disorder. This moves away from conceptions of disease as being the result of social or environmental factors and helps to obscure the social determinants of disease, especially among poor and marginalized communities. Moreover, this liberal emphasis leads to discourses of noncompliance and precision medicine, both of which assume that the individual is a lone actor and either the sole cause of a treatment's failure or the only necessary site of medical intervention. See Duana Fullwiley, *The Enculturated Gene: Sickle Cell Health Politics and Biological Difference in West Africa* (Princeton, N.J.: Princeton University Press, 2011); Susan McKinnon,

Neo-liberal Genetics: The Myths and Moral Tales of Evolutionary Psychology (Chicago: Prickly Paradigm Press, 2006); Michael J. Montoya, *Making the Mexican Diabetic: Race, Science, and the Genetics of Inequality* (Berkeley: University of California Press, 2011); Rose and Abi-Rached, *Neuro*.

49. Harry Triandis, *Individualism and Collectivism* (Boulder, Colo.: Westview Press, 1995).

50. Charles Taylor, *Hegel and Modern Society* (Cambridge: Cambridge University Press, 1979).

51. Human rights discourses are often based on a universal humanism that argues for the value in all human life, regardless of historical context. In this way, human rights discourses have been essential to the well-being of individuals and communities in the twentieth and early twenty-first centuries. But human rights discourses have recently been critiqued as exclusionary and harmful, embedded as they are in nineteenth-century ideas of humanism. For a variety of perspectives, particularly in the context of health, see Paul Farmer, *Pathologies of Power: Health, Human Rights, and the New War on the Poor* (Berkeley: University of California Press, 2003); Makau Mutua, *Human Rights: A Political and Cultural Critique* (Philadelphia: University of Pennsylvania Press, 2013); Miriam Ticktin, "Where Ethics and Politics Meet: The Violence of Humanitarianism in France," *American Ethnologist* 33, no. 1 (2006): 33–49.

52. Benedicte Boisseron, *Afro-Dog: Blackness and the Animal Question* (New York: Columbia University Press, 2018); Megan Glick, *Infrahumanisms: Science, Culture, and the Making of Modern Non-personhood* (Durham, N.C.: Duke University Press, 2018).

53. For Norbert Elias, the civilizing process is a culturally and historically variable process that is intended to separate humans from nonhuman animals through the inculcation of etiquette. In *The Civilizing Process*, which focuses on Western Europe in the twelfth through eighteenth centuries, he shows how there are changing expectations about what the threshold between nonhuman animals and humans is, including bodily comportment, utensil use, and norms around public and private bodily functions. He argues that a central fallacy to civilizational thinking is that the process of enculturation for each child is meant to reproduce the whole of that child's society's civilizing process—that is, each child moves from a state of savagery through barbarism to being fully civilized.

54. Stacy Simplican and Sunaura Taylor identify the conflation of animals and disabled people as being central to the conception of bodily and cognitive impairments. For Simplican, in the Western liberal tradition, this serves as a

mechanism to adduce who can be a participating member of society, whereas for Taylor the conflation between animals and humans enables exclusionary and violent practices that target disabled individuals and populations. See Simplican, *Capacity Contract*; Sunaura Taylor, *Beasts of Burden: Animal and Disability Liberation* (New York: New Press, 2017).

55. The discourse of neurodiversity has sparked debate in and beyond the autism community, largely due to the popularization of the concept. At its heart, neurodiversity is meant to describe the varieties of cognitive styles within the human population; it is also used as a human rights platform to include neurodivergent individuals who are representative of nonneurotypicality. The challenge has been that the popularization efforts around neurodiversity have largely focused on individuals who are able to labor or produce value in a capitalist neoliberal system. See Armstrong, *Neurodiversity*; Silberman, *Neurotribes*. For a typical critique of neurodiversity, see Twilah Hiari, "Neurodiversity Is Dead. Now What?," *Mad in America* (blog), April 8, 2018, https://www.madinamerica.com/. Beyond its demand of a disliberal subject—or speakers on the part of that individual—the implicit neuroreductivism in the concept is impoverished in the way it conceives of individuals and their capacities as productive of neoliberal subjectivity.

56. Lennard Davis, *Bending Over Backwards: Essays on Disability and the Body* (New York: New York University Press, 2002).

57. I draw my inspiration here from Gilles Deleuze and Félix Guattari's *A Thousand Plateaus*, trans. Brian Massumi, vol. 2, *Capitalism and Schizophrenia* (Minneapolis: University of Minnesota, 1987), in which they discuss "bodies without organs" as the basis of human existence. "Organs" for Deleuze and Guattari are meant to comprise all of those external processes and objects that facilitate specific forms of embodiment. This is similar to Bernard Stiegler's postphenomenological discussion of technics as technologies that produce particular temporalities and futures through their use, and which he uses as a way to discuss a wide variety of human capacities, institutions, and objects. See Stiegler, *Technics and Time 1: The Fault of Epimetheus*, trans. Richard Beardsworth (Stanford, Calif.: Stanford University Press, 1994).

58. Disability studies scholars have recently begun to address disability through the lens of posthumanism, particularly as a way to rethink the interrelations between the categories of disability and the human. See Luna Dolezal, "Representing Posthuman Embodiment: Considering Disability and the Case of Aimee Mullins," *Women's Studies* 46, no. 2 (2017): 60–75; Dan Goodley, Rebecca Lawthom, and Katherine R. Cole, "Posthuman Disability Studies," *Subjectivity* 7, no. 4 (2014): 342–61; Stuart Murray, "Reading Disability

in a Time of Posthuman Work: Speed and Embodiment in Joshua Ferris' *The Unnamed* and Michael Faber's *Under the Skin*," *Disability Studies Quarterly* 37, no. 4 (2017), http://dsq-sds.org/. Drawing on posthumanist traditions to think through the categories of disability and the human provides a means to engage with the roles of technology in everyday life and as a necessary part of the human social experience; posthumanism also provides a means to bring the human/nonhuman axis into relief in an effort to consider the qualities and capacities that are used to differentiate animals and persons.

59. Often prosthetics are taken as supplying a replacement for something that is lost or lacking; this view of prosthetics accepts them as compensatory and normalizing of an individual. For example, a person who is born without a leg is provided with an artificial leg in an effort to make their body whole. However, recent approaches have noted how prosthetics enable relations between individuals, social others, and environments, all of which point to the ways that prosthetics create social worlds. See Steven L. Kurzman, "Performing Able-Bodiedness: Amputees and Prosthetics in America" (PhD diss., University of California, Santa Cruz, 2003); Seth Messinger, "Incorporating the Prosthetic: Traumatic Limb-Loss, Rehabilitation and Refigured Military Bodies," *Disability and Rehabilitation* 31, no. 25 (2009): 2130–34; Seth Messinger, "Rehabilitating Time: Multiple Temporalities among Military Clinicians and Patients," *Medical Anthropology* 29, no. 2 (2010): 150–69; Zoe Wool, *After War: The Weight of Life at Walter Reed* (Durham, N.C.: Duke University Press, 2015).

60. Animal studies brings together approaches in posthumanist cultural studies, anthropology-based multispecies ethnography, and humanities approaches to representational arts and history. Scholars are interested in the human/nonhuman animal axis and how it has variously been affected by the politics of humanism, wherein humans are afforded some rights, agencies, and capacities and nonhuman animals are not. See John Hartigan, *Aesop's Anthropology: A Multispecies Approach* (Minneapolis: University of Minnesota Press, 2014); Eben Kirksey, ed., *The Multispecies Salon* (Durham, N.C.: Duke University Press, 2015); Susan J. Pearson, *The Rights of the Defenseless: Protecting Animals and Children in Gilded Age America* (Chicago: University of Chicago Press, 2011); Cary Wolfe, ed., *Zoontologies: The Question of the Animal* (Minneapolis: University of Minnesota Press, 2003); Cary Wolfe, *Animal Rites: American Culture, the Discourse of Species, and Posthumanist Theory* (Chicago: University of Chicago Press, 2003).

61. Davis reviews the critiques of dismodernism in "Dismodernism Reconsidered" in *The End of Normal: Identity in a Biocultural Era* (Ann Arbor: University of Michigan Press, 2014).

62. Anthropologists have been especially interested in the use of genomic science as the basis for identity and community. In its earliest, speculative iteration, genomic profiling of disease communities led Paul Rabinow to consider the possibility of an emerging biosociality, a form of belonging based on shared genetic profiles. See Rabinow, "Artificiality and Enlightenment: From Sociobiology to Biosociality," in *Essays on the Anthropology of Reason* (Princeton, N.J.: Princeton University Press, 1996), 91–111. In time, anthropologists turned to the use of "genetic citizenship" based on the activism of individuals and their families who advocate for state recognition of disease categories that find their basis in genetics. See Deborah Heath, Rayna Rapp, and Karen-Sue Taussig, "Genetic Citizenship," in *A Companion to the Anthropology of Politics*, ed. David Nugent and Joan Vincent (Malden, Mass.: Blackwell, 2005), 152–66. In both cases, individuals rely on an understanding of genetic difference as the basis for state recognition, and potentially identity claims.

63. One recurrent trope in disability studies is the equation of human difference with human value. The history of this line of reasoning is important and is based on the need to support nonnormative experiences, thereby serving as an explicitly antieugenic platform. See Bauman and Murray, *Deaf Gain*; Fleischer and Zames, *Disability Rights Movement*. The challenge, as some critics have elaborated, is that such claims play into biopolitical discourses around difference and value. Michele Friedner and Karen Weingarten's discussion in "Disability as Diversity: A New Biopolitics," *Somatosphere* (blog), May 23, 2016, http://somatosphere.net/, points to how liberal forms of differentiation rely on valuation of the less than fully human and dangerously reify difference as integral to biopolitics. The recourse to individual value was essential in the context of liberal biopolitics; moving away from liberalism and neoliberalism will necessitate new bases for an inclusive politics of difference.

64. Bioethics in the United States has long relied on a discourse of "quality of life" to make judgments about the necessity of medical treatments. See Martha Nussbaum and Amartya Sen, eds., *The Quality of Life* (Oxford: Oxford University Press, 1993); M. L. Tina Stevens, *Bioethics in America: Origins and Cultural Politics* (Baltimore, Md.: Johns Hopkins University Press, 2000). These discourses have been subject to a variety of critiques, with scholars interested in dismantling the ways that ableism is enshrined in quality-of-life discourses, serving as a basis for eugenic policies in the medical treatment of individuals, both born and unborn. See Lawrence C. Becker, "Reciprocity, Justice, and Disability," *Ethics* 116, no. 1 (2005): 9–39; Sara Goering, "'You Say You're Happy, But . . .': Contested Quality of Life Judgments in Bioethics and Disability Studies," *Journal of Bioethical Inquiry* 5, no. 2–3 (2008): 125–35;

Ayo Wahlberg, "The Vitality of Disease," in *The Palgrave Handbook of Biology and Society*, ed. Maurizio Meloni et al. (London: Palgrave Macmillan, 2018), 727–48.

65. Friedner and Weingarten, in "Disability as Diversity," argue that the efforts to recognize disability as a form of diversity tend to flatten the experience of individuals with disabilities while also subsuming disability as a form of token-seeking inclusion in the face of human diversity. As such, "disability as diversity" plays into the biopolitical regimes of contemporary politics in the North Atlantic that seek to have individuals claim their position as "diverse" rather than as "disabled," thereby casting biological differences as valuable variations within the human species.

66. Discourses of "high" and "low" functioning individuals have dogged discussions of autism since the inception of the category as a result of the inaugural difference between the two clinical populations that laid the basis for the diagnostic category, with one being verbal and the other nonverbal. For a history of the category, see Uta Frith, *Autism: Explaining the Enigma* (Malden, Mass.: Wiley-Blackwell, 2003). Many activists have worked to dismantle the distinction, arguing that such distinctions are ableist and serve to dehumanize nonverbal people diagnosed with autism and similar neurological disorders. See Leah Harris, "Why We Must Strike the Terms 'High Functioning' and 'Low Functioning' from Our Vocabulary," Mad in America (blog), March 3, 2015, https://www.madinamerica.com/.

67. Anthropologists have long stressed that value is socially constructed and symbolic. Following the kula exchange, a practice in which men from the Trobriand Islands circulate a collection of highly valued but otherwise useless necklaces and bracelets, Branislav Malinowski, Nancy Munn, and David Graeber have all shown how the value of the kula shells accumulates through their exchange as valuable objects. Through their exchange, they produce stories that create relationships between individuals and communities; they also produce a social world in which their value is symbolic rather than based on use. See Graeber, *Toward an Anthropological Theory of Value: The False Coin of Our Own Dreams* (New York: Palgrave, 2001); Malinowski, *Argonauts of the Western Pacific* (Prospect Heights, Ill.: Waveland Press, 1961); Munn, *The Fame of Gawa: A Symbolic Study of Value Transformation in a Massim Society* (Durham, N.C.: Duke University Press, 1992). The recognition that symbolic value often trumps use value borrows from Pierre Bourdieu and Marshall Sahlins, both of whom argue against the Marxist division of use and exchange value, which would seem to be the basis of the capitalist market. Instead, focusing on the symbolic helps to explain why consumers are willing to pay

more for an item that is virtually interchangeable with a similar item, with the difference being reducible to merely the brand of the more expensive item. See Pierre Bourdieu, *Language and Symbolic Power*, ed. John B. Thompson, trans. Gino Raymond (Cambridge, Mass.: Harvard University Press, 1991); Marshall Sahlins, *Culture and Practical Reason* (Chicago: University of Chicago Press, 1976). The leap from a consumable item to a person is not so great, as they both exist within symbolic constructions of value. This can be seen in the debate between Eva Kittay, Peter Singer, and Jeff McMahan, three philosophers invested in ideas about human capacities. Singer and McMahan argue that "radically cognitively limited" individuals are equivalent to or less than nonhuman animals precisely because of their lack of particular "psychological" or "cognitive" capacities. As the mother of a disabled child whom she describes as "completely dependent," Kittay argues that individuals with cognitive disabilities are valuable to society because they are important to individuals who are accepted as valuable to society; a child, whatever his or her cognitive capacities, is important to his or her mother, and that mother's care for the child is a fundamental relationship that is recognized by society as caring and valuable. What lies at the heart of Singer and McMahan's assessment of which lives matter and which do not is a question of capacities or whether an individual is appreciably different from a nonhuman animal. Their use of "dog or pig" as the basis for differentiating humans from nonhumans explicitly draws on the symbolic associations Americans have with those two animals; it puts Kittay in the position of having to symbolically differentiate her daughter from domesticated pets and farm animals. Singer and McMahan thereby build on a long history of symbolic associations between kinds of people and kinds of nonhuman animals that seek to establish humans as unique in their capacities—but precarious in that some individual claims to personhood need to be defended against dehumanizing efforts. For an overview of their debate, see Kittay, "The Personal Is Philosophical Is Political: A Philosopher and Mother of a Cognitively Disabled Person Sends Notes from the Battlefield," *Metaphilosophy* 40, no. 3–4 (2009): 606–27.

68. Neuroreductionism posits that human experiences and capacities are reducible to individual brains and their parts. Acting on the brain and its parts can produce specific effects, guided by conceptions of localization. See Marcus Jacobson, "Neuroreductionism," in *Foundations of Neuroscience* (Boston, Mass.: Springer, 1993), 97–149.

69. Localization depends on evidence that specific parts of the brain determine particular human capacities. In the late nineteenth and twentieth centuries, the Broca area was associated with capacities for language, and the

prefrontal cortex was seen as regulating behavior and providing the ability to make future-oriented plans. From there, there have been a series of associations drawn between parts of the brain and socially recognized capacities and behaviors. With a foundation in localization, material aberrations in the brain can be identified as the source of particular behaviors or lack of capacities. For a critical history of localization, see Malcolm Macmillan, *An Odd Kind of Fame: Stories of Phineas Gage* (Cambridge, Mass.: MIT Press, 2002). For criticisms of how localization has played into cultural understandings of difference between populations and individuals, see Joseph Dumit, *Picturing Personhood: Brainscans and Biomedical Identity* (Princeton, N.J.: Princeton University Press, 2003); Stephen Jay Gould, *The Mismeasure of Man* (New York: Norton, 1996).

70. Biological anthropologist Jonathan Marks has been especially critical of approaches that see human evolution as having stopped or slowed at the dawn of early modern humans, some quarter million years ago. For Marks and biologists who follow him, evolution is a constant process, and claims that it has stopped or slowed serve ideological purposes that support regressive views of human nature. See Agustin Fuentes et al., "On Nature and the Human," *American Anthropologist* 112, no. 4 (2010): 512–21; Jonathan Marks, *What It Means to Be 98% Chimpanzee: Apes, People, and Their Genes* (Berkeley: University of California Press, 2002).

71. Gregory Bateson was central to the first generation of cybernetics theory, having participated in the Macy Conferences, which brought together social scientists, philosophers, mathematicians, and laboratory scientists to develop models of complex individual–environment interactions and to seek ways to apply these theories of information transfer to emergent social phenomena. For Bateson and those who followed, cybernetics offered a way to describe complex human and nonhuman systems, but a significant portion of cyberneticists gravitated toward information theory as a way to approach nonhuman systems, particularly in relation to artificial intelligence and computing. See Robert Kline, *The Cybernetics Moment, or Why We Call Our Age the Information Age* (Baltimore, Md.: Johns Hopkins University Press, 2017).

72. Dumit, *Picturing Personhood*; Martin, *Bipolar Expeditions*; Rose and Abi-Rached, *Neuro*; Barry Saunders, *CT Suite: The Work of Diagnosis in the Age of Noninvasive Cutting* (Durham, N.C.: Duke University Press, 2008).

73. Contemporary understandings of the nervous system are deeply indebted to Humbert Maturana and Francisco Varela, who in *Autopoiesis and Cognition* (Boston, Mass.: Reidel, 1980) argue that the nervous system is a materially bounded feature of animal life.

74. Monadism sees the individual as materially circumscribed, leading to

a conception of the individual as existing within an environmental milieu but potentially unaffected by that milieu outside of one's perception of it. This philosophical tradition is laid out in René Descartes, *Discourse on Method and the Meditations*, trans. F. E. Sutcliffe (1641; New York: Penguin Classics, 1968); Gottfried Wilhelm Leibniz, *Discourse on Metaphysics*, trans. George Montgomery (1686; La Salle, Ill.: Open Court Publishing, 1991).

75. The study of kinship has been central to the discipline of anthropology since its inception and tends to follow culturally emphasized traditions of reckoning relationality between humans. Over time this has given way to accounting for kinship with nonhuman things, particularly in areas outside of the North Atlantic, and has focused on agents that are perceived as nonpersons in Western traditions (e.g. yams, spirits, nonhuman animals). In addition, anthropologists have increasingly attended to how emergent biotechnologies and social practices have changed the contours of kinship, which have included approaches to shared substance and experience. See Sarah Franklin, *Dolly Mixtures: The Remaking of Genealogy* (Durham, N.C.: Duke University Press, 2007); Stefan Helmreich, "Trees and Seas of Information: Alien Kinship and the Biopolitics of Gene Transfer in Marine Biology and Biotechnology," *American Ethnologist* 30, no. 3 (2003): 340–58; Jessaca Leinaweaver, "On Moving Children: The Social Implications of Andean Child Circulation," *American Ethnologist* 34, no. 1 (2007): 163–80; Claude Lévi-Strauss, *The Elementary Structures of Kinship* (1949; Boston, Mass.: Beacon Press, 1969); Rayna Rapp, Deborah Heath, and Karen-Sue Taussig, "Genealogical Dis-ease: Where Hereditary Abnormality, Biomedical Explanation, and Family Responsibility Meet," in *Relative Values: Reconfiguring Kinship Studies*, ed. Sarah Franklin and Susan McKinnon (Durham, N.C.: Duke University Press, 2001), 384–409; Gayle Rubin, "The Traffic in Women: Notes on the 'Political Economy' of Sex," in *Toward an Anthropology of Women*, ed. Rayna R. Reiter (New York: Monthly Review Press, 1975), 157–210; David Schneider, *American Kinship: A Cultural Account* (Chicago: University of Chicago Press, 1980); Strathern, *Reproducing the Future*; Kath Weston, *Families We Choose: Lesbians, Gays, Kinship* (New York: Columbia University Press, 1997); Sylvia Yanagisako, "Variance in American Kinship: Implications for Cultural Analysis," *American Ethnologist* 5, no. 1 (1978): 15–29.

76. Disability studies scholars have become increasingly interested in animacy as a function of material interactions between bodies. In this way they have drawn on recent turns in new materialist traditions that situate human and nonhuman, organic and inorganic actors in interdependent relationships. As Mel Chen points out in *Animacies: Biopolitics, Racial Mattering, and Queer*

Affect (Durham, N.C.: Duke University Press, 2012) and Taylor discusses in *Beasts of Burden*, animacy is a means to differentiate between different kinds of actors, humans and nonhuman, things and persons, and it often serves as the basis for recognizing some kinds of individuals as full persons and others as disabled. For additional approaches to animacy in disability studies, see Ryan Parrey, "Being Disoriented: Uncertain Encounters with Disability," *Disability Studies Quarterly* 36, no. 2 (2016), http://dsq-sds.org/; Julia Watts Belser, "Vital Wheels: Disability, Relationality, and the Queer Animacy of Vibrant Things," *Hypatia* 31, no. 1 (2016): 5–21.

77. Animal helpers or service animals are one site that brings together many of the concerns in disability studies, animal studies, and science and technology studies, yet they are sparingly discussed by scholars in any of those fields. See Olga Solomon, "What a Dog Can Do: Children with Autism and Therapy Dogs in Social Interaction," *Ethos* 38, no. 1 (2010): 143–66; Olga Solomon, "'But—He'll Fall!': Children with Autism, Interspecies Intersubjectivity, and the Problem of 'Being Social,'" *Culture, Medicine, and Psychiatry* 39, no. 2 (2015): 323–44; Taylor, *Beasts of Burden*. As Taylor discusses in the final chapter of *Beasts of Burden*, her service dog becomes disabled too, forcing a reassessment of their relationship and what each does for the other. Taylor is thus interested in the interdependence they share rather than on her dependence on the dog. Like Solomon's work with children diagnosed with autism and dogs, animals serve as both a person for their humans, as they are seen as having key capacities that allow for human–animal interactions, and as a conduit to facilitating human–human interactions. Service animals thereby blur the boundaries between animating media, facilitating technologies, and modulating institutions in that they are sometimes able to animate, facilitate, and modulate all at once for their humans.

78. Animal models are deployed by scientists to conduct research on a living being that is then extrapolated as relevant to human bodies and societies. However, animal models are merely models, and what might be explanatory for mice or monkeys does not necessarily apply to humans, particularly when sociotechnical environments are taken into consideration. See Donna Haraway, *Modest_Witness@Second_Millennium.FemaleMan©_Meets_OncoMouse™* (New York: Routledge, 1997); Sara Shostak, *Exposed Science: Genes, the Environment, and the Politics of Population Health* (Berkeley: University of California Press, 2013).

79. Gregory Bateson, *Naven: A Survey of the Problems Suggested by a Composite Picture of the Culture of a New Guinea Tribe Drawn from Three Points of View* (Palo Alto, Calif.: Stanford University Press, 1958).

80. Bateson, *Steps to an Ecology of Mind*.

81. Gregory Bateson, *Mind and Nature: A Necessary Unity* (New York: Bantam Books, 1988).

82. Oliver Sacks is well known for his humanistic approach to patients, most famously in *The Man Who Mistook His Wife for a Hat: And Other Clinical Tales* (1985; reprint, New York: Touchstone, 1998) and *Awakenings* (1990; reprint, New York: Vintage Books, 1999). Across his oeuvre, Sacks draws on his clinical experiences to humanize a variety of clinically recognized conditions. In doing so, Sacks draws on a long tradition of case-based medical knowledge production, discussed by Roy Porter in *The Greatest Benefit to Mankind: A Medical History of Humanity* (New York: Norton, 1999). This approach is sometimes viewed—especially within disability studies—as detached and imperial, and has been critiqued by Simi Linton in *Claiming Disability: Knowledge and Identity* (New York: New York University Press, 1998).

83. Imperial knowledge production is necessarily extractive and takes from the populations it studies without giving back. I follow in the decolonial tradition in my attempt to displace imperial knowledge production practices—particularly in scientific and social scientific traditions—by situating my analysis of scientists alongside equally powerful theory developers in the form of disorderly individuals and their families. For a discussion of decolonizing knowledge practices, see Linda Tuhiwai Smith, *Decolonizing Methodologies: Research and Indigenous Peoples* (London: Zed Books, 2012); Kim TallBear, *Native American DNA: Tribal Belonging and the False Promise of Genetic Science* (Minneapolis: University of Minnesota Press, 2013).

84. Jasbir Puar makes a similar observation in "The Cost of Getting Better: Ability and Debility," in Davis, *Disability Studies Reader*, ed. Lennard Davis, 4th ed. (New York: Routledge, 2013), 177–84. Puar suggests that "granting 'voice' to the subaltern comes into tension with the need, in the case of the human/animal distinction, to destabilize the privileging of communication/representation/language altogether. The ability to understand language is also where the human/nonhuman animal distinctions, as well as the human/technology distinctions, have long been drawn. . . . a nonanthropomorphic conception of the human is necessary to resituate language as one of many captures of the intensities of bodily capacities" (182–83).

85. There is a persistent bias in disability studies and the anthropology of disability that favors research that occurs with families over research that occurs with individual disabled people. This is an effect of human-subject protocols that seek to protect at-risk populations, of which individuals with disabilities are one; it is also an effect of the anthropological interests in the

relational effects of disability and the ways that individual diagnoses and interdependencies proliferate social connections that depend on families and social others. See Gelya Frank, *Venus on Wheels: Two Decades of Dialogue on Disability, Biography, and Being Female in America* (Berkeley: University of California Press, 2000); Benedicte Ingstad and Susan Reynolds Whyte, *Disability and Culture* (Berkeley: University of California Press, 1995); Matthew Kohrman, *Bodies of Difference: Experiences of Disability and Institutional Advocacy in the Making of Modern China* (Berkeley: University of California Press, 2005); Nancy Mairs, *Waist-High in the World: A Life among the Nondisabled* (Boston, Mass.: Beacon Press, 1997); Silverman, *Understanding Autism.*

86. Rose and Abi-Rached, *Neuro.*

87. Deaf studies comprises the study of a wide variety of experiences of deafness, including hereditary deafness, deafness caused by illness and exposure, and forms of hearing loss that are mitigated by hearing aids and other prosthetic devices. For a discussion of the varieties of deafness, see Bauman and Murray, *Deaf Gain.* The two cases I discuss here are of individuals who primarily communicate though spoken language and have near-total hearing loss. Both rely on lip reading as well as prosthetic technologies.

88. For discussions of my work with neuroscientists and psychiatrists and with psychoanalysts, see "Disclosure as Method, Disclosure as Dilemma," in *Disclosure in Health and Illness*, ed. Lenore Manderson and Mark Davis, (New York: Routledge, 2014), 104–19; "Our Master's Voice, the Practice of Melancholy, and Minor Sciences," *Cultural Anthropology* 30, no. 4 (2015): 670–91.

89. Science and technology studies scholars have shown how experiments shape and are shaped by knowledge production practices; rather than novel endeavors that create ruptures from earlier ways of knowing, experiments, as Hans-Jorg Rheinberger and Peter Galison demonstrate, tend to follow conservative knowledge practices that slowly widen scientific disciplines' epistemic objects and their means of being known. See Galison, "Trading Zone: Coordinating Action and Belief," in *The Science Studies Reader*, ed. Mario Biagioli (New York: Routledge, 1999), 137–60; Rheinberger, *Toward a History of Epistemic Things: Synthesizing Proteins in the Test Tube* (Stanford, Calif.: Stanford University Press, 1997).

90. Anthropologists of science have been especially interested in the ways that scientific claims of discovery are better conceptualized as inventions. They seek to point to the ways that knowledge is always culturally bound and that advancements in science only make sense in the context of a body of knowledge that makes discoveries legible. See Emily Martin, "The Egg and the

Sperm: How Science Has Created a Romance Based on Traditional Gender Stereotypes," *Signs* 16, no. 3 (1991): 485–501.

91. The relationship between language and subjectivity is most popularly captured in Judith Butler's work, which draws on philosophical traditions that depend on an understanding of the self as being forged through language. In developing this conception of the subject, Butler is explicitly logocentric and implicitly neuroreductive in that language capacities are associated with qualities of full personhood that are founded in an originary human capacity for language located in the brain. See especially Butler, *Excitable Speech: A Politics of the Performative* (New York: Routledge, 1997).

92. Objectivity has been the subject of sustained critique in science and technology studies, particularly from feminist scholars who see in claims to objectivity what Donna Haraway has referred to as a "god trick," enabling scientists to stand outside of the thing being observed while still being constituted by and through their observation. See Lorraine Daston and Peter Galison, *Objectivity* (New York: Zone Books, 2007); Haraway, *Modest_Witness@Second_Millennium.FemaleMan©_Meets_OncoMouse™*; Sandra Harding, *The Science Question in Feminism* (Ithaca, N.Y.: Cornell University Press, 1986). These critiques of objectivity have had profound effects on the social sciences, leading to a generation of scholars interested in a reflexive turn that seeks to situate the observer in the contexts of what is being observed. On this, see Ruth Behar, *The Vulnerable Observer: Anthropology That Breaks Your Heart* (Boston: Beacon Press, 1996); Briggs, *Never in Anger*; James Clifford and George Marcus, eds., *Writing Culture: The Poetics and Politics of Ethnography* (Berkeley: University of California Press, 1986); Delmos Jones, "Towards a Native Anthropology," *Human Organization* 29, no. 4 (1970): 251–59; Paul Rabinow, *Reflections on Fieldwork in Morocco* (Berkeley: University of California Press, 1977).

93. Avery Gordon has developed a sociology of "ghosts" that addresses the often purposefully obscured roles that women have played in the development of knowledge practices, particularly psychoanalysis. Gordon attends to the ways that women have been written out of history, rendering them ghostly presences in the knowledge practices that they have contributed to. In her archival research, Gordon recovers these ghosts and demonstrates the long-lasting effects they have had on the knowledge production they participated in. Gordon points to the implicit and obscured interdependence that has existed in social forms and their production. Gordon's project runs parallel to Kafer's critique of independence in *Feminist, Queer, Crip*. See Gordon, *Ghostly Matters: Haunting and the Sociological Imagination* (Minneapolis: University of

Minnesota Press, 1997). It is precisely these feminist projects that I am interested in in my theorization of ghostwriting in chapter 3.

94. Faye Ginsburg and Rayna Rapp, "Making Disability Count: Demography, Futurity, and the Making of Disability Publics," Somatosphere (blog), May 11, 2015, http://somatosphere.net/.

95. Chronic illnesses have provided scholars with the basis to conceptualize the temporal relationships that are engendered as an effect of a medical diagnosis that unfolds in predictable, yet sometimes surprising, ways. Chronic illnesses are marked by persistent, if changing, states, and enter individuals into long-term relationships with the medical–industrial complex, including relations with pharmaceutical treatments that manage symptoms without curing underlying conditions. See Lenore Manderson and Carolyn Smith-Morris, eds., *Chronic Conditions, Fluid States: Chronicity and the Anthropology of Illness* (New Brunswick, N.J.: Rutgers University Press, 2010); Todd Meyers, "A Turn towards Dying: Presence, Signature, and the Social Course of Chronic Illness in Urban America," *Medical Anthropology* 26, no. 3 (2007): 205–27; Carolyn Smith-Morris, *Diabetes among the Pima: Stories of Survival* (Tucson: University of Arizona Press, 2008); Matthew Wolf-Meyer, "Therapy, Remedy, Cure: Disorder and the Spatiotemporality of Medicine and Everyday Life," *Medical Anthropology* 33, no. 2 (2014): 144–59.

96. Susan Reynolds Whyte has long been interested in what she refers to as subjunctivity—that is, the subjective experience of gauging one's relationship to an unknown but sometimes predictable future. She attends to this process in the context of postcolonial sub-Saharan Africa and with individuals who have been diagnosed with chronic illnesses. This relation to futurity upends models of subjectivity that are primarily historically focused and situates subjectivity as a process of risk assessment and future formation. See Whyte, "Subjunctivity and Subjectivity: Hoping for Health in Eastern Uganda," in *Postcolonial Subjectivities in Africa*, ed. Richard Werbner (London: Zed Books, 2002), 171–90; Matthew Wolf-Meyer and Celina Callahan-Kapoor, "Chronic Subjunctivity, or How Physicians Use Diabetes and Insomnia to Manage Futures in the U.S.," *Medical Anthropology* 36, no. 2 (2017): 83–95.

97. Stiegler, in *Technics and Time 1*, argues against seeing loss as necessarily something that depends on a historical relationship. Instead, Stiegler sees human relationships to time as shaped by the anticipatory futures that are embedded in technologies that range from language to institutions, all of which he understands as prosthetics. In this way, he is providing a parallel to anthropological approaches to the medical and social uses of prosthetics.

98. Audre Lorde is well known for her claim that "the master's tools

will never dismantle the master's house." But rather than be cynical that the master's house will never be dismantled, Lorde is expressly committed to the decolonization of the university and knowledge production more generally. See Lorde, "The Master's Tools Will Never Dismantle the Master's House," in *Sister Outsider: Essays and Speeches* (Berkeley, Calif.: Crossing Press, 2007), 110–14. Since Foucault's development of micropolitics as the basis for contemporary power relations in *History of Sexuality*, many scholars have been motivated to conceptualize what forms resistance to dominant powers and institutions might take, especially in the context of conceptualizing a social field suffused with power relations. For some, this has led to a resigned relation to power, based on the conception of hegemonic power structures staging controllable forms of resistance that are ultimately only performed. For others, this has led to a renewed interest in social movements as the basis for developing new norms. See Lila Abu-Lughod, "The Romance of Resistance: Tracing Transformations of Power through Bedouin Women," *American Ethnologist* 17, no. 1 (1990): 41–55; Robyn Kliger, "'Resisting Resistance': Historicizing Contemporary Models of Agency," in *Essays on Controlling Processes*, ed. Laura Nader (Berkeley, Calif.: Kroeber Anthropological Society, 1996), 137–56; Robert McRuer, *Crip Times: Disability, Globalization, and Resistance* (New York: New York University Press, 2018). My interests here are precisely in using the master's tools—hence my engagement with dominant thinkers and scientists in their elaborations of the psychiatric and neurological basis of subjectivity. By perverting these traditions and modes of thought, the master's house can be refashioned from the inside, leaving it intact but irrevocably altering it.

1. Neurological Subjectivity

1. Martin, *Bipolar Expeditions*.

2. Silberman, *Neurotribes*.

3. Antonio Damasio, *Descartes' Error: Emotion, Reason, and the Human Brain* (New York: Penguin, 2005).

4. Antonio Damasio, *Self Comes to Mind: Constructing the Conscious Brain* (New York: Vintage, 2010).

5. Antonio Damasio, *Looking for Spinoza: Joy, Sorrow, and the Feeling Brain* (New York: Harcourt, 2003).

6. Damasio, *Descartes' Error*.

7. Walter Freeman was not the first lobotomist, but he was the most fervent one. Using what was functionally an ice pick, Freeman would damage the brain by inserting the tool into the frontal lobe. The effects were unpredictable,

but as a result of the damage, individuals would often lose a variety of behavioral capacities. See Freeman and Watts, *Psychosurgery*.

8. Macmillan, *Odd Kind of Fame*.

9. John M. Harlow, "Recovery from the Passage of an Iron Bar through the Head," in *Publications of the Massachusetts Medical Society* (Boston, Mass.: David Clapp & Son, 1868), 2:328–46.

10. Macmillan, *Odd Kind of Fame*, 116–19.

11. Mark Bear, Barry Connors, and Michael Paradiso, *Neuroscience: Exploring the Brain*, 4th ed. (Alphen aan den Rijn, Netherlands: Wolters Kluwer, 2015), 625.

12. Paul A. Young, Paul H. Young, and Daniel L. Tolbert, *Basic Clinical Neuroscience*, 3rd ed. (Alphen aan den Rijn, Netherlands: Wolters Kluwer, 2015), 218.

13. Neil R. Carlson, *Foundations of Behavioral Neuroscience*, 9th ed. (Essex: Pearson Education, 2014), 275.

14. Robert Stevenson, *The Strange Case of Dr. Jekyll and Mr. Hyde* (1886; Mineola, N.Y.: Dover, 1991).

15. Steven Shaviro, *Discognition* (London: Repeater Books, 2015).

16. Immanuel Kant, *Anthropology from a Pragmatic Point of View*, trans. Mary J. Gregor (1798; The Hague: Martinus Nijhoff, 1996).

17. Simplican, *Capacity Contract*.

18. Davis, *Enforcing Normalcy*.

19. Damasio, *Self Comes to Mind*, 29, 32, emphasis in original.

20. Damasio, *Self Comes to Mind*, 262.

21. Damasio, *Self Comes to Mind*, 49.

22. Sahlins, *Culture and Practical Reason*.

23. Damasio, *Self Comes to Mind*, 51, emphasis in original.

24. Damasio, *Self Comes to Mind*, 53.

25. Damasio, *Self Comes to Mind*, 85.

26. Damasio, *Self Comes to Mind*, 86.

27. Damasio, *Self Comes to Mind*, 87, emphasis in original.

28. Damasio, *Self Comes to Mind*, 88.

29. For many Japanese people, the heart is seen as the source of the self instead of the brain. This has impacts for concerns like life support and its termination, as well as for organ transplantation and the collection of organs from brain-dead individuals. See Margaret Lock, *Twice Dead: Organ Transplants and the Reinvention of Death* (Berkeley: University of California Press, 2002).

30. Alfred Gell offers a cross-cultural view of inanimate objects that are

treated as persons—or at least imbued with agency to shape the actions of human actors. Totems, rocks, and artworks are all accepted as agentive individuals outside Western traditions. Gell, *Art and Agency: An Anthropological Theory* (Oxford: Oxford University Press, 1998).

31. For examples of how age and personhood relate to one another, see Judy DeLoache and Alma Gottlieb, *A World of Babies: Imagined Childcare Guides for Seven Societies* (Cambridge: Cambridge University Press, 2000); Alma Gottlieb, "Where Have All the Babies Gone? Toward an Anthropology of Infants (and Their Caretakers)," *Anthropological Quarterly* 73, no. 3 (2000): 121–32.

32. The gift has been central to anthropological theorizing of social groups and of interpersonal relationships. See Strathern, *Reproducing the Future*, for a discussion of individuality and gift giving.

33. The literature on nonhuman agency is diverse and covers inanimate and animate actors, including mosquitoes, pharmaceuticals, microbes, nonhuman primates, and just about everything else. See, e.g., Michel Callon, "Some Elements of a Sociology of Translation: Domestication of the Scallops and the Fishermen of St. Brieuc Bay," in *Power, Action, and Belief: A New Sociology of Knowledge*, ed. John Law (New York: Routledge, 1986), 196–233; Hartigan, *Aesop's Anthropology*; Timothy Mitchell, *Rule of Experts: Egypt, Techno-politics, Modernity* (Berkeley: University of California Press, 2002); Heather Paxson, "Post-Pasteurian Cultures: The Microbiopolitics of Raw-Milk Cheese in the United States," *Cultural Anthropology* 23, no. 1 (2008): 15–47.

34. For a discussion of the scientific management of labor, see Mel van Elteren, *Managerial Control of American Workers: Methods and Technology from the 1880s to Today* (Jefferson, N.C.: McFarland, 2017). As scholars have shown, the arrangements of labor led to the development of particular sensibilities and subjectivities, profoundly shaping the experiences of individual workers and societies. See, e.g., Anson Rabinbach, *The Human Motor: Energy, Fatigue, and the Origins of Modernity* (Berkeley: University of California Press, 1990); Edward Palmer Thompson, *Customs in Common: Studies in Traditional Popular Culture* (New York: New Press, 1993).

35. In his history of changing social mores in Europe from the twelfth through eighteenth centuries, Norbert Elias shows how behavior moves from being something that is shaped by social demands placed on the individual by social others to what is seen as an expression of the self. By the early industrial age, individuals are taken to be in control of their behaviors, and those who do not act in accordance with social norms are perceived as willfully ignoring or

challenging these norms. See Elias's discussion of manners and their role in making the modern individual in *The Civilizing Process*.

36. As Jonathan Metzl shows in his study of a rural asylum in Michigan, blacks were disproportionately seen as experiencing schizophrenia as a means to medicalize their social experiences—and to treat them as patients rather than as social discontents. This allowed for the medicalization of their experiences, leading to lifetime institutionalization as well as psychosurgery and debilitating medication regimes. See Metzl, *Protest Psychosis*.

37. Roland Barthes, *The Semiotic Challenge*, trans. Richard Howard (Berkeley: University of California Press, 1988).

38. This view of human behavior is catalyzed in the work of B. F. Skinner, who divided behavior into respondent and operant behaviors. Respondent behaviors are instinctual; their enactment occurs in response to specific stimuli. Operant behaviors are behaviors that an individual learns over time and reliably reproduces in response to learned circumstances. See Skinner, *Science and Human Behavior* (New York: Free Press, 1953).

39. Sigmund Freud writes extensively about the death drive—the will toward destruction that motivates a wide variety of human actions. For Freud, the death drive is counterpoised to the pleasure principle—the human desire for enjoyment. Taken together, the urges to create and destroy are seen by Freud as motors for civilization, generally tamed by social norms but at times exacerbated to the point of the destruction of others, including whole societies. See his initial discussion in *Beyond the Pleasure Principle*, trans. James Strachey (1920; New York: Norton, 1961), and his later, more expansive use of the ideas in *Civilization and Its Discontents*, trans. James Strachey (1930; New York: Norton, 1961).

40. One might think here of recent discussion of the Anthropocene, the era of planetary change initiated by humans through their actions on the environment, from the building of large dams and earthworks to the pollution of the soil through industrial manufacturing. Over the last several decades, the effects of these actions have become increasingly apparent, yet individuals and whole societies are continually invested in practices that will lead to further environmental degradation. On the Anthropocene, see Christophe Bonneuil and Jean-Baptiste Fressoz, *The Shock of the Anthropocene: The Earth, History, and Us*, trans. David Fernbach (New York: Verso, 2016). On a more intimate scale, one might consider here the ways that individuals become invested in their addictions to illicit (and sometimes legal) drugs to the point of self-destruction. See Phillippe Bourgois and Jeffrey Schonberg, *Righteous Dopefiend* (Berkeley: University of California Press, 2009).

41. Gregory Bateson argues that dogs are able to indicate their desire for play by using gestures—a play bow—which allows other dogs to see that the inviting dog is not intending to be aggressive despite wrestling, biting, and verbal playacting. Similarly, primatologists have shown that nonhuman primates have verbal skills in communicating the presence of predators—and, potentially, particularly kinds of predators—thus calling for specific reactions (like climbing a tree when a lion is near or hiding in bushes when birds of prey fly overhead). See Bateson, *Steps to an Ecology of Mind*; Cheney and Seyfarth, *Baboon Metaphysics*.

42. Garfinkel, *Studies in Ethnomethodology*, deploys a similar tactic to call into question the cultural assumptions that individuals hold about everyday life and its ordering. By slightly perturbing others through the disruption of a shared assumption, Garfinkel demonstrates how the rules of social interaction can be broken for the purpose of demonstrating the institutionalized bases of interpretation and social norms.

43. Rhodes, "Changing the Subject."

44. In a series of experiments, Benjamin Libet attempts to show that the physiological impulse to act precedes an individual's intention to act, thereby potentially showing that free will, as it is commonly understood, is an illusion. Instead, he and his colleagues suggest, our understandings of our actions occur after the action has occurred, and we labor to retroactively make sense of why or how an action occurred. See Libet et al., "Time of Conscious Intention to Act in Relation to Onset of Cerebral Activity (Readiness-Potential): The Unconscious Initiation of a Freely Voluntary Act," *Brain* 106, no. 3 (1983): 623–42; Benjamin Libet, "Unconscious Cerebral Initiative and the Role of Conscious Will in Voluntary Action," *Behavioral and Brain Sciences* 8, no. 4 (1985): 529–39.

45. Generations of sociologists invested in symbolic interactionism have shown that actions are interpreted by an audience of others despite the intentions of the actor. This has ramifications for how individuals conduct themselves—usually in an effort to imagine how their actions will be interpreted by their audience. For an early text in this field, see Erving Goffman, *The Presentation of Self in Everyday Life* (New York: Anchor Books, 1959).

2. Symbolic Subjectivity

1. See, for example, Andre Leroi-Gourhan, *Gesture and Speech*, trans. Anna Bostock Berger (Cambridge, Mass.: MIT Press, 1964).

2. Linguistic anthropological approaches to communication focus on the ways that interpretation and communicative acts are shaped by language

ideologies that undergird the conventions of speech, gesture, and interaction. These approaches point to the ways that language is regimented in its referentiality through convention, implying that all linguistic action is necessarily historically institutionalized. See Silverstein, "Language Structure"; Gal and Irvine, "Language Ideology"; Gal, "Language Ideologies Compared."

3. Félix Guattari, *Molecular Revolution: Psychiatry and Politics*, trans. Rosemary Sheed (New York: Penguin, 1984).

4. The trilogy includes Josh Greenfeld, *A Child Called Noah: A Family Journey* (New York: Harcourt Brace, 1972); *A Place for Noah* (New York: Holt, Rinehart and Winston, 1978); *A Client Called Noah: A Family Journey Continued* (New York: Harcourt Brace, 1986).

5. "Noah's Story: Family Struggles with a Brain-Damaged, Autistic Son," *60 Minutes*, May 9, 2000, http://www.cbsnews.com/.

6. Greenfeld, *Child Called Noah*, 18–19.

7. Quoted in Greenfeld, *Child Called Noah*, 59.

8. Greenfeld, *Child Called Noah*, 64.

9. Greenfeld, *Child Called Noah*, 103.

10. Greenfeld, *Child Called Noah*, 99–100.

11. Greenfeld, *Child Called Noah*, 102.

12. Greenfeld, *Child Called Noah*, 117–18.

13. Greenfeld, *Client Called Noah*.

14. I see language as a kind of technology, following Stiegler's discussion of technics in *Technics and Time 1*. For Stiegler, technologies are imbued with particular temporalities, pasts and futures that impel their users. In conceptualizing technologies in this way, Stiegler attempts to move away from phenomenological approaches to an embodiment that sees humans as without qualities when compared to nonhuman animals. Humans, Stiegler argues, are defined by their use of technologies that create particular futures. Although this view is anthropocentric, I find Stiegler's attention to the temporal quality of technologies to be useful in conceptualizing how language, communicative forms, gesture, and speech create emergent socialities that are shaped by history and that potentially produce emergent social formations with new possibilities for personhood, subjectivity, and society.

15. Linguistic anthropologists have long pointed to the determinative powers of interpretive structures in understanding language and being able to respond as a knowing, full communicator. Two representative examples are Charles L. Briggs, "Learning How to Ask: Native Metacommunicative Competence and the Incompetence of Fieldworkers," *Language in Society* 13, no. 1 (1984): 1–28; Judith Irvine, "Shadow Conversations: The Indeterminacy

of Participant Roles," in *Natural Histories of Discourse*, ed. Michael Silverstein and Greg Urban (Chicago: University of Chicago Press, 1996), 131–59. In both cases, the competence of speakers and the spoken to are predicated on the ability to inhabit a historically constructed—and agreed-on—set of strategies for interpretation and communication.

16. On some of the pathological types in neoliberal capitalism, see John Marlovits, "Give Me Slack: Depression, Alertness, and Laziness in Seattle," *Anthropology of Consciousness* 24, no. 2 (2013): 137–57.

17. For a discussion of how the discourse of compliance works to shape the subjectivities of medical professionals and patients, see Kalman Applbaum and Michael Oldani, "Towards an Era of Bureaucratically Controlled Medical Compliance?," *Anthropology and Medicine* 17, no. 2 (2010): 113–27.

18. Greenfeld, *Child Called Noah*, 127.

19. Greenfeld, *Child Called Noah*, 139.

20. Greenfeld, *Child Called Noah*, 169.

21. Greenfeld, *Child Called Noah*, 115.

22. Henry Kisor, *What's that Pig Outdoors? A Memoir of Deafness* (New York: Penguin, 1990), 15.

23. Douglas Baynton, *Forbidden Signs: American Culture and the Campaign against Sign Language* (Chicago: University of Chicago Press, 1998).

24. Kisor, *What's that Pig Outdoors?*, 15.

25. Kisor, *What's that Pig Outdoors?*, 25.

26. Doris Mirrielees, *Education of the Young Deaf Child: Special Subjects and Methods* (Chicago: University of Chicago Press, 1947).

27. For a history of mainstreaming in U.S. schools, particularly with reference to disabilities, see Robert Osgood, *The History of Inclusion in the United States* (Washington, D.C.: Gallaudet University Press, 2005).

28. Kisor, *What's That Pig Outdoors?*, 73.

29. Kisor, *What's That Pig Outdoors?*, 242.

30. Kisor, *What's That Pig Outdoors?*, 137.

31. Kisor, *What's That Pig Outdoors?*, 75.

32. Kisor, *What's That Pig Outdoors?*, 139.

33. Kisor, *What's That Pig Outdoors?*, 227–28.

34. For a history of the cochlear implant, see Albert Mudry and Mara Mills, "The Early History of the Cochlear Implant: A Retrospective," *JAMA Otolaryngology–Head and Neck Surgery* 139, no. 5 (2013): 446–53.

35. Kisor, *What's That Pig Outdoors?*, 146.

36. For a discussion of how technology has shaped the experience of deafness, see Mara Mills, "Do Signals Have Politics? Inscribing Abilities in

Cochlear Implants," in *The Oxford Handbook of Sound Studies*, ed. Trevor Pinch and Karin Bijsterveld (Oxford: Oxford University Press, 2011), 320–46.

37. Kisor, *What's That Pig Outdoors?*, 152.

38. The question of whether technology drives history has long animated historians of science and technology, who see either that technological developments make new social forms possible or that the invention of new technologies has negligible effects on society. On one side of the debate, technology is seen as pushing human societies toward greater efficiencies and capabilities in mastering the environment; on the other side of the debate, technologies are seen as outgrowths of already existing power relations, often entrenching social forms. See Donald MacKenzie and Judy Wajcman, eds., *The Social Shaping of Technology: How the Refrigerator Got Its Hum* (Bristol, Pa.: Open University Press, 1985); Merritt Roe Smith and Leo Marx, eds., *Does Technology Drive History? The Dilemma of Technological Determinism* (Cambridge, Mass.: MIT Press, 1994).

39. Kisor, *What's That Pig Outdoors?*, 152.

40. Kisor, *What's That Pig Outdoors?*, 152–53.

41. Kisor, *What's That Pig Outdoors?*, 262.

42. Kisor, *What's That Pig Outdoors?*, 263.

43. Wolf-Meyer, "Our Master's Voice."

44. See Sigmund Freud's discussion of the Oedipal complex in *The Interpretation of Dreams*, trans. Joyce Crick (1899; Oxford: Oxford University Press, 1999).

45. Sigmund Freud, *Totem and Taboo* (1913), trans. James Strachey (New York: Norton, 1950).

46. Sigmund Freud, "Project for a Scientific Psychology" (1895), in *The Complete Psychological Works of Sigmund Freud*, trans. James Strachey, vol. 1 (London: Vintage Classics, 2001).

47. Since the 1990s, Mark Solms has been working at the intersection of laboratory neuroscience—using various monitoring technologies—and psychoanalysis. His work on dreams is deeply influenced by psychoanalytic approaches and might be seen as an inheritor to Freud's early neurological work. See Solms, *The Neuropsychology of Dreams: A Clinico-anatomical Study* (New York: Routledge, 2015).

48. Freud's biological determinism is most clearly seen in his discussion of human sexuality. He sees the possibility for the development of a wide range of sexualities (generally pathological in nature), but they are ultimately undergirded by an obligatory heterosexuality, which is reinforced by social norms. See Sigmund Freud, *Three Essays on the Theory of Sexuality* (1905), trans. James Strachey (New York: Basic Books, 2000).

49. Freud, *Interpretation of Dreams*.

50. Sigmund Freud, *Jokes and Their Relation to the Unconscious* (1905), trans. James Strachey (New York: Penguin, 1991).

51. See the work of Terrance Deacon, who argues that the evolution of the human brain has been dependent on language and the human use of symbols in ways that exceed nonhuman animal forms of communication. See Deacon, *The Symbolic Species: The Co-evolution of Language and the Brain* (New York: Norton, 1998).

52. Jacques Lacan discussed the symbolic order throughout his work, particularly in relation to the formation of the subject and the relationship between the subject and society. See his discussions of the subject and the symbolic in *The Four Fundamental Concepts of Psychoanalysis* (1973), trans. Alan Sheridan (New York: Norton, 1998).

53. Jacques Lacan, *The Language of the Self: The Function of Language in Psychoanalysis* (1968), trans. Anthony Wilden (Baltimore, Md.: Johns Hopkins University Press, 1981).

54. Medical semiotics depend on the ability to correlate symptoms—a bump, a cough—with a category that a given set of symptoms fit into, generally for diagnosis and treatment. Early discussions of these processes can be found in Barthes, *Semiotic Challenge*; Foucault, *Birth of the Clinic*.

55. On the subject of the emerging world of microbial medicine, see Amber Benezra, "Datafying Microbes: Malnutrition at the Intersection of Genomics and Global Health," *BioSocieties* 11, no. 3 (2016): 334–51.

56. Neuroplasticity has become the subject of a wide variety of analyses, including social scientists interested in critiquing the idea as a function of neoliberalism, philosophers invested in how neuroplasticity upends ideas about the self, and self-help practitioners selling methods for improving one's brain. See Rose and Abi-Rached, *Neuro*. For an example of the philosophical use of plasticity, see Catherine Malabou, *What Should We Do with Our Brain?*, trans. Sebastian Rand (New York: Fordham University Press, 2008).

57. See the discussion of poverty and brain development in Kimberly G. Noble et al., "Family Income, Parental Education and Brain Structure in Children and Adolescents," *Nature Neuroscience* 18, no. 5 (2015): 773–78.

58. This claim has famously been made by Bruno Bettelheim in his psychoanalytically informed study of autism, *The Empty Fortress: Infantile Autism and the Birth of the Self* (New York: Free Press, 1967). His claims have long since been debunked. Even at the time of their publication, his ideas were subject to wide derision and scrutiny.

59. The latter-day psychoanalysts Nicolas Abraham and Maria Torok argue that trauma—and human experience more generally—can be transmitted from generation to generation, informing the experiences of the living. Although parallel in some ways to Marxian understandings of historical materialism, this psychoanalytic view depends on a deeply symbolic understanding of experience and its transmissions. See their *The Shell and the Kernel: Renewals of Psychoanalysis*, trans. Nicholas Rand (Chicago: University of Chicago Press, 1994).

60. This echoes an argument made by Lennard Davis: essentially, we are all disabled. As controversial as that claim may be, it is based in part on Davis's understanding that the world we live in is not built for each of us individually but has been standardized to meet the needs of most people most of the time. The call to action that Davis makes is to individually attempt to negotiate with the makers of our lived spaces and institutions to meet our individual needs, thereby expanding the category of the normal by deploying disability in this way. See Davis, *Bending Over Backwards*.

61. Charles Sanders Peirce suggested that the semiotic process is fundamentally threefold, comprising a sign, its object, and the interpretant who interprets the sign in its communicative milieu. In making this argument, Peirce's conception of semiotics highlights the role of subjectivity in making sense of communicative acts as well as the representational arts. Inasmuch as objects are partially determinative of signs, they do not totally circumscribe the interpretant's interpretational powers. I find this interpretive function to be fundamental to all symbolic interaction, whether verbal or gestural. See Peirce, *The Essential Peirce: Selected Philosophical Writings, Volume 2 (1893–1913)* (Bloomington: Indiana University Press, 1998).

62. Bateson, *Steps to an Ecology of Mind*.

63. Benveniste, "Subjectivity in Language"; Butler, *Psychic Life of Power*; Emmanuel Levinas, *Otherwise than Being or Beyond Essence*, trans. Alphonso Lingis (Pittsburgh, Pa.: Duquesne University Press, 1998).

64. There is a debate about the emergence of this term; see Elizabeth J. (Ibby) Grace, "Important Correction Re: Origin of 'Neurotypical,'" Tiny Grace Notes (Ask an Autistic) (blog), July 23, 2013, http://tinygracenotes.blog spot.com/.

65. Witold Gombrowicz, *Operetta* (1968), in *Three Plays*, trans. Krystyna Griffith-Jones, Catherine Robins, and Louis Iribarne (New York: Marion Boyars, 1998).

66. Nicolas Philibert, *La Moindre Des Choses* (International Film Circuit, 1997).

67. Félix Guattari, "La Borde: A Clinic Unlike Any Other," in *Chaosophy* (New York: Semiotext(e), 1995), 188.

68. Guattari uses the term "psychotics" in ways that would seem politically incorrect to modern readers, largely due to the stigma associated with the term—rather than the more polite "mentally ill," "disabled," or "autistic." But Guattari has two aims in using such a term. The first is to unsettle people. The second is to argue for a commonality across the human experiences of capitalism. He explores both of these goals in his work with Gilles Deleuze, namely *Anti-Oedipus*, trans. Robert Hurley (Minneapolis: University of Minnesota Press, 1983); Deleuze and Guattari, *Thousand Plateaus*, vol. 2, *Capitalism and Schizophrenia*.

69. Guattari's use of "seriality" is derived from the philosophy of Jean-Paul Sartre, who develops the idea to describe the conditions of everyday life in the context of existentialism. See Sartre, *Critique of Dialectical Reason* (1960), trans. Alan Sheridan-Smith (New York: Verso, 2004).

70. Guattari, "La Borde," 191.

71. Félix Guattari, "Institutional Practice and Politics," in *The Guattari Reader*, ed. Gary Genosko, trans. Baker Lang (Cambridge, Mass.: Blackwell, 1996), 128–29.

72. Guattari, *Molecular Revolution*, 42.

73. Guattari, *Molecular Revolution*, 161.

74. For a discussion of Guattari's use of "concrete machines," see Charles J. Stivale, *The Two-Fold Thought of Deleuze and Guattari: Intersections and Animations* (New York: Guilford, 1998).

75. Guattari, "Institutional Practice and Politics," 195.

76. The antipsychiatry movement developed in the 1960s as a critique of then-dominant models of psychiatric care, especially psychoanalysis, institutionalization, and psychosurgery. The basic tenet of those working in this tradition was that psychiatry was a pseudoscience, more the product of power relations in society than a medical practice intended to reduce psychiatric symptoms. Psychiatry, in this idiom, was a means to medicalize people and treat them as patients, ignoring the social conditions that produced their abnormal behaviors. See David Cooper, ed., *Psychiatry and Anti-psychiatry* (New York: Ballantine Books, 1971); Thomas Szasz, *Ideology and Insanity: Essays on the Psychiatric Dehumanization of Man* (Syracuse, N.Y.: Syracuse University Press, 1991).

77. Quoted in Gary Genosko, *Félix Guattari: An Aberrant Introduction* (New York: Continuum, 2002), 95.

78. Guattari, "La Borde," 208.

3. Materialist Subjectivity

1. Peyton Goddard, Diane Goddard, and Carol Cujec, *I Am Intelligent: From Heartbreak to Healing—A Mother and Daughter's Journey through Autism* (Augusta, Ga.: Skirt, 2012), xi.

2. Peyton Goddard, Peyton Goddard (blog), "I Am Hungry to Free My Lip," August 30, 2013, http://peytongoddard.com/.

3. Goddard, Goddard, and Cujec, *I Am Intelligent*, 53.

4. Goddard, Goddard, and Cujec, *I Am Intelligent*, 46–47.

5. Goddard, Goddard, and Cujec, *I Am Intelligent*, 129.

6. Goddard, Goddard, and Cujec, *I Am Intelligent*, 130.

7. Goddard, Goddard, and Cujec, *I Am Intelligent*, 130.

8. Goddard, Goddard, and Cujec, *I Am Intelligent*, 53.

9. Goddard, Goddard, and Cujec, *I Am Intelligent*, 65.

10. Goddard, Goddard, and Cujec, *I Am Intelligent*, 65–66.

11. Goddard, Goddard, and Cujec, *I Am Intelligent*, 94.

12. Goddard, Goddard, and Cujec, *I Am Intelligent*, 113.

13. Goddard, Goddard, and Cujec, *I Am Intelligent*, 145.

14. Goddard, Goddard, and Cujec, *I Am Intelligent*, 172.

15. Goddard, Goddard, and Cujec, *I Am Intelligent*, 172.

16. Goddard, Goddard, and Cujec, *I Am Intelligent*, 182.

17. Goddard, Goddard, and Cujec, *I Am Intelligent*, 182.

18. Goddard, Goddard, and Cujec, *I Am Intelligent*, 198.

19. Goddard, Goddard, and Cujec, *I Am Intelligent*, 230.

20. Goddard, Goddard, and Cujec, *I Am Intelligent*, 205–7.

21. Goddard, Goddard, and Cujec, *I Am Intelligent*, 205.

22. Goddard, Goddard, and Cujec, *I Am Intelligent*, 206.

23. Goddard, Goddard, and Cujec, *I Am Intelligent*, 78–81.

24. Goddard, Goddard, and Cujec, *I Am Intelligent*, 107.

25. Goddard, Goddard, and Cujec, *I Am Intelligent*, 188.

26. Goddard, Goddard, and Cujec, *I Am Intelligent*, 189.

27. Goddard, Goddard, and Cujec, *I Am Intelligent*, 211.

28. Goddard, Goddard, and Cujec, *I Am Intelligent*, 212.

29. Goddard, Goddard, and Cujec, *I Am Intelligent*, 213.

30. Goddard, Goddard, and Cujec, *I Am Intelligent*, 252.

31. Goddard, Goddard, and Cujec, *I Am Intelligent*, 259.

32. Goddard, Goddard, and Cujec, *I Am Intelligent*, 260.

33. CeCe Bell, *El Deafo* (New York: Amulet Books, 2014).

34. Bell, *El Deafo*, 29.

35. Bell, *El Deafo*, 31–32.
36. Bell, *El Deafo*, 40.
37. Bell, *El Deafo*, 43, ellipses and italics in original.
38. Bell, *El Deafo*, 36.
39. Bell, *El Deafo*, 46–47.
40. Bell, *El Deafo*, 67.
41. Bell, *El Deafo*, 70.
42. Bell, *El Deafo*, 84.
43. The idea of the "supercrip" is that through one's disability, secondary capacities are developed—in some cases, capacities that far exceed "normal" people. Bell's superhearing is an iteration of this, but more mundane claims attribute emergent sensory powers to those who lose a sensorial capacity. For a review of the uses of supercrip figures, see Sami Schalk, "Reevaluating the Supercrip," *Journal of Literary and Cultural Disability Studies* 10, no. 1 (2016): 71–86.
44. Bell, *El Deafo*, 174.
45. Bell, *El Deafo*, 174.
46. Bell, *El Deafo*, 211.
47. José Delgado, *Physical Control of the Mind: Toward a Psychocivilized Society* (New York: Harper Colophon, 1971).
48. For a discussion of the history of institutional review boards and the shaping of scientific research, see Laura Stark, *Behind Closed Doors: IRBs and the Making of Ethical Research* (Chicago: University of Chicago Press, 2012).
49. Delgado, *Physical Control of the Mind*, 166.
50. Delgado, *Physical Control of the Mind*, 45.
51. Delgado, *Physical Control of the Mind*, 45.
52. Delgado, *Physical Control of the Mind*, 215.
53. Delgado, *Physical Control of the Mind*, 104.
54. Delgado, *Physical Control of the Mind*, 18.
55. Delgado, *Physical Control of the Mind*, 144.
56. Delgado, *Physical Control of the Mind*, 93.
57. Delgado, *Physical Control of the Mind*, 191.
58. Delgado, *Physical Control of the Mind*, 59.
59. Delgado, *Physical Control of the Mind*, 59.
60. Delgado, *Physical Control of the Mind*, 221.
61. Delgado, *Physical Control of the Mind*, 220–21.
62. Delgado, *Physical Control of the Mind*, 221.
63. Delgado, *Physical Control of the Mind*, 249.
64. Delgado, *Physical Control of the Mind*, 216.

65. For an overview of the social study of infrastructure see Brian Larkin, "The Politics and Poetics of Infrastructure," *Annual Review of Anthropology* 42 (2013): 327–43. In relation to language as a form of infrastructure, see Julia Elyachar, "Phatic Labor, Infrastructure, and the Question of Empowerment in Cairo," *American Ethnologist* 37, no. 3 (2010): 452–64.

66. Such a claim echoes those who have been inspired by the work of Jacques Derrida, particularly Vicki Kirby. In Derrida's and Kirby's deconstructive approach to texts, they argue for a capacious understanding of writing as a way to conceptualize all of the intentionally (and potentially unintentionally) crafted institutions, forms of embodiment, and styles of interaction that humans participate in and through. To the extent that writing can serve as an analog for human activity in this way, I agree that it is a useful way to conceptualize how individuals interpret and facilitate the actions of one another. See Jacques Derrida, *Writing and Difference* (1967), trans. Alan Bass (Chicago: University of Chicago Press, 1980); Vicki Kirby, *Telling Flesh: The Substance of the Corporeal* (New York: Routledge, 1997).

67. For a history of historical materialism as a founding understanding of sociological analyses of the impact of conditions on the lives of individuals, see Perry Anderson, *In the Tracks of Historical Materialism* (London: Verso, 1983). The central proposition of Marxian historical materialism is that the actions of individuals will be overdetermined by the power structures that they find themselves subject to—a situation that can be difficult, if not impossible, to break free from. For Karl Marx, and for many on the political left throughout the twentieth century, capitalism is taken as working in this way to subjugate the working classes (and really everyone) to ensure that as a system it continues despite its dehumanizing effects. See Karl Marx, *Capital: A Critique of Political Economy* (1867), trans. Ben Fowkes (New York: Penguin, 1990).

68. On the subject of the agencies of pharmaceuticals, see, e.g., Joseph Dumit, *Drugs for Life: How Pharmaceutical Companies Define Our Health* (Durham, N.C.: Duke University Press, 2012); Nicolas Rasmussen, *On Speed: The Many Lives of Amphetamine* (New York: New York University Press, 2009).

69. For a discussion of play and its integral function in human sociality, see Roger Caillois, *Man, Play, and Games*, trans. Barash Meyer (Urbana: University of Illinois Press, 2001).

70. Caillois, "Mimicry and Legendary Psychesthenia."

4. Cybernetic Subjectivity

1. Ron Suskind, *Life, Animated: A Story of Sidekicks, Heroes, and Autism* (New York: Kingswell, 2014), 13.

2. For a discussion of Floortime as a pedagogical method in autism treatment, see Stanley Greenspan and Serena Wieder, *Engaging Autism: Using the Floortime Approach to Help Children Relate, Communicate, and Think* (Philadelphia, Pa.: Da Capo Press, 2006). Rather than strict behavioralism, as in the case of earlier models of treatment, Floortime approaches attempt to engage children with the things that they find interesting and use these interests as leverage points into developing normative capacities.

3. Suskind, *Life, Animated*, 15.

4. Suskind, *Life, Animated*, 15.

5. Suskind, *Life, Animated*, 16.

6. Suskind, *Life, Animated*, 19.

7. Suskind, *Life, Animated*, 23–24.

8. Suskind, *Life, Animated*, 37.

9. Suskind, *Life, Animated*, 55.

10. Suskind, *Life, Animated*, 60.

11. Suskind, *Life, Animated*, 72.

12. Suskind, *Life, Animated*, 72.

13. Suskind, *Life, Animated*, 73.

14. Suskind, *Life, Animated*, 73.

15. Suskind, *Life, Animated*, 73.

16. Suskind, *Life, Animated*, 81–82.

17. Suskind, *Life, Animated*, 81.

18. Suskind, *Life, Animated*, 82.

19. Suskind, *Life, Animated*, 88–90.

20. Suskind, *Life, Animated*, 89.

21. Suskind, *Life, Animated*, 220.

22. Suskind, *Life, Animated*, 351.

23. Suskind, *Life, Animated*, 352.

24. Suskind, *Life, Animated*, 353.

25. Suskind, *Life, Animated*, 176.

26. Suskind, *Life, Animated*, 158.

27. Suskind, *Life, Animated*, 322.

28. Suskind, *Life, Animated*, 322.

29. Suskind, *Life, Animated*, 320.

30. Suskind, *Life, Animated*, 320.

31. Nancy Ordover, *American Eugenics: Race, Queer Anatomy, and the Science of Nationalism* (Minneapolis: University of Minnesota Press, 2003).

32. Suskind, *Life, Animated*, 335.

33. Paul Karasik and Judy Karasik, *The Ride Together: A Brother and*

Sister's Memoir of Autism in the Family (New York: Washington Square Press, 2003).

34. Karasik and Karasik, *Ride Together*, 32–33.

35. Karasik and Karasik, *Ride Together*, 90–91.

36. Quoted in Karasik and Karasik, *Ride Together*, 94.

37. Karasik and Karasik, *Ride Together*, 95.

38. Karasik and Karasik, *Ride Together*, 96.

39. Karasik and Karasik, *Ride Together*, 96.

40. Karasik and Karasik, *Ride Together*, 110.

41. Karasik and Karasik, *Ride Together*, 117.

42. Karasik and Karasik, *Ride Together*, 76.

43. Quoted in Karasik and Karasik, *Ride Together*, 80.

44. Karasik and Karasik, *Ride Together*, 81.

45. Karasik and Karasik, *Ride Together*, 134.

46. Karasik and Karasik, *Ride Together*, 178.

47. Karasik and Karasik, *Ride Together*, 181.

48. Karasik and Karasik, *Ride Together*, 181.

49. Karasik and Karasik, *Ride Together*, 184.

50. Karasik and Karasik, *Ride Together*, 137.

51. Karasik and Karasik, *Ride Together*, 136.

52. Karasik and Karasik, *Ride Together*, 139.

53. Karasik and Karasik, *Ride Together*, 79–80.

54. Quoted in Karasik and Karasik, *Ride Together*, 80.

55. Karasik and Karasik, *Ride Together*, 151.

56. Karasik and Karasik, *Ride Together*, 24–25.

57. Karasik and Karasik, *Ride Together*, 15.

58. Karasik and Karasik, *Ride Together*, 34.

59. Karasik and Karasik, *Ride Together*, 62–67.

60. Karasik and Karasik, *Ride Together*, 63, ellipses in original.

61. Karasik and Karasik, *Ride Together*, 160, ellipses in original.

62. Karasik and Karasik, *Ride Together*, 158, ellipses in original.

63. The concept of framing is developed by Gregory Bateson as a means to understand communicative acts, originally derived from how nonhuman animals indicate the desire to play with one another. It was later developed in a variety of ways to conceptualize how communicative acts are produced within interpretive regimes. For two discussions of framing, see Bateson, *Steps to an Ecology of Mind*; Erving Goffman, *Forms of Talk* (Philadelphia: University of Pennsylvania Press, 1981).

64. Karasik and Karasik, *Ride Together*, 148.

65. Harry F. Harlow, *Learning to Love* (New York: Jason Aronson, 1974), 38.

66. Harlow, *Learning to Love*, 39.

67. Harlow, *Learning to Love*, 131.

68. Harry F. Harlow and Clara Mears, *The Human Model: Primate Perspectives* (New York: John Wiley & Sons, 1979).

69. Harlow and Mears, *Human Model*, 169.

70. For a discussion of early cybernetics and feedback, see Kline, *Cybernetics Moment*.

71. Harlow and Mears, *Human Model*, 286.

72. Harlow and Mears, *Human Model*, 286.

73. Harlow and Mears, *Human Model*, 287.

74. Harlow and Mears, *Human Model*, 287.

75. Harlow and Mears, *Human Model*, 287.

76. Harlow and Mears, *Human Model*, 287–88.

77. Harlow and Mears, *Human Model*, 227.

78. Harlow and Mears, *Human Model*, 228.

79. Harlow and Mears, *Human Model*, 228.

80. Harlow, *Learning to Love*, 56.

81. The theory of "theory of mind" is a psychological one that holds that part of the developmental process for children is the eventual understanding that other individuals have interior experiences much like the child's. In this way, a child can come to understand not just that another child is sad, but that that child is sad because the first child took a toy away from him or her. In this way, theory of mind is fundamental to intersubjective experiences. The lack of theory of mind has been associated with autism; see Baron-Cohen, *Mindblindness*.

82. Harlow, *Learning to Love*, 55.

83. Harlow, *Learning to Love*, 68.

84. Harlow and Mears, *Human Model*, 288–89.

85. Harlow and Mears, *Human Model*, 183.

86. Harlow and Mears, *Human Model*, 184.

87. Harlow and Mears, *Human Model*, 167.

88. Mony Elkaïm, *If You Love Me, Don't Love Me: Undoing Double Binds and Other Methods of Change in Couple and Family Therapy*, trans. Hendon Chubb (Northvale, N.J.: Aronson, 1997), 59–61.

89. See, e.g., Maturana and Varela, *Autopoiesis and Cognition*, xv.

90. See Humbert Maturana and Francisco Varela, *Tree of Knowledge: The Biological Roots of Human Understanding* (Boulder, Colo.: Shambhala, 1987), 163.

91. Elkaïm, *If You Love Me*, 61–62.

92. Elkaïm, *If You Love Me*, 69.

93. Bateson, *Steps to an Ecology of Mind*, 65–66.

94. Bateson, *Steps to an Ecology of Mind*, 66.

95. Bateson, *Steps to an Ecology of Mind*, 206–7.

96. Bateson, *Steps to an Ecology of Mind*, 215.

97. Bateson, *Steps to an Ecology of Mind*, 242.

98. Bateson, *Steps to an Ecology of Mind*, 242.

99. Bateson, *Steps to an Ecology of Mind*, 318.

100. Bateson, *Steps to an Ecology of Mind*, 319.

101. Bateson, *Steps to an Ecology of Mind*, 459.

102. Structural functionalism held sway over sociology and anthropology for nearly a century, the theoretical assumption being that societies tend toward homeostasis and that the organization of society—and the social functions of individuals—is intended to preserve the historical organization of a given society. See, e.g., Talcott Parsons, *The Social System* (London: Routledge, 1951).

103. On autism in this respect, see Grinker, *Unstrange Minds*. On schizophrenia, see Tanya Luhrmann et al., "Hearing Voices in Different Cultures: A Social Kindling Hypothesis," *Topics in Cognitive Science* 7, no. 4 (2015): 646–63.

104. On autism in this respect, see Eyal et al., *Autism Matrix*. On schizophrenia, see Myers, *Recovery's Edge*.

105. On deinstitutionalization—the erosion of state funding for medical residential facilities and the return of clients to their home communities—see Phil Brown, *Transfer of Care: Psychiatric Deinstitutionalization and Its Aftermath* (New York: Routledge Kegan & Paul, 1988); E. Fuller Torrey, *American Psychosis: How the Federal Government Destroyed the Mental Illness Treatment System* (Oxford: Oxford University Press, 2013).

5. Facilitated Subjectivity, Affective Bioethics, and the Nervous System

1. Diane Ackerman, *One Hundred Names for Love: A Memoir* (New York: Norton, 2011), 56–57.

2. Paul West, *The Shadow Factory* (Santa Fe, N.M.: Lumen Books, 2008), 162–63.

3. West, *Shadow Factory*, 88–89.

4. Ackerman, *One Hundred Names for Love*, 19.

5. Ackerman, *One Hundred Names for Love*, 135.

6. Ackerman, *One Hundred Names for Love*, 62.

7. Ackerman, *One Hundred Names for Love*, 79–80.

8. Ackerman, *One Hundred Names for Love*, 99.

9. Ackerman, *One Hundred Names for Love*, 110.

10. Ackerman, *One Hundred Names for Love*, 135.

11. Ackerman, *One Hundred Names for Love*, 41.

12. Ackerman, *One Hundred Names for Love*, 87.

13. West, *Shadow Factory*, 50.

14. West, *Shadow Factory*, 108.

15. Ackerman, *One Hundred Names for Love*, 37.

16. West, *Shadow Factory*, 75.

17. Ackerman, *One Hundred Names for Love*, 98.

18. West, *Shadow Factory*, 171.

19. West, *Shadow Factory*, 104.

20. West, *Shadow Factory*, 109.

21. Ackerman, *One Hundred Names for Love*, 45.

22. Ackerman, *One Hundred Names for Love*, 103.

23. Quoted in Ackerman, *One Hundred Names for Love*, 294.

24. Michael Schiavo and Michael Hirsch, *Terri: The Truth* (New York: Dutton, 2006), 123–24.

25. Schiavo and Hirsch, *Terri*, 206.

26. Schiavo and Hirsch, *Terri*, 3.

27. Schiavo and Hirsch, *Terri*, 27.

28. Quoted in Schiavo and Hirsch, *Terri*, 59–60.

29. Quoted in Schiavo and Hirsch, *Terri*, 74.

30. Schiavo and Hirsch, *Terri*, 205.

31. Schiavo and Hirsch, *Terri*, 99.

32. Schiavo and Hirsch, *Terri*, 99.

33. Schiavo and Hirsch, *Terri*, 99.

34. Schiavo and Hirsch, *Terri*, 163.

35. Schiavo and Hirsch, *Terri*, 154–55.

36. Schiavo and Hirsch, *Terri*, 162.

37. Schiavo and Hirsch, *Terri*, 65.

38. Schiavo and Hirsch, *Terri*, 69.

39. Schiavo and Hirsch, *Terri*, 310.

40. Schiavo and Hirsch, *Terri*, 313.

41. Michael Lambek, *Ordinary Ethics: Anthropology, Language, and Action* (New York: Fordham University Press, 2010).

42. Joel Robbins, "Beyond the Suffering Subject: Toward an Anthropology of the Good," *Journal of the Royal Anthropological Institute* 19, no. 3 (2013): 447–62.

43. Catherine Lutz, "Emotion, Thought, and Estrangement: Emotion as a Cultural Category," *Cultural Anthropology* 1, no. 3 (1986): 287–309; Renato Rosaldo, *Culture and Truth: The Remaking of Social Analysis* (Boston: Beacon Press, 1993).

44. Mary Johnson, "After Terri Schiavo: Why the Disability Rights Movement Spoke Out, Why Some of Us Worried, and Where Do We Go from Here?," Ragged Edge Online (blog), April 2, 2005, http://www.ragged edgemagazine.com/.

45. Schiavo and Hirsch, *Terri*, 207.

46. Dumit, *Picturing Personhood*; Gould, *Mismeasure of Man*; Saunders, *CT Suite*.

47. Schneider, *American Kinship*.

48. Weston, *Families We Choose*.

49. Yanagisako, "Variance in American Kinship."

50. In her review of the literature on grief, Sara Ahmed highlights the ways that grief has been used to denote a relationship with something that has been lost. Drawing on Sigmund Freud and Judith Butler, Ahmed is primarily concerned with the historical aspect of loss—that is, something has been lost. Grief denotes the emotional experience of working through and living with that loss. Additionally, she focuses on how grief is impossible in the context of queer loss—those persons and experiences that are not recognized as valuable or acceptable within a society. Her discussion of grief therefore points to how it might also be used to conceptualize lost possibilities for individuals, communities, and society generally. Sara Ahmed, *The Cultural Politics of Emotion*, 2nd ed. (New York: Routledge, 2015).

51. Bateson, *Steps to an Ecology of Mind*, 318.

INDEX

Matthew J. Wolf-Meyer is associate professor of anthropology at Binghamton University. He is author of *The Slumbering Masses: Sleep, Medicine, and Modern American Life* and *Theory for the World to Come: Speculative Fiction and Apocalyptic Anthropology*, both published by the University of Minnesota Press.

Made in the USA
Middletown, DE
02 February 2021

32931879R00186